Common Musculoskeletal Problems in the Ambulatory Setting

Editor

MATTHEW L. SILVIS

MEDICAL CLINICS
OF NORTH AMERICA

www.medical.theclinics.com

Consulting Editors
DOUGLAS S. PAAUW
EDWARD R. BOLLARD

July 2014 • Volume 98 • Number 4

ELSEVIER

1600 John F. Kennedy Boulevard • Suite 1800 • Philadelphia, Pennsylvania, 19103-2899

http://www.theclinics.com

MEDICAL CLINICS OF NORTH AMERICA Volume 98, Number 4
July 2014 ISSN 0025-7125, ISBN-13: 978-0-323-31165-6

Editor: Jessica McCool
Developmental Editor: Yonah Korngold

Medical Clinics of North America (ISSN 0025-7125) is published bimonthly by Elsevier Inc., 360 Park Avenue South, New York, NY 10010-1710. Months of publication are January, March, May, July, September, and November. Business and editorial offices: 1600 John F. Kennedy Boulevard, Suite 1800, Philadelphia, PA 19103-2899. Periodicals postage paid at New York, NY, and additional mailing offices. Subscription prices are USD $255.00 per year (US individuals), $471.00 per year (US institutions), $125.00 per year (US Students), $320.00 per year (Canadian individuals), $612.00 per year (Canadian institutions), $200.00 per year (Canadian and foreign students), $390.00 per year (foreign individuals), and $612.00 per year (foreign institutions). To receive student/resident rate, orders must be accompanied by name of affiliated institution, date of term, and the signature of program/residency coordinator on institution letterhead. Orders will be billed at individual rate until proof of status is received. Foreign air speed delivery is included in all Clinics' subscription prices. All prices are subject to change without notice. **POSTMASTER:** Send address changes to *Medical Clinics of North America*, Elsevier Health Sciences Division, Subscription Customer Service, 3251 Riverport Lane, Maryland Heights, MO 63043. **Customer Service: Telephone: 1-800-654-2452** (U.S. and Canada); **1-314-447-8871** (outside U.S. and Canada). **Fax: 314-447-8029. E-mail: journalscustomerserviceusa@elsevier.com** (for print support); **journalsonlinesupport-usa@elsevier.com** (for online support).

Reprints. For copies of 100 or more of articles in this publication, please contact the Commercial Reprints Department, Elsevier Inc., 360 Park Avenue South, New York, NY 10010-1710. Tel.: 212-633-3874; Fax: 212-633-3820; E-mail: reprints@elsevier.com.

Medical Clinics of North America is also published in Spanish by McGraw-Hill Interamericana Editores S. A., P.O. Box 5-237, 06500 Mexico, D.F., Mexico.

Medical Clinics of North America is covered in *MEDLINE/PubMed (Index Medicus), Current Contents, ASCA, Excerpta Medica, Science Citation Index, and ISI/BIOMED.*

PROGRAM OBJECTIVE
The goal of the *Medical Clinics of North America* is to keep practicing physicians up to date with current clinical practice by providing timely articles reviewing the state of the art in patient care.

LEARNING OBJECTIVES
Upon completion of this activity, participants will be able to:
1. Review evaluation and treatment of chronic hand conditions
2. Recognize knee pain including anterior knee pain and acutely injured knee pain.
3. Discuss the types and indications of musculoskeletal imaging.

ACCREDITATION
The Elsevier Office of Continuing Medical Education (EOCME) is accredited by the Accreditation Council for Continuing Medical Education (ACCME) to provide continuing medical education for physicians.

The EOCME designates this enduring material for a maximum of 15 *AMA PRA Category 1 Credit*(s)™. Physicians should claim only the credit commensurate with the extent of their participation in the activity.

All other health care professionals requesting continuing education credit for this enduring material will be issued a certificate of participation.

DISCLOSURE OF CONFLICTS OF INTEREST
The EOCME assesses conflict of interest with its instructors, faculty, planners, and other individuals who are in a position to control the content of CME activities. All relevant conflicts of interest that are identified are thoroughly vetted by EOCME for fair balance, scientific objectivity, and patient care recommendations. EOCME is committed to providing its learners with CME activities that promote improvements or quality in healthcare and not a specific proprietary business or a commercial interest.

The planning committee, staff, authors and editors listed below have identified no financial relationships or relationships to products or devices they or their spouse/life partner have with commercial interest related to the content of this CME activity:
April D. Armstrong, BSc(PT), MD, MSc, FRCSC; Dov A. Bader, MD; Edward R. Bollard, MD, DDS, FACP; Douglas Comeau, D.O., CAQSM, FAAFP; Deanna Lynn Corey, MD; Michael Darowish; Eric Emanski, MD; Robert A. Gallo, MD; Eugene Hong, MD; Allyson S. Howe, MD, CAQ, FAAFP; Brynne Hunter; Bret C. Jacobs, DO, MA; Christopher Karrasch, MD; Mark Knaub, MD; Michael C. Kraft, MD; Sandy Lavery; Justin A. Lee, MD; Jessica McCool; Jill McNair; Cayce A. Onks, DO, MS, ATC; Lindsay Parnell; Nathan Patrick, MD; Michael E. Pitzer, MD; Santha Priya; George GA Pujalte, MD; Peter H. Seidenberg, MD, FAAFP, FACSM; Jyoti Sharma; Matthew L. Silvis, MD; Matt A. Varacallo, MD; John R. Wawrzyniak, MA, ATC, PT, CSCS.

The planning committee, staff, authors and editors listed below have identified financial relationships or relationships to products or devices they or their spouse/life partner have with commercial interest related to the content of this CME activity:
Edward J. Fox, MD is on speakers bureau for Eli Lilly; spouse has employment affiliation and stock ownership with GSK.

Scott A. Lynch, MD has stock ownership with Ridonk, LLC.

UNAPPROVED/OFF-LABEL USE DISCLOSURE
The EOCME requires CME faculty to disclose to the participants:
1. When products or procedures being discussed are off-label, unlabelled, experimental, and/or investigational (not US Food and Drug Administration (FDA) approved); and
2. Any limitations on the information presented, such as data that are preliminary or that represent ongoing research, interim analyses, and/or unsupported opinions. Faculty may discuss information about pharmaceutical agents that is outside of FDA-approved labelling. This information is intended solely for CME and is not intended to promote off-label use of these medications. If you have any questions, contact the medical affairs department of the manufacturer for the most recent prescribing information.

TO ENROLL
To enroll in the *Medical Clinics of North America* Continuing Medical Education program, call customer service at 1-800-654-2452 or sign up online at http://www.theclinics.com/home/cme. The CME program is available to subscribers for an additional annual fee of USD $267

METHOD OF PARTICIPATION

In order to claim credit, participants must complete the following:

1. Complete enrolment as indicated above.
2. Read the activity.
3. Complete the CME Test and Evaluation. Participants must achieve a score of 70% on the test. All CME Tests and Evaluations must be completed online.

CME INQUIRIES/SPECIAL NEEDS

For all CME inquiries or special needs, please contact elsevierCME@elsevier.com.

MEDICAL CLINICS OF NORTH AMERICA

RELATED INTEREST

Primary Care: Clinics in Office Practice, December 2013, (Vol 40, No. 4)
Orthopedics
George Pujalte, *Editor*
http://www.primarycare.theclinics.com/

Contributors

CONSULTING EDITORS

DOUGLAS S. PAAUW, MD, MACP
Professor, Division of General Internal Medicine, Department of Medicine; Rathmann Family Foundation Endowed Chair for Patient-Centered Clinical Education; Medicine Student Programs, University of Washington School of Medicine, Seattle, Washington

EDWARD R. BOLLARD, MD, DDS, FACP
Professor of Medicine; Associate Dean for Graduate Medical Education; Designated Institutional Official (DIO), Penn State–Milton S. Hershey Medical Center, Hershey, Pennsylvania

EDITOR

MATTHEW L. SILVIS, MD
Program Director, Penn State Primary Care Sports Medicine Fellowship, Hershey; Associate Professor, Departments of Family and Community Medicine and Orthopedics and Rehabilitation, Penn State–Milton S. Hershey Medical Center, Hershey, Pennsylvania

AUTHORS

APRIL ARMSTRONG, BSc(PT), MD, MSc, FRCSC
Professor, Department of Orthopaedics and Rehabilitation, Bone and Joint Institute, Penn State–Milton S. Hershey Medical Center, Hershey, Pennsylvania

DOV A. BADER, MD
Assistant Professor of Orthopaedics and Rehabilitation, Penn State Hershey Bone and Joint Institute; Team Physician, Penn State University, State College, Pennsylvania

DOUGLAS COMEAU, DO, CAQSM, FAAFP
Medical Director, Sports Medicine; Director, Primary Care Sports Medicine Fellowship, Ryan Center for Sports Medicine, Boston Medical Center, Boston University; Assistant Professor, Family Medicine, Boston University School of Medicine; Head Team Physician, Boston University, Boston, Massachusetts; Team Physician, Boston College, Boston, Massachusetts

DEANNA LYNN COREY, MD
Fellow, Primary Care Sports Medicine, Boston Medical Center, Boston University, Boston, Massachusetts

MICHAEL DAROWISH, MD
Assistant Professor, Penn State Bone and Joint Institute, Penn State–Milton S. Hershey Medical Center, Hershey, Pennsylvania

ERIC EMANSKI, MD
Department of Orthopaedic Surgery, Penn State–Milton S. Hershey Medical Center, Hershey, Pennsylvania

ED J. FOX, MD
Resident Physician, Penn State Hershey Department of Orthopaedics and Rehabilitation, College of Medicine, Hershey, Pennsylvania

ROBERT A. GALLO, MD
Assistant Professor, Department of Orthopaedics, Penn State–Milton S. Hershey Medical Center, Hershey, Pennsylvania

EUGENE HONG, MD, CAQSM, FAAFP
Hamot and Sturgis Endowed Chair and Professor; Chief, Division of Sports Medicine, Drexel University College of Medicine, Philadelphia, Pennsylvania

ALLYSON H. HOWE, MD, FAAFP
Assistant Professor, Tufts School of Medicine Faculty, Family Medicine Residency, Primary Care Sports Medicine Fellowship Faculty, University of Southern Maine, Portland, Maine

BRET C. JACOBS, DO, MA
Assistant Professor, Departments of Family and Community Medicine and Orthopaedics and Rehabilitation, Penn State–Milton S. Hershey Medical Center, Hershey, Pennsylvania

CHRISTOPHER KARRASCH, MD
Department of Orthopaedic Surgery, Penn State–Milton S. Hershey Medical Center, Pennsylvania State University College of Medicine, Hershey, Pennsylvania

MARK A. KNAUB, MD
Assistant Professor, Department of Orthopaedic Surgery; Chief of Adult Spine Service, Penn State–Milton S. Hershey Medical Center, Hershey, Pennsylvania

MICHAEL C. KRAFT, MD
Division of Sports Medicine, Drexel University College of Medicine, Philadelphia, Pennsylvania

JUSTIN A. LEE, MD
Clinical Assistant Professor, Department of Family Medicine, Brody School of Medicine, East Carolina University, Greenville, North Carolina

SCOTT LYNCH, MD
Associate Professor, Department of Orthopaedic Surgery, Penn State–Milton S. Hershey Medical Center, Hershey, Pennsylvania

CAYCE A. ONKS, DO, MS, ATC
Assistant Professor, Department of Family and Community Medicine; Department of Orthopaedics and Rehabilitation, Penn State–Milton S. Hershey Medical Center, Hershey, Pennsylvania

NATHAN PATRICK, MD
Department of Orthopaedic Surgery, Penn State–Milton S. Hershey Medical Center, Hershey, Pennsylvania

MICHAEL E. PITZER, MD
Primary Care Sports Medicine Fellow, Penn State Hershey Bone and Joint Institute; Team Physician, Penn State University, State College, Pennsylvania

GEORGE G.A. PUJALTE, MD, FACSM
Assistant Professor, Departments of Family and Community Medicine, and Orthopaedics and Rehabilitation, Penn State–Milton S. Hershey Medical Center, Hershey, Pennsylvania

PETER H. SEIDENBERG, MD, FAAFP, FACSM
Program Director, Penn State Primary Care Sports Medicine Fellowship; Associate Professor of Orthopaedics and Rehabilitation, Penn State Hershey Bone and Joint Institute; Team Physician, Penn State University, State College, Pennsylvania

JYOTI SHARMA, MD
Resident, Penn State Bone and Joint Institute, Penn State–Milton S. Hershey Medical Center, Hershey, Pennsylvania

MATTHEW L. SILVIS, MD
Program Director, Penn State Primary Care Sports Medicine Fellowship, Hershey; Associate Professor, Departments of Family and Community Medicine, and Orthopaedics and Rehabilitation, Penn State–Milton S. Hershey Medical Center, Hershey, Pennsylvania

MATTHEW A. VARACALLO, MD
Professor, Penn State Hershey Department of Orthopaedics and Rehabilitation, College of Medicine, Hershey, Pennsylvania

JOHN WAWRZYNIAK, MA, ATC, PT, CSCS
Department of Orthopaedics and Rehabilitation, Therapy Services, Penn State–Milton S. Hershey Medical Center, Hershey, Pennsylvania

Contents

health care system are emphasized to highlight the need for increased knowledge and awareness of its complications if left untreated or treated incorrectly. Special attention is given to hip fracture and vertebral compression fracture, stressing the importance of diagnosing osteoporosis before fragility fractures occur. Models for improved care of fragility fractures during follow-up in the outpatient setting and the use of pharmacologic agents are discussed.

Overuse injuries of the lateral and medial elbow are common in sport, recreational activities, and occupational endeavors. They are commonly diagnosed as lateral and medial epicondylitis; however, the pathophysiology of these disorders demonstrates a lack of inflammation. Instead, angiofibroblastic degeneration is present, referred to as tendinosis. As such, a more appropriate terminology for these conditions is epicondylosis. This is a clinical diagnosis, and further investigations are only performed to rule out other clinical entities after conventional therapy has failed. Yet, most patients respond to conservative measures with physical therapy and counterforce bracing. Corticosteroid injections are effective for short-term pain control but have not demonstrated long-term benefit.

Running is often recommended by physicians to maintain a healthy lifestyle. As more individuals participate in running-related activities, clinicians must be increasingly aware of common injuries. Training errors leading to overuse are the most common underlying factors in most running-related injuries. Clinicians need to keep in mind that the presenting injury is frequently the result of an inability to compensate for a primary dysfunction at another site. Although imaging may be helpful in differentiating among diagnoses with similar clinical presentations, a detailed history and physical examination are essential in making a correct diagnosis.

Physical therapy was first noted in the time of Hippocrates. The physical therapy visit includes a complete history, physical examination, and development of a treatment plan. Health care providers usually initiate a referral based on physical examination, symptoms, or a specific diagnosis. Physical therapy has been shown to be particularly helpful for musculoskeletal ailments, and has a growing body of evidence for use.

There are various treatments for musculoskeletal-related conditions, including the use of durable medical equipment (DME). Numerous DME devices are currently available. This article addresses several of the common DME devices used for treating upper and lower extremity orthopedic conditions.

Musculoskeletal imaging includes radiographs, computed tomography scans, bone scans, magnetic resonance imaging, and musculoskeletal ultrasonography. Each modality has its advantages and disadvantages. This article presents general guidelines regarding which imaging modality to order when evaluating patients with musculoskeletal complaints. However, it must be remembered that imaging is not meant to replace a thorough history and physical examination, but instead should be seen as a suite of methods to confirm suspected diagnoses.

Foreword

Common Musculoskeletal Problems in the Ambulatory Setting

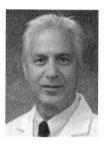

Edward R. Bollard, MD, DDS, FACP
Consulting Editor

Musculoskeletal complaints are one of the most common reasons patients seek care from their primary care physicians. Of these presenting complaints, it is estimated that 90% of the nonsurgical orthopedic conditions can be managed in the primary care setting. In this issue of the *Medical Clinics of North America*, Dr Matthew Silvis and his colleagues address many of these common musculoskeletal conditions that make up the 10% to 15% of all visits to primary care offices.[1] Reviews have previously noted the inadequate examinations and inappropriate ordering of tests and procedures that often occur when a comprehensive understanding of a focused history, musculoskeletal examination, and diagnostic approach is not undertaken. As we continue to emphasize the need for exercise and physical activity in our patients with the reality that we are asking this of a population that continues to advance in age, the skills of the primary care physician to appropriately diagnose and efficiently treat these conditions will be essential. The ultimate goal for our patients will be the return to functional status and management of symptoms that will allow them to re-engage in the activities that will promote their overall wellness.

Edward R. Bollard, MD, DDS, FACP
Penn State–Milton S. Hershey Medical Center
500 University Drive
P.O. Box 850 (Mail Code H039)
Hershey, PA 17033-0850, USA

E-mail address:
ebollard@hmc.psu.edu

Med Clin N Am 98 (2014) xv–xvi
http://dx.doi.org/10.1016/j.mcna.2014.04.006
0025-7125/14/$ – see front matter © 2014 Elsevier Inc. All rights reserved.

medical.theclinics.com

REFERENCE

1. Praemer A, Furner S, Rice DP. Musculoskeletal conditions in the United States. Rosemont (IL): American Academy of Orthopedic Surgeons; 1992.

Preface

Common Musculoskeletal Problems in the Ambulatory Setting

 CrossMark

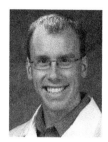

Matthew L. Silvis, MD
Editor

In this issue of *Medical Clinics of North America*, the focus is on the outpatient evaluation and management of common musculoskeletal complaints. Why is this information important to a busy practitioner? Musculoskeletal complaints and injuries comprise 15 to 30% of all primary care visits in the United States and Canada. The overarching goal of this issue is to provide a ready resource for busy clinicians managing these common musculoskeletal disorders.

The authors of this issue are all directly involved in patient care of the covered conditions, whether on the sidelines, clinic, or operating room. All articles encompass a succinct review of recent literature and each author has added clinical "pearls" to their assigned material. Topics covered are reflective of clinical practice in primary care, diverse in nature, and broad in scope.

This issue would not have been possible without the dedication, time, and effort of my contributing authors. Thanks to each of you.

It is my pleasure to share this work with you. I hope you enjoy reading this issue as much as I did assembling it.

Matthew L. Silvis, MD
Departments of Family and Community Medicine
and Orthopedics and Rehabilitation
Penn State–Milton S. Hershey Medical Center, H154
500 University Drive
Hershey, PA 17078, USA

E-mail address:
msilvis@hmc.psu.edu

Med Clin N Am 98 (2014) xvii
http://dx.doi.org/10.1016/j.mcna.2014.04.005
0025-7125/14/$ – see front matter © 2014 Elsevier Inc. All rights reserved.

Evaluating Anterior Knee Pain

Engene Hong, MD, CAQSM, FAAFP*, Michael C. Kraft, MD

KEYWORDS

- Anterior knee pain • Bursitis • Patellar pain • Patellar fractures
- Patellar tendinopathy • Patellofemoral pain syndrome • Patellar subluxation
- Chondromalacia • Osgood Schlatter's disease

KEY POINTS

- Patellofemoral osteoarthritis and chondromalacia are common causes of anterior knee pain and may be overlooked as the etiology (especially if the radiology report reads "normal").
- Quadriceps and patellar tendinopathy often occur in patients where there is repetitive stress placed on the anterior knee, such as in jumping and running sports.
- Patellar dislocation and subluxation is a common problem with incidence of 5.8 per 100,000 persons and increasing to 29 per 100,000 persons in the age range of 10 to 17 years old.
- Bursitis of the knee commonly occurs in the pre-patellar bursa or the pes anserine bursa.
- Patellofemoral pain syndrome can be described as patellar tracking dysfunction, and is a common cause of anterior knee pain.
- A bipartite patella is the result of a secondary ossification center that did not completely fuse to the primary site.
- Osgood-Schlatter is a condition that typically presents at the beginning of a growth spurt.
- Sinding-Larsen-Johannson syndrome is a traction apophysitis of the inferior pole of the patella.
- Osteochondritis dissecans is an uncommon but important cause of anterior knee pain in adolescents.
- Plicae are remnants of embryologic tissue.
- Patellar fractures can account for up to 1% of all fractures seen.
- Fat pad impingement syndrome can be an unusual cause of anterior knee pain.

Division of Sports Medicine, Drexel University College of Medicine, 10 Shurs Lane, Ste 301, Philadelphia, PA 19127, USA
* Corresponding author.
E-mail address: Eugene.Hong@DrexelMed.edu

Med Clin N Am 98 (2014) 697–717
http://dx.doi.org/10.1016/j.mcna.2014.03.001
0025-7125/14/$ – see front matter © 2014 Elsevier Inc. All rights reserved.

INTRODUCTION

Musculoskeletal complaints account for about 20% to 30% of all primary care office visits; of these visits, discomfort in the knee, shoulder, and back are the most prevalent musculoskeletal symptoms. Having pain or dysfunction in the front part of the knee is a common presentation and reason for a patient to see a health care provider.

A good history and thorough physical examination are essential to an accurate diagnosis of the cause of anterior knee symptoms. In turn, an accurate diagnosis is essential to optimal management and best possible outcome for the patient. As with other musculoskeletal conditions, the overall goals in management of anterior knee pain are to improve comfort, restore function, maximize function, and to preserve function.

There are a number of pathophysiological etiologies to anterior knee pain. This article describes some of the common and less common causes, and includes sections on diagnosis and treatment for each condition, as well as key points.

PATELLOFEMORAL OSTEOARTHRITIS AND CHONDROMALACIA

Key points for patellofemoral osteoarthritis (OA) and chondromalacia

1. Patellofemoral OA and chondromalacia are common causes of anterior knee pain and may be overlooked as the etiology (especially if the radiology report reads "normal").

2. Physical examination findings may largely be nonspecific, but an important finding is tenderness over the lateral or medial patella facet.

3. Radiologic evaluations can be very helpful aides in diagnosing this condition. The Merchant or skyline view is helpful when evaluating isolated patellofemoral OA.

4. Nonoperative management may include ideal body weight maintenance, physical therapy, oral medication and supplements, corticosteroid and viscosupplementation injections, and bracing.

5. The overall goal of treatment is to improve and maximize patient comfort and function.

Introduction

Isolated patellofemoral OA is not an uncommon disease process; it can be an etiology of anterior knee pain or simply an incidental finding on radiographs without clinical significance. In a study conducted by Davies and colleagues,[1] of 206 knees of patients older than 60 presenting with symptomatic knee pain, 15.4% of men and 13.6% of women had isolated patellofemoral osteoarthritis. In another study, of 240 asymptomatic knees of patients 55 years and older, 19% of men and 34% of women had radiologic evidence of isolated patellofemoral osteoarthritis.[2] Patellofemoral osteoarthritis, defined as a loss of the cartilage in the trochlear groove and retro-patella surface, is found in approximately half of patients who are diagnosed with degenerative arthritis of the knee.[3] Chondromalacia is a softening of the patellofemoral cartilage, and may be a precursor to degenerative joint disease in this compartment of the knee. For the purposes of this article, both chondromalacia and OA can be the cause of anterior knee pain related to the cartilage in this knee compartment.

Diagnosis

Patients with patellofemoral OA or chondromalacia will typically present with anterior knee pain. There is no one single defining symptom that is characteristic of patellofemoral OA. The presenting anterior knee discomfort may be exacerbated by kneeling or squatting, walking up or down hills or inclines, climbing or descending stairs, rising from a seated position, or being in one position for too long (typically sitting).[3] There may be crepitus or a cracking sensation. Often, patients will complain of stiffness in the knee, especially in the morning on first waking; occasionally there may be a sensation of locking (which is really a pseudo locking) or catching, secondary to irritation between the patella and trochlea groove when friction occurs between the bones.[3] Iwano and colleagues[4] tried to assess a patient's activities of daily living (ADLs) to further support a diagnosis of patellofemoral OA. In this scale, the highest attainable score was 14 points. Iwano and colleagues[4] had found that a score of 4.1 was more predictive of patellofemoral OA combined with femorotibial OA; however, a score of 9.4 was more predictive of isolated patellofemoral OA. Iwano and colleagues[4] used the following 7 items to help predict the presence and type of OA: (1) Clarke test (positive when patients complained of pain during knee extension with patella compression), (2) limitation of patellar mobility, (3) pain on compression of the patella, (4) peripatellar tenderness, (5) crepitation during knee movement, (6) crepitation on grinding of the patella, and (7) pain on grinding the patella. Each item was given a score of 0 to 2 points. Two points equaled maneuvers completed without any problem, 1 point equaled maneuvers completed with some difficultly, and 0 equaled maneuvers completed with great difficulty.

Evaluating a patient with suspected patellofemoral OA or chondromalacia may be challenging for the busy primary care provider. The physical examination may often have nonspecific findings. Leslie and Bentley[5] found retro patellar crepitus, effusion, and quadriceps wasting greater than 2 cm as the most important findings for detection of chondromalacia of the patella. According to Grelsamer,[6] the most important sign for patellofemoral OA is tenderness over the medial or lateral patellar facet. Often radiographic evidence can largely aid in diagnosis. One of the most important views that should be obtained is the Merchant or skyline view (45° angle). Radiographically, patellofemoral joint arthritis can be classified into 4 stages of severity. The stages are as follows: stage 1, mild with more than 3 mm of joint space preserved; stage 2, moderate with less than 3 mm of joint space preserved but no bony contacts; stage 3, severe with the bony surfaces in contact with less than one-quarter of the joint surface; and stage 4, very severe with bony contact throughout the entirety of the joint.[7]

Treatment

In patients who have symptomatic patellofemoral OA or chondromalacia, there are a number of options to improve comfort and maximize function. An ideal body weight will decrease the load on the anterior knee. Physical therapy will help with the management by focusing on stabilizing the patella and includes strengthening the entire lower kinetic chain. Oral medications and supplements include nonsteroidal anti-inflammatory agents, as well as glucosamine (an over-the-counter supplement, 1500 mg/d). Intra-articular steroid injections may also be useful in alleviating symptoms[3] intermittently. Consider adding hyaluronic acid (viscosupplementation) injections intra-articularly. Although not used routinely, a patella stabilization brace or an unloading knee brace may be helpful in pain relief[8,9] and improving function. Operative treatments should be reserved when 3 to 6 months of nonoperative treatment is not effective in improving comfort and function of the patient. Surgical options may include realignment of the extensor mechanism, osteotomies of the tibial tubercle, patellectomy, patellofemoral replacement, and total knee arthroplasty.[3]

QUADRICEPS AND PATELLAR TENDINOPATHY

Key points for quadriceps and patellar tendinopathy

1. Quadriceps and patellar tendinopathy often occur in patients where there is repetitive stress placed on the anterior knee, such as in jumping and running sports.

2. Physical examination will typically show tenderness to palpation of the affected tendon, usually at or near its insertion onto the patella. Consider evaluating for tendon rupture in the appropriate clinical situation.

3. If imaging is needed ultrasound and magnetic resonance imaging (MRI) are the most sensitive to evaluate the tendon.

4. Aggressive nonoperative management is key and may include activity modification, topical ice, oral or topical medications, bracing, and physical therapy that includes stretching and *eccentric strengthening.*

5. Consider referral for the patient whose symptoms or dysfunction persist or worsen, or if the diagnosis is unclear.

Introduction

Quadriceps and patellar tendinopathy (also known as Jumper's Knee) are common conditions seen in sports medicine offices, and were first described by Blazina and colleagues.[10] These conditions are most often a result of overuse: repetitive stresses on the tendon overwhelm the tissue's ability to heal itself, resulting in symptoms and dysfunction. This section does not discuss the acute traumatic rupture of either tendon. Patellar tendinopathy can be broken down into 4 stages: Blazina stages I to IV. The stages are broken down in the following manner (**Box 1**).

Most patients encountered with this diagnosis will be the skeletally mature athlete from high school age to middle age, although it is possible to encounter these conditions in the younger and older populations. Oftentimes this will be seen in sports or activities that require repetitive stresses on the patellar and quadriceps tendons (eg, jumping). Some obvious examples of "at-risk" sports are basketball and volleyball,[11-17] but we have seen these conditions in nearly every sport, including soccer, football, wrestling, and lacrosse.

Diagnosis

The patient population will typically be composed of the demographics previously described. These patients will typically complain of an aching pain in the anterior portion of the knee, and may be able to localize the source as below or above the

---

Box 1
The Blazina stages of patellar tendinopathy

Blazina Stage	Presenting Symptoms
I	Pain only after sports activity
II	Pain at the beginning of sports activity, disappearing after warm-up and reappearing at fatigue
III	Constant pain at rest and during activity. Athlete unable to compete at previous level
IV	Complete rupture of patellar tendon

patella. Ask the patient if he or she can put a finger on the location of the anterior knee pain. The pain can be further classified into the Blazina stages, which will affect the treatment. Palpating the tendon should elicit discomfort in these conditions. Strength testing may also cause discomfort. This is a clinical diagnosis, that is, a thorough history and good knee physical examination is typically all that is needed for diagnosis. An important maneuver if concerned for an acute rupture of either tendon is to look for an extension lag, that is, the ability, or lack thereof, to easily bring the knee into full extension from a flexed starting position; compared with the other leg, any asymmetry could be consistent with a disruption of the affected knee extensor mechanism.

Imaging can be useful when the diagnosis is uncertain, to evaluate for other diagnoses or a tendon rupture, or occasionally to monitor progress. MRI or ultrasound are the most sensitive imaging tests for supporting a diagnosis of quadriceps or patellar tendinopathy.[18–21] Musculoskeletal ultrasound may have several advantages, including real-time dynamic evaluation (useful for partial tear evaluation) and sensitive measurements of tendinosis changes (tendon thickening, signal heterogeneity, calcifications, enthesophyte formation, and neovascularization).[22,23]

Treatment

Treatment for quadriceps or patellar tendinopathy is primarily nonoperative in nature and can be managed by the primary care provider. Aggressive nonoperative management may include activity modifications (decreasing the stress on the quadriceps and patellar tendon), cryotherapy (20–30 minutes of topical ice 3–4 times a day), stretching (including the extensors/flexors of the hip and knee, and the iliotibial band), strengthening (including all extensors/flexors of hip and knee).[24,25] Eccentric strengthening exercises are key to good rehabilitation for these conditions, and good physical therapy plays an important part of the management. Corticosteroid should NOT be injected into either tendon; the quadriceps and patellar tendons are load-bearing tendons and have a higher risk of rupture after steroid injection than non–load-bearing tendons. Oral nonsteroidal anti-inflammatory medications may be used also to improve comfort and function. Topical application of nitroglycerin has shown some promise for chronic tendinosis by improving blood flow and stimulating fibroblastic activity in the affected area. A counterforce brace is useful for patellar tendinopathy; the brace reduces the stress of the proximal patella on its insertion of the distal patella.

Invasive management options for chronic quadriceps or patellar tendinopathy include percutaneous tenotomy, platelet-rich plasma injections, prolotherapy, and surgical debridement.

PATELLAR DISLOCATIONS AND SUBLUXATIONS

Key points for patellar dislocations and subluxations

1. Patellar dislocation and subluxation is a common problem with incidence of 5.8 per 100,000 persons and increasing to 29 per 100,000 persons in the age range of 10 to 17 years old.

2. The patella will most often dislocate laterally.

3. Initial imaging should be plain films with the following views: anteroposterior, lateral, and axial (Merchant or sunrise).

4. Initial management should consist of protecting the knee and restricting its range of motion.

Introduction

The incidence of patellar dislocations with the general population is 5.8 per 100,000 persons; for ages 10 to 17 years, the incidence increases to 29 per 100,000 persons.[26] Most often, the dislocation or subluxation is lateral. This can occur as a result of direct trauma to the knee, or just as frequently by indirect trauma (for example, a pivoting mechanism without a direct blow to the knee). The patients who present with an indirect trauma history may have predisposing mechanical factors, such as a hypermobile patella, patella alta (high riding patella), a shallow trochlear groove, or a systemic collagen tissue disorder (eg, Marfan syndrome).[27]

Diagnosis

A patient will present complaining of anterior knee pain and may report hearing a pop or snap at the time of injury; the patient may describe feeling as if the knee itself dislocated. The patella can spontaneously reduce itself before the patient presents in the office; otherwise a manual reduction of the dislocated patella is necessary. A good history and physical are essential to the diagnosis. It is important to ascertain whether or not this has previously occurred, either in the same or contralateral knee. Reoccurrence can be as high as a sixfold increase.[26]

On physical examination, a patient will typically have tenderness over the medial retinaculum and there may be an intra-articular effusion in the acute setting as well as a positive apprehension sign. The apprehension sign is when the examiner tries to displace the reduced patella in the direction of the previous dislocation (typically laterally), and the patient exhibits apprehension with the maneuver because of concern of dislocation. If the effusion is aspirated, a hemarthrosis should raise the suspicion of an osteochondral fracture and warrant further evaluation for such.[26] The initial imaging should be plain radiographs that include anteroposterior, lateral, and axial (Merchant or sunrise) views. Look for patella tilting on the axial x-rays, that is, asymmetry to the way the patella sits in the femoral trochlear groove. Up to 95% of patients with first-time dislocations may have some damage to the articular cartilage from the injury.[28] MRI may be obtained if there is concern for significant osteochondral injury, to evaluate the extent of cartilage damage or other injury to the knee, or if the diagnosis is unclear.

Treatment

Nonoperative treatment for patellar dislocation and subluxation should focus on restoring stability to the anterior knee. In a lateral patella dislocation, the medial retinaculum and the medial patellofemoral ligament are disrupted. If there is an intra-articular effusion present, knee aspiration can be considered but is not always required; consider performing it if suspicious for a hemiarthrosis or to provide the patient with symptom relief. Postinjury management for a true patella dislocation involves protecting the knee and restricting the range of motion; consider placing the knee in a postoperative brace and restricting the motion to 0 to 30° initially. Crutches can be used for comfort and the patient is allowed to weight-bear as tolerated on the injured splinted leg. Topical ice and oral nonsteroidal anti-inflammatory medications can be used to reduce swelling and for pain control. Protecting the knee and restricting motion will allow the anterior medial structures (retinaculum and ligament) to heal.[26] The patient should be reevaluated every 2 to 3 weeks. Consider 4 to 6 weeks of relative immobilization for the first-time dislocation episode, before increasing the allowed range of motion and starting physical therapy. The goal of rehabilitation is to restore motion and regain function of the knee and lower leg.

Indications for referral to orthopedic surgery include an osteochondral fracture, the presence of intra-articular loose bodies, or persistent symptoms or dysfunction after aggressive nonoperative management. For the active patient with a history of recurrent patella dislocation, consider surgical consult for surgical stabilization, including medial patellofemoral ligament reconstruction.

PREPATELLAR AND PES ANSERINE BURSITIS

Key points for prepatellar and pes anserine bursitis

1. Bursitis of the knee commonly occurs in the prepatellar bursa or the pes anserine bursa.

2. Consider the possibility of a septic bursitis, especially with prepatellar bursitis, and manage accordingly.

3. Clinical presentation will include pain with aggravating activities, and localized swelling and tenderness on examination.

4. A thorough history and a good physical examination are essential for diagnosis; ultrasound can confirm the presence of a bursal effusion.

5. Initial management includes activity modification, rest, ice, and anti-inflammatory medication; it may also include physical therapy, aspiration, and corticosteroid injection.

Introduction

Bursitis about the knee usually occurs in 1 of 2 bursa, the prepatellar and the pes anserine. The prepatellar bursa is located anterior to the extensor mechanism between the subcutaneous tissue and the patella. The pes anserine bursa overlies the medial tibial metaphysis just inferior to the tibial plateau; the bursa is just deep to the insertion of sartorius, semitendinous, and gracilis muscles on to the proximal tibia. Bursitis can be caused by direct trauma, infections, and repetitive overuse. The prepatellar bursa in particular can be susceptible to an infectious septic bursitis due to its superficial location. The exact incidence of both prepatellar and pes anserine bursitis is currently unknown because many patients may not seek out treatment.[29] Patients whose occupations or passions may predispose them to prepatellar bursitis include coal miners, carpet layers, gardeners, roofers, housekeepers, and athletes such as wrestlers.[29,30] Pes anserine bursitis can affect patients of all ages and pursuits; in athletes, the more commonly affected may be middle-aged and older female long-distance runners.[31,32]

Diagnosis

For both prepatellar and pes anserine bursitis, pain is typically present with direct pressure or activity at first. Local swelling over the involved bursa also is a typical finding, especially in prepatellar bursitis.[33–35] In acute bursitis, the area may be swollen, tender, and warm to the touch. In cases of chronic bursitis, a patient may have a history of swelling and pain that waxes and wanes; this may be seen in occupations that require prolonged or repetitive kneeling on hard surfaces.[29] In making the diagnosis of aseptic prepatellar or pes anserine bursitis, a good history and physical is all that is needed. Further imaging is not needed to confirm the diagnosis of bursitis; imaging may be used if the diagnosis is unclear or to evaluate for other causes of pain or dysfunction. Pes anserine bursitis will typically present with anterior and medial pain that may worsen with the use of stairs, pain at night or morning pain, and stiffness lasting more than an hour.[32]

Significant erythema, warmth, tenderness of the prepatellar bursa, or accompa-
nying systemic signs, such as a fever, nausea, or malaise, should raise the suspicion
of a septic bursitis. In this case, consider a diagnostic aspiration, sending the aspirate
for Gram stain, cell count, and culture; also consider treating empirically with antibiotics covering gram-positive organisms from skin flora while awaiting laboratory
results.

Treatment

Initial treatment for both prepatellar and pes anserine bursitis starts with activity modification, rest, topical ice and nonsteroidal anti-inflammatory drugs (NSAIDs).[31,32,36,37]
Activity modification for prepatellar bursitis consists of avoiding prolonged kneeling
postures or pain-precipitating activities[29,36]; for pes anserine bursitis, the inciting activity may need to be modified; for example, reducing the duration, frequency, and intensity of running in a marathoner. Physical therapy may be helpful. Consider
aspirating a significant effusion with prepatellar bursitis, not only for diagnosis, as
mentioned previously, but also for improved comfort and function. Corticosteroid injections may be helpful in treating either bursitis; of course, if septic bursitis is suspected, corticosteroid injections should be avoided. Surgical excision, bursectomy,
is reserved for refractory cases for both prepatellar and pes anserine bursitis and is
rarely needed.[29,32]

PATELLOFEMORAL PAIN SYNDROME (PATELLAR TRACKING DYSFUNCTION)

Key points for patellofemoral pain syndrome (patellar tracking dysfunction)

1. Patellofemoral pain syndrome can be described as patellar tracking dysfunction, and is a common cause of anterior knee pain.
2. Three contributing factors include overactivity, malalignment of the lower extremity, and muscular imbalance of the lower extremity.
3. Common symptoms include anterior knee pain with prolonged rest and strenuous activity that causes an increased load on the patellofemoral joint, such as squatting, jumping, and running.
4. A good history and thorough physical examination are essential to the diagnosis; on physical examination, pain can often be reproduced in the office with 1-legged squatting.
5. Initial therapy includes activity modification, topical ice, and good physical therapy that addresses the entire kinetic chain; bracing, orthotics, and injections also can be considered.

Introduction

Patellofemoral pain syndrome is a common cause of anterior knee pain. The authors
prefer to describe the condition as patellar tracking dysfunction; this more accurately
describes the underlying mechanical etiology of this condition. An appropriate analogy
is that the patella is like a train, and the trochlear groove is like a train track; in patellar
tracking dysfunction, the train is having difficulty staying on the track as it moves up
and down with knee flexion and extension.

The patients may describe a multitude of symptoms, including diffuse, aching anterior knee pain that worsens with activities, with intermittent sharp discomfort in
the knee. Women may be at higher risk for patellar tracking dysfunction because of
the normal female anatomy of a wider pelvis leading to an increased Q angle at the

knee. Overactivity, malalignment of the lower extremity, and muscular imbalance of the lower extremity seem to be 3 contributing factors.[38]

Diagnosis

Patients present with a variety of symptoms; however, there are a few common symptoms that present a little more frequently. These include pain with both prolonged rest and strenuous activity; the strenuous activity is usually one that increases the load on the weight-bearing knee, such as jumping, climbing stairs, or running. Crepitus may be reported by the patient, as well as found on physical examination. Occasionally patients may even complain of the knee giving way or buckling; it may be helpful to differentiate between this not uncommon pseudo buckling complaint in patellar tracking dysfunction, and true buckling such as is found with an anterior cruciate ligament tear.

On physical examination, findings can include tenderness (articular surface of the patella or peripatellar tenderness), discomfort with displacement of the patella medially or laterally (apprehension maneuver), inhibition sign (Clark test), and crepitus with flexion and extension. Occasionally, a clinician might find asymmetry of the vastus medialis. In making the diagnosis, the pain is typically reproducible in the office setting with squatting.[39] Have the patient stand on the affected leg and slowly go down into a 1-legged squat as far as possible, looking for reproduction of the anterior knee pain in deep flexion. Occasionally this may be the only "positive" finding on office examination: the one physical examination maneuver that reproduces the patient's pain. Look for evidence of hip abductor weakness by seeing if the knee deviates medially with 1-legged squat; if the patient is not able to maintain a straight up and down alignment because of hip weakness, this should be corrected with good physical therapy as part of the management. Also evaluate for pes planovalgus on examination; this can be corrected with orthotic inserts and needs to be considered as part of the overall treatment plan for patellar tracking dysfunction.

Physical examination has shown to be more useful than radiographs[40] in making the diagnosis; however, imaging may be important to rule out other causes of anterior knee pain as clinically indicated.

Treatment

Treatment of patellar tracking dysfunction is primarily nonoperative, and surgery is very rarely indicated. Initial therapy should be focused on pain relief for the patient, which can be achieved with rest, ice, and analgesics. Patients also should focus on activity modification, often this includes reduction of jumping, squatting, kneeling, and climbing activities (to decrease the patellofemoral load). A patellar sleeve knee brace with a lateral buttress (a patellar stabilization brace) may prove to be helpful in reducing pain in these patients by assisting a more functional and less painful tracking of the patella in the trochlear groove.[41] Physical therapy also may be of benefit to recovery with keeping the following key factors in mind: flexibility, strength, endurance, proprioception, functional training, and gradual progression of exercise load.[38] Specific goals of therapy can include strengthening the muscles of the entire lower leg (including the hip and quadriceps, as mentioned previously) to aid in more functional patellar tracking. Orthotics (as mentioned previously), corticosteroid injections, and viscosupplementation also can be considered for treatment.

Surgery is rarely used for this condition, and outcomes are mixed with patellar realignment surgical procedures. The goal of operative and nonoperative management for patellar tracking dysfunction is restoring and maximizing the patients comfort and function.

BIPARTITE PATELLA

Key points for bipartite patella

1. A bipartite patella is the result of a secondary ossification center that did not completely fuse to the primary site.

2. Three types of bipartite patella have been described based on the location of the accessory fragment: type 1, 5% of cases, is within the inferior pole; type 2, 20% of cases, is within the lateral margin; and type 3, 75% of cases, is within the superolateral pole.

3. Active young men are at a higher risk of developing a painful bipartite patella; however, only 2% of all bipartite patellas become symptomatic.

4. Plain radiographs can be used as the initial modality for imaging; the skyline view with weight-bearing and non–weight-bearing views may also be helpful in diagnosis.

5. Aggressive nonoperative management should initially be attempted, including ice, activity modification, NSAIDs, stretching of the quadriceps, and a patellar sleeve brace.

Introduction

A bipartite patella is a less common cause of anterior knee pain. The patella will typically ossify from 1 center (77% of the time), but 23% of the time it will ossify from 2 to 3 centers in children.[42] These ossification centers will typically fuse mutually, but in about 2% to 6% will remain separated.[43] When the secondary ossification centers fail to amalgamate, a bipartite patella is formed.[44] Bipartite patella is more common in men compared with women, at a ratio of 9:1 and is seen bilaterally in 50% of the cases.[45] Three types of bipartite patella have been described based on the accessory fragment position: type 1, 5% of cases, is within the inferior pole; type 2, 20% of cases, is within the lateral margin; and type 3, 75% of cases, is within the superolateral pole.[46]

Diagnosis

Most cases of bipartite patella are incidental findings on radiographs or on physical examination and remain asymptomatic. However, approximately 2% of bipartite patellas becomes symptomatic and painful.[47] Most of the patients who present with a painful bipartite patella are men younger than 20 years of age and who are active in sports.[42,47] On rare occasions, patients may present as adults participating in strenuous activity or from a traumatic fracture.[45] A direct trauma history or indirect injury while cycling or hill climbing may be obtained in the history.[48] The patient will usually report increased pain with most activities the involve knee extension, but the most significant pain is often in a squatting position.[45]

Physical examination often only shows a patella that has localized tenderness over the accessory fragment,[45] usually in the upper outer quadrant. Initial imaging should include plain films with anteroposterior and skyline views. This is often enough to determine if indeed a bipartite patella exists. If the patient is symptomatic, an additional weight-bearing skyline view in the squatting position may be helpful.[49] If the bipartite patella is the source of pain, there may be a greater degree of separation of the ossification centers on the weight-bearing portion compared with the non–weight-bearing view.[49] An MRI, if obtained, also may show bone marrow edema within the accessory fragment.[50]

Treatment

Initial treatment of a symptomatic bipartite patella consists of 2 to 4 weeks of rest, activity modification, NSAIDs, quadriceps muscle stretching to decrease the load, and a patellar sleeve brace to aide in patellar support.[51] If the patient is acutely painful, for example from direct trauma, an immobilizing brace may be helpful with the brace locked at less than 30° of flexion to alleviate the superolateral tension of the vastus lateralis[45] for an additional short period of time (1–2 weeks). Most patients will respond nicely to this treatment regimen and will be able to return to play. If the patient has been unable to return to play within 6 months of nonoperative management, some surgeons may consider surgical excision of the offending accessory fragment.[45]

ADOLESCENT CAUSES OF ANTERIOR KNEE PAIN
Osgood-Schlatter Disease

Key points for Osgood-Schlatter disease

1. Osgood-Schlatter is a condition that typically presents at the beginning of a growth spurt.
2. Adolescents who are affected by this are typically the ones who engage in running, cutting and jumping sports.
3. On examination, tenderness can be localized to the (prominent) tibial tubercle.
4. This condition is often self-limited, and nonoperative therapy is the cornerstone of management.
5. When nonoperative therapy fails or complications arise, it is recommended to refer to a specialist.

Introduction

Osgood-Schlatter disease is a common cause of anterior knee pain in the adolescent. It is an apophysitis of the tibial tubercle, thus found only in the skeletally immature in acute cases. Patients usually present at the beginning of their growth spurt with this pain. In boys, this tends to be 10 to 15 years of age and in girls, 8 to 13 years of age. Boys also seem to be more affected than girls.[52] Most adolescents are patients who are active in sports with running and cutting involved, such as soccer, basketball, and lacrosse.[53] With the tibial apophyses undergoing repetitive stress from the patellar tendon constantly pulling on it, this can lead to the condition and presentation of the patient.

Diagnosis

Patients are brought in by parents complaining of swelling, warmth, and pain within the anterior portion of the knee.[52] Most will point to the tibial tuberosity when asked where the pain is located; however, some may report a vague anterior knee pain that is made worse with squatting or stairs. The tibial tubercle may appear prominent in fact. Recent trauma should be ruled out during the initial evaluation. On physical examination, there is often an enlarged tender tibial tubercle at the distal patellar tendon insertion. This is often bilateral. Imaging studies are not necessary to make the diagnosis, unless the clinician has a high suspicion for infection, neoplasm, or occult trauma.[52] If the pain is acute in onset or prolonged in nature, radiographs can help rule out an avulsion fracture or significantly displaced apophyses.

Treatment

Most patients respond well to appropriate nonoperative therapy. Icing, decreasing or avoiding aggravating activities, and anti-inflammatory medications are the cornerstones of treatment.[54] Reassurance is also a part of management of the adolescent and parents; this is typically a self-limited disease, although it may last months to several years until the patient stops growing. Steroid injections are NOT indicated.[53,54] Padding the anterior knee may be helpful; the tibial tubercle can be sensitive to direct trauma in sports. The authors will usually let the adolescent engage in most activities, recommending that their symptoms be their guide to sports and that they modify their activities if there is significant discomfort or dysfunction. If there is a significantly displaced apophysis or fracture, or prolonged symptoms, consider referral to an orthopedic surgeon for possible fixation.[53]

Sinding-Larsen-Johannson Syndrome

Key points for Sinding-Larsen-Johannson syndrome

1. Sinding-Larsen-Johannson syndrome is a traction apophysitis of the inferior pole of the patella.

2. This disease is typically seen in active adolescents with age range of 10 to 13 years.

3. Patients typically present with pain at the inferior pole of the patella that is exacerbated with activities that increase the patellofemoral load.

4. Physical examination will have tenderness at the inferior pole of patella, along with quadriceps and hamstring tightness.

5. As with other traction apophysitis locations, activity modification is the cornerstone of treatment.

Introduction

Sinding-Larsen-Johannson syndrome is a traction apophysitis of the inferior pole of the patella. It is typically seen in boys 10 to 13 years of age; however, active girls also may present with this. It is caused by repetitive stress on the patella at the proximal insertion of the patellar tendon.[55] The pain can range from mild to severe and the duration of these symptoms can be from 3 to 18 months.[55] Patients will usually be involved in sports or exercise that requires a fair amount of running or jumping.

Diagnosis

Patients will usually present pain with any activity that increases the patellofemoral joint load (eg, running, jumping, climbing, stairs, squatting/kneeling).[55,56] On physical examination, there is focal tenderness at the patella's inferior pole; there also may be localized soft tissue swelling. There should not be significant tenderness elsewhere in the patellofemoral compartment, and inhibition testing and apprehension testing are usually unremarkable or equivocal.[56] The quadriceps may have decreased flexibility when compared with the unaffected side, as does the hamstring on the injured side.[56] Imaging is not required for diagnosis, but can be obtained for confirmation of the patella apophyses, and to rule out significant apophyseal displacement.

Treatment

The mainstay of treatment is activity modification and rest from aggravating activities, such as running, jumping, and climbing.[55,56] A period of 2 to 4 weeks of avoiding any aggravating activities, followed by 4 to 6 weeks of gradual reintroduction of sports and exercise is a reasonable first step. Anti-inflammatory medications and application of topical ice daily may be used to decrease the acute inflammation of the apophysitis. A patellar tendon counterforce strap or patella knee sleeve can be helpful with symptoms during activity.[55] Physical therapy also can be helpful in symptom reduction and to address hamstring and quadriceps tightness.[56] Physical therapy may help with a faster and more successful return to sports and exercise. Surgery intervention, for example, ossicle excision or tubercleplasty, can be considered for persistent symptoms but is rarely indicated; surgery can be considered for an apophysis that is significantly displaced.[56]

Osteochondritis Dissecans

Key points for osteochondritis dissecans

1. Osteochondritis dissecans (OCD) is an uncommon but important cause of anterior knee pain in adolescents.

2. OCD can be linked to an injury, but also may occur with repetitive micro-injuries to the subchondral bone, leading to an area of focal necrosis.

3. Plain radiographs are essential to the diagnosis, and include tunnel views in addition to the standard anteroposterior, lateral, and sunrise views.

4. After x-ray confirmation, MRI should be obtained for evaluation of stability. MRI also can be considered if radiographs are negative but an OCD is still clinically suspected.

5. Unstable OCD lesions need surgical intervention; stable lesions may be considered for nonoperative management first. Non–weight-bearing status should be considered on initial high suspicion of the presence of an OCD lesion pending further evaluation with imaging.

Introduction

OCD is a relatively uncommon diagnosis in adolescents, but an important one to recognize. However, when it is diagnosed there seems to be predominance in the male population and the age range is typically in those 10 to 23 years old.[57] OCD is defined as a focal area of necrosis within the subchondral bone.

Diagnosis

The typical patient profile is a male, 10 to 23 years old, and involved with organized sports. The patient will report most commonly pain related to the sports or activity, and may also report sensations of giving way (buckling or pseudo buckling) or painful catching. The pain is often poorly localized and weight bearing worsens the pain.[58,59] On a detailed history, up to 21% of patients can associate the pain with an injury.[58] Physical examination findings are often nonspecific; there may be an effusion and crepitus.[60] The provider needs to have a high index of suspicion and consider this possible diagnosis in the appropriate clinical setting; OCD, however, needs imaging to confirm the diagnosis.[61]

Initial imaging should be plain radiographs and include lateral, tunnel, and anteroposterior views of the knee.[61] If anteroposterior views are the only films used to evaluate this suspected diagnosis, it is possible to miss lesions of the posterior aspect of the medial femoral condyle, a not uncommon place for OCD lesions to occur.[62] Tunnel views are not standard, and should be requested specifically; in a tunnel view, the knee is flexed 45°, the beam is shot posterior to anterior, and there is an improved visualization of the trochlear groove, femoral condyles, and tibial spine in this plane. Some of the indications for ordering a tunnel view are suspected OCD lesion, loose bodies, or arthritis.

It is important to remember that up to 30% of OCD injuries are bilateral; if the OCD diagnosis is confirmed, the contralateral knee should be evaluated and imaged.[63] If OCD is confirmed on plain radiographs, an MRI should be obtained to evaluate the stability of the injury and to stage the lesion.[61] MRI can also be considered if the radiographs are unremarkable but there is still a clinical suspicion of an OCD lesion. Prognosis and management will differ based on the stage of the OCD lesion; stages 1 to 4 have been described.[61] MRI has been shown to have 97% sensitivity at detecting unstable lesions.[64,65]

Treatment

Treatment for OCD lesions can largely be differentiated on whether the lesion is felt to be stable or unstable. Grades 1 and 2 are thought to be more stable, with a lower risk of displacement of the lesion into the joint and with a higher likelihood of healing and good functional outcome. If the OCD lesion is deemed unstable, surgery may be considered. For the stable OCD lesion, grades 1 and 2, generally a nonoperative approach is used.[61] In the skeletally immature, the goal of management is to have the lesion heal before the physes closing.[61] In the skeletally mature adult, the goal of therapy is to preserve as much function as possible and prevent early-onset degenerative joint disease.[63] In all patients, the overall goal of management is to preserve the integrity of the joint and articular cartilage surfaces as much as possible.

With aggressive nonoperative management of the stable OCD lesion in the skeletally immature patient, consider making the patient non–weight bearing from the time of initial diagnosis or even with a suspected OCD lesion. Given the potential risk for a poor outcome with an OCD lesion, as well as the increased risk for surgical intervention with this condition, consider a referral to a specialist, sports medicine or orthopedic surgery, for confirmed or suspected OCD lesions in a patient of any age for further evaluation and management.

OTHER CAUSES OF ANTERIOR KNEE PAIN
Patellar Fracture

Key points for patellar fracture

1. Patellar fractures can account for up to 1% of all fractures seen.

2. Patellar fractures may be obtained from either direct (ie, dashboard injury) or indirect (ie, extensor load greater than patella tensile strength) trauma.

3. Open and closed fractures have different approaches, but the extensor mechanism should always be assessed.

4. Anteroposterior and lateral views should be obtained to help guide the management and assess if the fracture is displaced or nondisplaced.

5. Nonsurgical management is an acceptable approach in a patient with a nondisplaced fracture and intact extensor mechanism.

Introduction

Patellar fractures can account for up to 1% of all fractures seen. The patient will typically present after some sort of trauma, whether direct or indirect.[66] Often the direct trauma is from a fall directly onto the anterior knee, or the knee hitting the dashboard in a motor vehicle accident. With an indirect trauma history, the patella can fracture as a result of load failure with increasing extensor mechanism tension.[67,68]

Diagnosis

A detailed history and physical are key to making the diagnosis. If in the history a direct blow from high energy (eg, a dashboard injury) is obtained, the provider should also have a suspicion for associated injuries, such as posterior wall acetabular fracture and femoral neck fracture.[66] Always examine the joint above and below the one that the patient reports being symptomatic. Open patella fractures should be referred to orthopedics immediately. In the case of closed patellar fractures, inspection and palpation may show the following abnormalities: a palpable defect or step off within the patella, an effusion from hemarthrosis, and patella bony tenderness.[66] It is important to decipher if the extensor mechanism of the lower limb is still intact, as this will help guide treatment; perform an extension lag test to assess for integrity of the entire extensor mechanism of the knee.[66] Anteroposterior and lateral radiographs at a minimum are obtained for radiographic support and confirmation of a patellar fracture.

Treatment

There are 2 ways to classify patellar fractures. The more useful classification is displaced versus nondisplaced fracture. The other is the Orthopedic Trauma Association classification; this classification takes into account the number of fragments of fracture and the degree of articular involvement, and is beyond the scope of this review.[69] A fracture is displaced depending on 2 factors: the degree of step-off and a fracture gap. A displaced fracture has a step-off greater than 2 to 3 mm and a fracture gap greater than 1 to 4 mm.[67] A nonsurgical approach is appropriate if the patient has a nondisplaced fracture and the extensor mechanism is intact, or if the patient has significant comorbidities and the fracture is displaced.[66] In the nonsurgical approach, consider immobilization with protected weight bearing (6–8 weeks), and then physical therapy to restore motion and strength; also consider periodic radiographs every 2 to 3 weeks while immobilized until there is radiographic evidence of healing.[70,71] If the patient does not meet the 2 indications for nonsurgical management, of if the fracture is open, consider referring to orthopedic surgery.

Plica Syndrome

Key points for plica syndrome

1. Plicae are remnants of embryologic tissue.

2. Three types of plicae exist, including mediopatellar, suprapatellar, and infrapatellar, all of which can present differently.

3. MRI is the test of choice for imaging, although musculoskeletal ultrasound may be considered.

4. Nonoperative management should be attempted, including activity modification, physical therapy, topical ice, oral NSAIDs, and injections.

Introduction

Plica syndrome is a less common cause of anterior knee pain in children but in adults it has an estimated incidence of 20%.[72] Plica syndrome is persistent anterior knee pain that is caused by plicae (synovial folds) that have become thickened, fibrotic, and sometimes hemorrhagic.[73] Plicae are thought to become symptomatic by repetitive stress and microtraumas. There are 3 different locations of plicae that can cause pain, the most common is the mediopatellar plica. The other 2 types are the infrapatellar plica, which rarely causes pain, and the suprapatellar, which may present with symptoms similar to chondromalacia patellae or a suprapatellar bursitis.[72,74]

Diagnosis

Most patients will present to the office complaining of anterior knee pain; however, they also may report locking or pseudo locking, clicking during flexion and extension, and an uncomfortable intermittent catching sensation.[72] There may be an acute onset of pain after a significant increase of their typical activities, sports, exercise, or hobbies.[75] Ask the patient if there has been any change to footwear, running surface, orthotics, or any new strenuous activity attempted.[72] Patients may complain of pain with stairs or sitting with legs flexed for a prolonged period. On physical examination, there may be some nodularity or focal thickening on the anterior medial joint, typically without an intra-articular effusion.[75] However, the patient may have crepitus, loss of motion, some effusion, and quadriceps atrophy.[74] With regard to imaging, radiographs are not usually indicated; MRI can be considered.[72,74] Dynamic musculoskeletal ultrasound has proven to be useful in diagnosis, with one study having 90% sensitivity and 83% specificity[76] of identifying symptomatic plica syndrome.

Treatment

As with other causes of anterior knee pain, aggressive nonoperative therapy is the mainstay of treatment and should be attempted before surgical intervention. Nonoperative management focuses on decreasing the repetitive microtraumas by modifying the exacerbating activities, and in aiding recovery of comfort and function by using physical therapy and anti-inflammatory treatments as appropriate.[72] Corticosteroid injection of the offending plica also can be considered. If the patient fails nonoperative management, or has chronic disabling persistent symptoms, the patient can be referred to an orthopedist for possible surgical excision.[72]

Fat Pad Impingement Syndrome

Key points for fat pad impingement syndrome

1. Fat pad impingement syndrome can be an unusual cause of anterior knee pain.
2. Three main fat pads are implicated: the anterior suprapatellar, posterior suprapatellar, and infrapatellar.
3. Patients may complain of swelling and an uncomfortable catching sensation; anterior pain is often the primary complaint, as the fat pads tend to be well innervated and vascularized.
4. MRI is the best imagining modality for supporting the diagnosis.
5. Nonoperative treatment, including ice, NSAIDs, activity modification, injections, and improving extensor mechanism flexibility via physical therapy, should be part of management.

Introduction

Fat pad impingement syndrome is a less common cause of anterior knee pain and can be very debilitating to the patient. Because of the vascularization and innervation, the fat pads of the knee can be some of the most sensitive structures.[77] Often the fat pad impingement syndrome results from repetitive microtraumas, major trauma, or patellofemoral instability that causes hemorrhage, fibrosis, inflammation, or degradation of the knee fat pads.[78,79] The 3 main fat pads that are affected include the anterior suprapatellar, infrapatellar, and posterior suprapatellar, all of which can experience a symptomatic impingement.[80]

Diagnosis

Often the diagnosis of fat pad impingement syndrome is one that is initially missed and can be difficult to diagnose, making an early diagnosis paramount because of the debilitating nature of the disease.[77] Typically patients will present with some effusion within the knee and complain of an uncomfortable catching sensation.[81] The pain may be worse with prolonged standing and knee extension. It is important to decipher the location and extent of the injury, as well as any predisposing factors; this can be accomplished with several imaging modalities.[78,82] MRI and computed tomography (CT) are the most used modalities; however, with the increase in ultrasound training, dynamic ultrasound may be of use. The finding that is often associated with fat pad impingement syndrome is an enlarged, edematous fat pad.[83] This finding is best seen on MRI; the CT may not be as sensitive in revealing early inflammatory changes with the fat pad. Dynamic ultrasound scanning may be helpful in detecting fat pad edema and hyperemia but visualization can be limited by the overlying suprapatellar bursa.[78]

Treatment

Treatment is primarily nonoperative; the goals are to decrease fat pad inflammation and to decrease the amount of impingement. Nonoperative treatment includes topical ice, NSAIDs, and activity modification. Physical therapy that includes stretching of the quadriceps and hip flexors can help decrease the downward pressure of the patella on the fat pad.[77] An injection of anesthetic, with or without corticosteroid, into the offending fat pad can be considered if the provider is comfortable with this procedure; the injection can be diagnostic as well as therapeutic. If the patient continues to have persistent pain, surgical excision of the fat pad can be considered.

SUMMARY

There is no "one-size-fits-all" approach to the patient with anterior knee pain. The provider must be familiar with the relevant anatomy, elicit a good history that sets the foundation for evaluation, and perform a thorough examination that guides the provider through the differential diagnosis. Imaging and injections can be added as diagnostic tools as clinically indicated. And, of course, the provider should be aware of, if not comfortable with, the numerous possible pathophysiologic etiologies to anterior knee pain.

That being said, evaluating anterior knee pain well is certainly within the clinical acumen and scope of the interested primary care provider. In assessing a patient with anterior knee pain, there is ample room for both the science and the art of medicine. Important factors for successful management, for example, include the patient's expectations for comfort and function in work and at home, and in sports, exercise, and hobbies. Evaluating and managing the patient with anterior knee pain can be challenging and rewarding; the intent of this article was to provide a resource for the busy primary care provider to care for these patients. Remember that the goals of treatment are to improve comfort, restore function, maximize function, and preserve function.

REFERENCES

1. Davies AP, Vince AS, Shepstone L, et al. The radiologic prevalence of patellofemoral osteoarthritis. Clin Orthop Relat Res 2002;402:206–12.
2. McAlindon TE, Snow S, Cooper C, et al. Radiographic patterns of osteoarthritis of the knee joint in the community: the importance of the patellofemoral joint. Ann Rheum Dis 1992;51(7):844–9.
3. Kim YM, Joo YB. Patellofemoral osteoarthritis. Knee Surg Relat Res 2012;24(4): 193–200.
4. Iwano T, Kurosawa H, Tokuyama H, et al. Roentgenographic and clinical findings of patellofemoral osteoarthrosis. With special reference to its relationship to femorotibial osteoarthrosis and etiologic factors. Clin Orthop Relat Res 1990;252:190–7.
5. Leslie IJ, Bentley G. Arthroscopy in the diagnosis of chondromalacia patellae. Ann Rheum Dis 1978;37(6):540–7.
6. Grelsamer RP. Patellar malalignment. J Bone Joint Surg Am 2000;82-A(11): 1639–50.
7. Merchant AC, Mercer RL, Jacobsen RH, et al. Roentgenographic analysis of patellofemoral congruence. J Bone Joint Surg Am 1974;56(7):1391–6.
8. Fulkerson JP. Alternatives to patellofemoral arthroplasty. Clin Orthop Relat Res 2005;436:76–80.
9. Gobbi A, Karnatzikos G, Mahajan V, et al. Platelet-rich plasma treatment in symptomatic patients with knee osteoarthritis: preliminary results in a group of active patients. Sports Health 2012;4(2):162–72.
10. Blazina ME, Kerlan RK, Jobe FW, et al. Jumper's knee. Orthop Clin North Am 1973;4(3):665–78.
11. Cook JL, Kiss ZS, Khan KM, et al. Anthropometry, physical performance, and ultrasound patellar tendon abnormality in elite junior basketball players: a cross-sectional study. Br J Sports Med 2004;38(2):206–9.
12. Cook JL, Khan KM, Kiss ZS, et al. Reproducibility and clinical utility of tendon palpation to detect patellar tendinopathy in young basketball players. Victorian Institute of Sport tendon study group. Br J Sports Med 2001;35(1):65–9.
13. Cook JL, Khan KM, Kiss ZS, et al. Prospective imaging study of asymptomatic patellar tendinopathy in elite junior basketball players. J Ultrasound Med 2000; 19(7):473–9.
14. Busch MT. Sports medicine in children and adolescents. In: Morrissy RT, editor. Lovell and Winter's pediatric orthopaedics. Philadelphia: Lippincott-Raven; 1990. p. 1091–128.
15. Ferretti A, Ippolito E, Mariani P, et al. Jumper's knee. Am J Sports Med 1983; 11(2):58–62.
16. Lian Ø, Refsnes PE, Engebretsen L, et al. Performance characteristics of volleyball players with patellar tendinopathy. Am J Sports Med 2003;31(3): 408–13.
17. Ferretti A. Epidemiology of jumper's knee. Sports Med 1986;3(4):289–95.
18. Hamilton B, Purdam C. Patellar tendinosis as an adaptive process: a new hypothesis. Br J Sports Med 2004;38(6):758–61.
19. Gisslén K, Alfredson H. Neovascularisation and pain in jumper's knee: a prospective clinical and sonographic study in elite junior volleyball players. Br J Sports Med 2005;39(7):423–8 [discussion: 423–8].
20. Johnson DP, Wakeley CJ, Watt I. Magnetic resonance imaging of patellar tendonitis. J Bone Joint Surg Br 1996;78(3):452–7.

21. Khan KM, Bonar F, Desmond PM, et al. Patellar tendinosis (jumper's knee): findings at histopathologic examination, US, and MR imaging. Victorian Institute of Sport Tendon Study Group. Radiology 1996;200(3):821–7.
22. Warden SJ, Kiss ZS, Malara FA, et al. Comparative accuracy of magnetic resonance imaging and ultrasonography in confirming clinically diagnosed patellar tendinopathy [Best Evidence]. Am J Sports Med 2007;35(3):427–36.
23. Alfredson H, Ohberg L. Neovascularisation in chronic painful patellar tendinosis—promising results after sclerosing neovessels outside the tendon challenge the need for surgery. Knee Surg Sports Traumatol Arthrosc 2005;13(2):74–80.
24. Hyman G. Jumper's knee. eMedicine. New York: Medscape; 2013. Available at: http://emedicine.medscape.com/article/89569-overview. Accessed October 1, 2014.
25. Fredberg U, Bolvig L, Pfeiffer-Jensen M, et al. Ultrasonography as a tool for diagnosis, guidance of local steroid injection and, together with pressure algometry, monitoring of the treatment of athletes with chronic jumper's knee and Achilles tendinitis: a randomized, double-blind, placebo-controlled study. Scand J Rheumatol 2004;33(2):94–101.
26. Mehta VM, Inoue M, Nomura E, et al. An algorithm guiding the evaluation and treatment of acute primary patellar dislocations. Sports Med Arthrosc 2007;15(2):78–81.
27. Dalton JF, Davies M, DellaValle CJ, et al. Patellofemoral instability and malalignment. In: Griffin LY, editor. Essentials of musculoskeletal care. 3rd edition. Rosemont (IL): American Academy of Orthopaedic Surgeons; 2005. p. 541–5.
28. Nomura E, Inoue M, Kurimura M. Chondral and osteochondral injuries associated with acute patellar dislocation. Arthroscopy 2003;19(7):717–21.
29. Mcfarland EG, Mamanee P, Queale WS, et al. Olecranon and prepatellar bursitis: treating acute, chronic, and inflamed. Phys Sportsmed 2000;28(3):40–52.
30. Reid CR, Bush PM, Cummings NH, et al. A review of occupational knee disorders. J Occup Rehabil 2010;20(4):489–501.
31. Alvarez-nemegyei J, Canoso JJ. Evidence-based soft tissue rheumatology IV: anserine bursitis. J Clin Rheumatol 2004;10(4):205–6.
32. Helfenstein M, Kuromoto J. Anserine syndrome. Rev Bras Reumatol 2010;50(3): 313–27.
33. Mcafee JH, Smith DL. Olecranon and prepatellar bursitis. Diagnosis and treatment. West J Med 1988;149(5):607–10.
34. Bussières AE, Taylor JA, Peterson C. Diagnostic imaging practice guidelines for musculoskeletal complaints in adults—an evidence-based approach. Part 1. Lower extremity disorders. J Manipulative Physiol Ther 2007;30(9):684–717.
35. Forbes JR, Holmo CA, Janzen DL. Acute pes anserine bursitis: MR imaging. Radiology 1995;194(2):525–7.
36. Aaron DL, Patel A, Kayiaros S, et al. Four common types of bursitis: diagnosis and management. J Am Acad Orthop Surg 2011;19(6):359–67.
37. Butcher JD, Salzman KL, Lillegard WA. Lower extremity bursitis. Am Fam Physician 1996;53(7):2317–24.
38. Thomeé R, Augustsson J, Karlsson J. Patellofemoral pain syndrome: a review of current issues. Sports Med 1999;28(4):245–62.
39. Patellofemoral pain syndrome. In: DynaMed [database online]. EBSCO Information Services. Updated July 10, 2013. Available at: http://web.ebscohost.com. ezproxy2.library.drexel.edu/dynamed/detail?vid=3&sid=00775f38-eecb-4067-b515-d60be9009aab%40sessionmgr13&hid=22&bdata=JnNpdGU9ZHluYW1lZC1saXZlJnNjb3BlPXNpdGU%3d#db=dme&AN=116002. Accessed October 1, 2013.

40. Haim A, Yaniv M, Dekel S, et al. Patellofemoral pain syndrome: validity of clinical and radiological features. Clin Orthop Relat Res 2006;451:223–8.
41. Finestone A, Radin EL, Lev B, et al. Treatment of overuse patellofemoral pain. Prospective randomized controlled clinical trial in a military setting. Clin Orthop Relat Res 1993;(293):208–10.
42. Green WT. Painful bipartite patellae. A report of three cases. Clin Orthop Relat Res 1975;(110):197–200.
43. Carter SR. Traumatic separation of a bipartite patella. Injury 1989;20(4):244.
44. Thomas AL, Wilson RH, Thompson TL. Quadriceps avulsion through a bipartite patella. Orthopedics 2007;30(6):491–2.
45. Rajinder SG, Kapoor S, Rysavy M. Contemporary management of symptomatic bipartite patella. Orthopedics 2011;32(11):843–9. http://dx.doi.org/10.3928/01477447-20090922-20. Available at: http://search.proquest.com/docview/919979135?accountid=10559.
46. Ireland ML, Chang JL. Acute fracture bipartite patella: case report and literature review. Med Sci Sports Exerc 1995;27(3):299–302.
47. Weaver JK. Bipartite patella as a cause of disability in the athlete. Am J Sports Med 1977;5(4):137–43.
48. Iossifidis A, Brueton RN. Painful bipartite patella following injury. Injury 1995; 26(3):175–6.
49. Ishikawa H, Sakurai A, Hirata S. Painful bipartite patella in young athletes. The diagnostic value of skyline views taken in squatting position and the results of surgical excision. Clin Orthop Relat Res 1994;(305):223–8.
50. Vanhoenacker FM, Bernaerts A, Van de Perre S, et al. MRI of painful bipartite patella. JBR-BTR 2002;85(4):219.
51. Grogan DP, Carey TP, Leffers D, et al. Avulsion fractures of the patella. J Pediatr Orthop 1990;10(6):721–30.
52. Osgood-Schlatter Disease. In: DynaMed [database online]. EBSCO Information Services. Updated July 10, 2013. Available at: http://web.ebscohost.com. ezproxy2.library.drexel.edu/dynamed/detail?vid=3&sid=519df60b-bfb8-4294-8771-268acbcfa8ed%40sessionmgr12&hid=22&bdata=JnNpdGU9ZHluYW1lZC1saXZlJnNjb3BlPXNpdGU%3d#db=dme&AN=115095. Accessed October 15, 2013.
53. Wall EJ. Osgood-Schlatter disease: practical treatment for a self-limiting condition. Phys Sportsmed 1998;26(3):29–34.
54. Bloom OJ, Mackler L, Barbee J. Clinical inquiries. What is the best treatment for Osgood-Schlatter disease? J Fam Pract 2004;53(2):153–6.
55. Buschbacher R. Musculoskeletal, sports, and occupational medicine. New York: Demos Medical Publishing; 2010.
56. Gerbino P. Adolescent anterior knee pain. Oper Tech Sports Med 2006;14: 203–11.
57. Osteochondritis dissecans. In: DynaMed [database online]. EBSCO Information Services. Updated July 10, 2013. Available at: http://web.ebscohost.com. ezproxy2.library.drexel.edu/dynamed/detail?vid=3&sid=b5dc6b1c-2aa9-40e2-ac5b-2336946d5570%40sessionmgr12&hid=22&bdata=JnNpdGU9ZHluYW1lZC1saXZlJnNjb3BlPXNpdGU%3d#db=dme&AN=114731. Accessed October 1, 2013.
58. Hughston JC, Hergenroeder PT, Courtenay BG. Osteochondritis dissecans of the femoral condyles. J Bone Joint Surg Am 1984;66:1340–8.
59. Schenck RC Jr, Goodnight JM. Osteochondritis dissecans. J Bone Joint Surg Am 1996;78:439–56.

60. Williamson LR, Albright JP. Bilateral osteochondritis dissecans of the elbow in a female pitcher. J Fam Pract 1996;43:489–93.
61. Hixon AL, Gibbs LM. Osteochondritis dissecans: a diagnosis not to miss. Am Fam Physician 2000;61(1):151–6, 158.
62. Obedian RS, Grelsamer RP. Osteochondritis dissecans of the distal femur and patella. Clin Sports Med 1997;16:157–74.
63. Clanton TO, DeLee JC. Osteochondritis dissecans: history, pathophysiology and current treatment concepts. Clin Orthop 1982;167:50–64.
64. De Smet AA, Ilahi OA, Graf BK. Reassessment of the MR criteria for stability of osteochondritis dissecans in the knee and ankle. Skeletal Radiol 1996;25:159–63.
65. Dipaola JD, Nelson DW, Colville MR. Characterizing osteochondral lesions by magnetic resonance imaging. Arthroscopy 1991;7:101–4.
66. Melvin JS, Mehta S. Patellar fractures in adults. J Am Acad Orthop Surg 2011; 19(4):198–207.
67. Carpenter JE, Kasman R, Matthews LS. Fractures of the patella. J Bone Joint Surg Am 1993;75:1550–61.
68. Nord RM, Quach T, Walsh M, et al. Detection of traumatic arthrotomy of the knee using the saline solution load test. J Bone Joint Surg Am 2009;91(1):66–70.
69. Marsh JL, Slongo TF, Agel J, et al. Fracture and dislocation classification compendium: 2007. Orthopaedic Trauma Association Classification, Database and Outcomes Committee. J Orthop Trauma 2007;21(Suppl 10):S1–133.
70. Bostrom A. Fracture of the patella: a study of 422 patellar fractures. Acta Orthop Scand Suppl 1972;143:1–80.
71. Braun W, Wiedemann M, Ruter A, et al. Indications and results of nonoperative treatment of patellar fractures. Clin Orthop Relat Res 1993;(289):197–201.
72. Duri ZA, Patel DV, Aichroth PM. The immature athlete. Clin Sports Med 2002; 21(3):461–82, ix.
73. Peace KA, Lee JC, Healy J. Imaging the infrapatellar tendon in the elite athlete. Clin Radiol 2006;61(7):570–8.
74. Tindel NL, Nisonson B. The plica syndrome. Orthop Clin North Am 1992;23(4): 613–8.
75. Calmbach WL, Hutchens M. Evaluation of patients presenting with knee pain: part II. Differential diagnosis. Am Fam Physician 2003;68(5):917–22.
76. Paczesny L, Kruczynski J. Medial plica syndrome of the knee: diagnosis with dynamic sonography. Radiology 2009;251(2):439–46.
77. Brukner P, Khan K. Anterior knee pain. Clinical sports medicine. 3rd edition. New York: McGraw-Hill; 2006. p. 464–94.
78. Faletti C, De Stofano N, Giudice G, et al. Knee Impingement syndromes. Eur J Radiol 1998;27(Suppl 1):S60–9.
79. Saddik D, McNally EG, Richardson M. MRI of Hoffa's fat pad. Skeletal Radiol 2004;33(8):433–44.
80. Resnick DL, Khang HS, Pretterklieber ML. Internal derangements of joints. 2nd edition. Philadelphia: Elsevier; 2007. Chapter 25.
81. Jacobson JA, Lenchik L, Ruhoy MK, et al. MR imaging of the infrapatellar fat pad of Hoffa. Radiographics 1997;17(3):675–91.
82. Chung CB, Skaf A, Roger B, et al. Patellar tendon-lateral femoral condyle friction syndrome: MR imaging in 42 patients. Skeletal Radiol 2001;30(12):694–7.
83. Kim YM, Shin HD, Yang JY, et al. Prefemoral fat pad impingement and a mass-like protrusion on the lateral femoral condyle causing mechanical symptoms. A case report. Knee Surg Sports Traumatol Arthrosc 2007;15(6):786–9.

The Acutely Injured Knee

Christopher Karrasch, MD, Robert A. Gallo, MD*

KEYWORDS

- Knee pain • Effusion • Ligament tear

KEY POINTS

- Detailed history, including age, onset of symptoms, history of trauma or overuse, duration of symptoms, rheumatologic conditions, and previous therapy, is important in narrowing the differential diagnosis.
- Physical examination and radiographic imaging are important in identifying conditions, such as extensor mechanism injuries and tibial plateau fractures, that require prompt referral to an orthopedic surgeon.
- Due to its high sensitivity and specificity in detecting common injuries, magnetic resonance imaging has become the diagnostic modality of choice in diagnosing soft tissue abnormalities of the knee.
- Initial treatment centers on analgesia and includes nonsteroidal anti-inflammatory drugs and cryotherapy and, if necessary, brief periods of immobilization.
- Timely diagnosis is important because time to operative intervention can have a significant effect on surgical outcomes, patient recovery, and satisfaction.

INTRODUCTION

Active lifestyles, including participation in athletic activities, have been promoted as a means of improving physical and mental health. However, engaging in athletic activity is not without peril. Musculoskeletal-related injuries are a leading source of morbidity among physically active individuals. Musculoskeletal ailments are responsible for nearly 21.5% of visits presenting to primary care offices[1] and 13.8% of emergency room visits.[2]

Symptoms within the knee prompt more visits to ambulatory clinics than any other musculoskeletal region except the lumbar spine and account for 1.5% of all ambulatory care visits.[3] In a study conducted by the US Department of Health and Human Services, knee symptoms cause more visits than headaches, depression, and hypertension and equal those due to chest pain.[3]

Although a large percentage of knee pain can be attributed to chronic conditions such as osteoarthritis, acute knee pain is a common ailment treated in primary care

Department of Orthopaedic Surgery, Penn State Milton S. Hershey Medical Center, Pennsylvania State University College of Medicine, 30 Hope Drive, Hershey, PA 17033, USA
* Corresponding author. Bone and Joint Institute, Milton S. Hershey Medical Center, Pennsylvania State University College of Medicine, 30 Hope Drive, PO Box 859, Hershey, PA 17033.
E-mail address: rgallo@hmc.psu.edu

Med Clin N Am 98 (2014) 719–736
http://dx.doi.org/10.1016/j.mcna.2014.03.002
0025-7125/14/$ – see front matter © 2014 Elsevier Inc. All rights reserved.

clinics. The differential diagnosis can be broad and ranges from tibial plateau and patella fractures to ligamentous or tendinous ruptures to meniscal and articular cartilage injuries. Several of these injuries, such as injuries to the extensor mechanism (quadriceps/patellar tendon ruptures, patella fractures), require prompt treatment by an orthopedic surgeon to avoid permanent dysfunction. A general knowledge of the diagnosis of these entities and overall treatment strategy is imperative to avoid long-term disability caused by delay in appropriate treatment of these injuries.

HISTORY

A comprehensive history helps narrow the differential diagnosis. A detailed history should include the following aspects: patient age, nature and location of pain, effusion and its onset, mechanical symptoms (ie, locking and/or catching), ability to bear weight, history of a traumatic event, documented dislocation requiring reduction, recent alterations in activity level, previous musculoskeletal injuries and/or surgeries, underlying rheumatologic and medical conditions, and systemic symptoms.

Onset of symptoms is important to assist in diagnosis and triage. Any penetrating injury should be identified and, if there is any question of joint involvement, further investigation preferably at an emergency department should be performed to prevent possible later development of septic arthritis. A history of a specific traumatic event, especially when associated with an effusion or swelling, should raise the suspicion for fracture or injury to a ligament, tendon, meniscus, and/or articular cartilage and should prompt more urgent referral to an orthopedic surgeon. Meanwhile, pain developing after a more insidious history such as recent increase in exercise or overuse more likely results in tendinopathy, patellofemoral symptoms, or stress fracture. Sudden fevers and overall malaise associated with an effusion often indicates septic arthritis, especially if a recent infection elsewhere. In elderly patients without a known traumatic event, osteoarthritis is likely the cause of pain. **Table 1** presents specific injuries with commonly reported mechanisms.

PHYSICAL EXAMINATION

Although the literature often focuses on provocative tests for specific pathologic abnormalities, physical examination should begin with the basics of any musculoskeletal

Table 1	
Common acute knee injuries and their usual mechanism	
Injury	**Mechanism**
ACL tear	Noncontact twisting injury with acute effusion and pain
Posterior cruciate ligament (PCL) tear	"Dashboard" injury when tibia struck, or fall onto tibia with foot plantarflexed
Medial collateral ligament (MCL) strain/tear	"Clipping" injury when lateral blow to knee causes valgus stress
Patella fracture	"Dashboard" injury when patella directly struck, or fall onto tibia with foot dorsiflexed
Meniscal tear	Twisting or squatting injury associated with specific medial or lateral pain and catching/locking
Quadriceps or patellar tendon rupture	Sudden hyperflexion causing sudden forceful quadriceps contraction and immediate inability to perform straight-leg raise

evaluation: observation, palpation, range of motion, motor strength, sensation, vascular, ligamentous testing/stability, and provocative maneuvers. The culmination of examination findings is much more reliable than specific testing alone.[4] The injured knee should always be compared with the contralateral limb.

Before evaluation of the affected limb, general overall ligamentous laxity should be assessed. The ability to touch thumbs to the forearm, hyperextend the elbow, and knee recurvatum are signs of increased laxity, which predisposes affected individuals to patellar dislocations and other generalized sprains.[5]

Inspection is ideally performed with full exposure of bilateral lower extremities. If the patient is able, gait and alignment should be assessed with shoes and socks removed for full appreciation of ankle and foot position. An obvious deformity that appeared after a recent traumatic event is concerning for a condition requiring prompt treatment, such as a fracture or dislocation. The skin should be carefully inspected for previous surgical scars, which offer insight to previous procedures. Localized swelling, ecchymosis, and effusion clue the examiner into location of injury. Localized swelling and ecchymosis can result from a direct blow or underlying injury, while an effusion heralds an intra-articular process such as an ACL tear. ACL tears account for greater than 70% of injuries among those with an acute effusion and a history of a noncontact twisting injury.[6]

Because of the superficial location of many important structures about the knee, palpation plays a large diagnostic role in the assessment of knee injuries. Palpation around the knee joint should proceed systematically and include all bony prominences. Joint line tenderness, according to some studies, is the most accurate predictor of a meniscal tear.[7] Extensor mechanism injuries can be diagnosed solely on physical examination: an inability to extend the knee actively and a palpable defect at the superior or inferior pole of the patella is pathognomonic for quadriceps and patellar tendon ruptures, respectively, and can eliminate the need for magnetic resonance imaging (MRI).

Range of motion of the hip and knee should be measured actively and passively. Normal knee motion with the patient supine ranges from 0° to 10° of hyperextension to 125° to 135° of flexion. Hip rotation is limited when the knee is extended, but, when the knee is flexed to 90°, normal hip internal and external rotation measure 30° and 45°, respectively. Acute loss of passive knee motion suggests a significant structural injury, such as a tibial plateau fracture or ligamentous rupture, while loss of active but not passive motion signals an injury to the dynamic musculotendinous unit.

Neurovascular testing should be performed bilaterally and include specific testing of major arteries and peripheral nerves, including femoral, superficial, deep peroneal, and tibial nerves. Specific testing for each peripheral nerve is presented in Table 2. A peroneal nerve palsy, commonly manifested as a drop foot, is frequently associated with an injury to the lateral collateral ligament (LCL). Strength or sensory testing that does not correspond to a specific nerve distribution may correspond to an underlying lumbar radiculopathy. The popliteal, dorsalis pedis, and posterior tibialis pulses

Table 2
Motor and sensory testing for major peripheral nerves of lower extremity

Nerve	Motor	Sensory
Femoral	Knee extension	Medial leg and foot (saphenous)
Deep peroneal	Ankle and great toe dorsiflexion	Dorsal first web space
Superficial peroneal	Hindfoot eversion	Dorsal lateral foot
Tibial nerve	Ankle plantarflexion	Plantar surface foot

should be palpated and any discrepancy warrants further investigation. Posterior knee pain, foot swelling, or calf tenderness is concerning for deep vein thrombosis and venous duplex should be considered.

Stability and provocative tests form the core of knee physical examination. Commonly used tests are described in **Table 3**. Ligamentous stress tests are performed with the knee relaxed and are gauged by the amount of excursion/laxity and quality of the end point.

DIAGNOSTIC TEST/IMAGING

Orthogonal radiographs are currently the preferred initial imaging study to evaluate acute knee injuries. Radiographs, which are more readily available and relatively inexpensive, are important to identify fractures that would require immediate treatment or referral to an orthopedic surgeon. Weight-bearing as tolerated is generally safe without risking further derangement if no femoral or tibial fracture is defined on radiographs. Radiographic assessment should include anteroposterior and lateral views at

Table 3
Commonly used knee physical examination tests

Structure	Test	Description
ACL	Lachman	Anteriorly directed force on the tibia applied with the knee flexed to 30°.
	Anterior drawer	Anteriorly directed force on the tibia applied with the knee flexed to 90°.
PCL	Posterior drawer	Posteriorly directed force on the tibia applied with the knee flexed to 90°.
	Quadriceps active	Patient actively contracts quadriceps while lying supine, hip flexed to 45°, and knee flexed to 90°. Tibia shifts anteriorly with an insufficient PCL.
MCL	Valgus stress	Laterally directed force applied to tibia. Test is performed at 0 and 30° of knee flexion. Laxity at 30° of flexion indicates injury to MCL, whereas laxity at 0° of flexion suggests injury to medial structures.
LCL	Varus stress	Medially directed force applied to tibia. Test is performed at 0 and 30° of knee flexion. Laxity at 30° of flexion indicates injury to LCL, whereas laxity at 0° of flexion suggests injury to lateral structures.
Patellar instability	Patellar apprehension	Laterally directed force applied to patella causes apprehension and feeling that patella is subluxing/dislocating.
	Patellar translation	Laterally directed force applied to patella. Lateral translation of the medial border of the patella to the lateral edge of the trochlear groove or further is usually considered abnormal but should be compared with contralateral patella.
Meniscal tear	Apley's compression	Reproducible pain in medial or lateral joint line when combined compressive and rotational force (varus/external rotation for medial meniscus; valgus/internal rotation for lateral meniscus) applied with patient in the prone position and knee flexed to 90°.

Table 4 Sensitivity and specificity of MRI in detecting common acute knee injuries		
Injury	Sensitivity (%)	Specificity (%)
ACL tears	78–91	85–100
PCL tears	100	97
Medial meniscal tears	91–100	52–90
Lateral meniscal tears	56–82	83–99

Data from Refs.[11,13,14]

a minimum. Merchant views offer an axial image of the patella and can provide useful information following patellar dislocations but require knee flexion angles of 45°.

The Ottawa rules have been developed to guide primary care clinicians in appropriate ordering of radiographs following development of acute knee symptoms.[8] Based on the Ottawa rules, radiographs should be obtained in those presenting with acute knee pain if (1) patient age is greater than 55 years old, (2) there is tenderness at the fibular head, (3) there is patellar tenderness, (4) there is an inability to flex knee to at least 90°, (5) there is an inability to bear weight for a minimum of 4 steps.[8] If one or more of these findings are present, the sensitivity of detecting a fracture is 1.0 and specificity of 0.54 according to the sentinel study.[8]

MRI has the ability to image meniscal, ligamentous, tendinous, and chondral structures optimally within the knee joint (**Table 4**) and is considered the gold standard imaging study for detecting soft tissue injuries within the knee. In addition, bone bruises on MRI have the ability to provide insight on injury pattern (**Fig. 1**). Given that most injuries in the knee involve soft tissue structures, some have advocated for the routine use of MRI early in management. Recent studies have suggested that obtaining a limited MRI at the time of initial evaluation shortens the time to completion of diagnostic workup, reduces the number of additional diagnostic procedures, improves quality of life in the first 6 weeks, and may reduce costs associated with lost productivity.[9,10] No significant advantage has been attained with the use of a 3-T MRI versus 1.5-T MRI in detecting common acute knee injuries.[11] Intra-articular contrast may

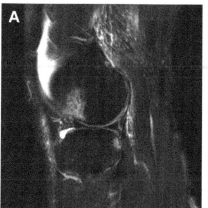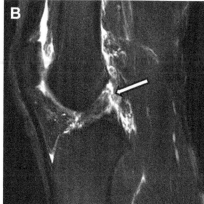

Fig. 1. Bone bruising patterns can assist in identifying injury patterns. For example, bone contusions involving the center of the lateral femoral condyle and posterior lateral tibial plateau (*A*) suggest a pivot-shift mechanism, which often results in an ACL tear (*B*). *Arrow* indicates site of ACL tear.

improve the characterization of meniscal tears,[12] but, due to the accuracy of conventional MRI in detecting injury, is generally deemed unnecessary.

Within the knee, computerized tomography (CT) is largely reserved to define fractures detected using plain radiographs further. Three-dimensional imaging has become an important component for preoperative management of tibial plateau fractures (**Fig. 2**). This imaging modality delineates a fracture that is underestimated in severity in 43%[15] and modifies treatment in 60%[16] when added to standard radiographic imaging.

Although ultrasonography has gained recent popularity because of its increasing availability, lack of ionizing irradiation, and decreased cost compared with MRI, its use in the knee has been limited because of the difficulty imaging around bony structures. Historically, the primary use of ultrasound in the management of acute knee injury has been to confirm injuries to the quadriceps and patellar tendons. However, one recent report has demonstrated the high reliability of ultrasonography in detecting meniscal tears.[17]

DIFFERENTIAL DIAGNOSIS

Knowledge of the knee anatomy and function can assist in formulating the differential diagnosis for a patient presenting with acute knee pain. Because of the relative simplicity of the knee's hinged design and superficial location, thorough history and thoughtful physical examination based on knowledge of known anatomic structures can narrow the potential diagnoses before imaging studies are obtained. Subjective and objective pain localized to a specific area of the knee often indicates injury adjacent to the sight of the described pain. **Table 5** lists differential diagnoses of acute injuries based on location.

Knee effusions and hemarthroses are common findings following acute knee injury and portend an increased probability of ultimate surgical intervention. In a recent study of an adolescent population, an acute knee effusion was associated with a 41% chance of surgery.[18] Injuries, such as tibial plateau and patellar fractures, cruciate

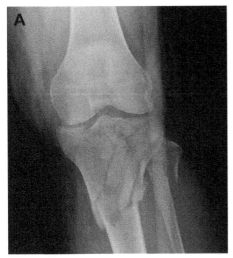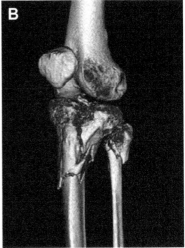

Fig. 2. Although radiographs are useful in identifying a tibial plateau fracture (*A*), CT scan, especially those with 3-dimensional reconstruction, provide more detail of fracture pattern (*B*).

Table 5
Differential diagnoses of acute knee injury based on location

Medial	Lateral	Anterior
Medial meniscal tears	Lateral meniscal tears	Patellar or quadriceps tendon rupture
Chondral/osteochondral injuries of medial femoral condyle	Chondral/osteochondral injuries of lateral femoral condyle	Chondral/osteochondral injuries of trochlea or patella
MCL sprains/tears	LCL sprains	Patellar or quadriceps tendon tendinitis
Distal pes anserinus tendon strains	Distal biceps femoris/popliteus tendon strains	Patella fractures
MPFL sprains/tears	Lateral retinacular tears	
Medial tibial plateau fractures	Lateral tibial plateau fractures	

ligament tears, peripheral meniscal tears, and traumatic patellar dislocations, involve vascularized intra-articular structures and are often associated with intra-articular effusions secondary to hemarthroses. Septic arthritis should be considered in any acute effusion associated with a fever and no significant traumatic event. Meanwhile, extra-articular injuries (eg, collateral ligament injuries) tend to cause focal swelling more than global effusions.

TREATMENT

The most important purpose of evaluation is efficiently differentiating between injuries that (1) require prompt surgical evaluation and treatment by an orthopedic surgeon, (2) need less urgent evaluation by an orthopedic surgeon, and (3) can be managed effectively by a primary care physician. Displaced intra-articular fractures (eg, tibial plateau fractures and patellar fractures) and tendon ruptures (eg, quadriceps and patellar tendon tears) are often treated surgically within 7 to 10 days and therefore benefit from immediate referral to an orthopedic surgeon for management. Differentiating these maladies from other less urgent entities is crucial in ensuring appropriate management of acute knee injuries.

Although the differential diagnosis for acute knee injury can be broad, initial treatment does not vary significantly between injuries. Regardless of ultimate diagnosis, those patients presenting with an acute knee effusion or moderate or severe pain often benefit from temporary immobilization in full extension using either a knee immobilizer or a hinged knee brace. Immobilizers, which are designed to prevent knee flexion, are often less costly initially. However, hinged braces can be locked in extension or unlocked to allow motion, which may be beneficial later in the treatment course. The period of immobilization should be balanced between need for stability versus potential for muscle atrophy,[19] arthrofibrosis, and altered ligamentous healing.[20,21] For most injuries, immobilization of the knee should be limited to 1 week unless the knee is grossly unstable due to fracture or multiligamentous injury. If the injury is serious enough to require prolonged immobilization, prompt referral to an orthopedic surgeon is appropriate. Studies have indicated that an immobilization period as short as 5 days is associated with muscle atrophy.[22]

In addition to immobilization, pain from knee effusions can be managed with nonsteroidal anti-inflammatory drugs (NSAIDs), ice, and aspiration. NSAIDs have both analgesic and anti-inflammatory properties but also have antiplatelet activity and potentially can cause increased bleeding, which may be detrimental in conditions at risk for compartment syndrome, such as tibial plateau fractures. Cryotherapy has been shown to produce significant decreases in pain,[23,24] but clinicians should caution patients about the potential for frostbite with inappropriate use.[25,26] Aspiration of an acute hemarthosis remains a controversial practice. Although some advocate aspiration of a hemarthosis to aid in diagnosis, alleviate pain, and facilitate rehabilitation,[27] others have questioned the practice because of the potential for infection and lack of efficacy. A review of 267 papers was unable to provide a definitive answer of the effectiveness of aspiration.[28]

Most patients with an acute knee injury can be allowed to progressively weight-bear as tolerated with or without bracing depending on the injury. The decision to allow weight-bearing, however, should be based on the results of initial radiographs: those with a known or suspected intra-articular fracture of the weight-bearing surfaces of the knee (ie, tibial plateau fractures, femoral condyle fractures) should avoid weight-bearing to prevent displacement of the fracture.

Although most acute knee injuries can be initially treated with a similar protocol centered on pain control, the ultimate treatment of these injuries varies based on the condition. A brief discussion of overall treatment strategies for common acute knee injuries is presented.

ACL Tears

ACL ruptures are associated with an acute hemarthosis, which limits knee motion within the first 2 weeks. Regardless of the eventual treatment plan, initial treatment measures are directed at restoring painless range of motion and preserving quadriceps strength. Physical therapy has been shown to be beneficial to accomplish these goals, especially among those wishing to proceed with surgical reconstruction.[29]

Not all who sustain ACL tears will develop clinical instability. Therefore, the decision to undergo surgical reconstruction of the ACL is based on several factors. Many patients without meniscal, acute chondral, or concomitant ligamentous injury are "copers" and have minimal functional difficulty after recovering from the initial trauma following ACL tear, or are "adapters" and modify their activities to prevent instability episodes.[30] Those patients opting for nonoperative management of an ACL tear must be aware of the potential long-term ramifications of their treatment choice. Several studies have demonstrated an increased risk of irreparable medial meniscal tears and osteochondral injuries[31,32] and therefore concerns for increased potential for progression to osteoarthritis long-term.[33]

Surgical treatments have metamorphasized considerably over the past 3 decades. Historical studies assessing direct ACL repairs reported high rates of decreased activity levels and unacceptable function.[34] Therefore, surgical reconstruction, not surgical repair, is the preferred treatment of ACL insufficiency (**Fig. 3**). Various graft options, including autografts and allografts, exist and each graft's benefits and risks must be weighed to provide optimal treatment. Although allografts do not suffer from problems associated with graft harvest, they are associated with higher rerupture rates, especially in younger populations.[35] Patellar tendon, hamstring tendon, and quadriceps tendon autografts have acceptable rerupture rates and initial strength[36]; however, they are limited by donor-site morbidity, such as anterior knee pain, posterior thigh pain, and quadriceps weakness, respectively.

Postoperative arthrofibrosis is an uncommon but major concern following ACL reconstruction. Therefore, most surgeons advocate delaying ACL reconstruction until the acute hemarthrosis has resolved and range of motion has been restored following the initial injury.[37] Furthermore, aggressive postoperative rehabilitation initiated within

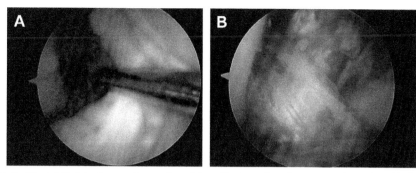

Fig. 3. Most ACL injuries are femoral avulsions that produced an empty lateral wall of the notch (*A*). In the past, repair was attempted but its poor long-term results have made reconstructions (*B*) the favored surgical treatment of ACL reconstructions.

the first 2 to 3 weeks has been shown to improve ultimate outcomes and decrease postoperative stiffness.[38]

Posterior Cruciate Ligament

A key to treating PCL injuries is to identify the entire injury pattern. Although isolated PCL injuries can successfully be treated nonoperatively,[39] PCL ruptures associated with other ligamentous knee injuries are more significant entities often treated operatively. Careful examination of the entire lower extremity is critical to avoid missing a potential limb-threatening injury, such as a popliteal artery tear.

Nonoperative treatment of isolated PCL injuries includes a therapy program that focuses on quadriceps strengthening, which assists anterior translation of the tibia. Long-term studies of nonoperatively managed PCL ruptures report increased rates of degenerative arthritis in the patellofemoral and medial compartments.[40]

Several surgical options exist for treatment of symptomatic PCL injuries. With the exception of bony avulsions, which are treated with open reduction and internal fixation, most PCL ruptures treated operatively are reconstructed. Reconstructions can be performed arthroscopically using a tunnel through the tibia or open through a posterior approach and using an inlay technique. The debatable biomechanical advantage of the inlay technique must be balanced by its increased potential morbidity.[41]

Postoperative rehabilitation progresses much more slowly than ACL reconstructions. In particular, hamstring contraction, which tends to exert a posterior force on the tibia, is deferred for up to 4 months postoperatively.

Medial Collateral Ligament

Often considered to be the most commonly injured knee ligament, the MCL rarely requires surgical intervention even if associated with an ACL injury. Most MCL injuries can be successfully treated with early mobilization and bracing using a hinged knee brace. Unlike the ACL, which is exposed to synovial fluid, the MCL is considered to have a robust blood supply and thought to be capable of adequate healing.

The decision for surgical intervention is based on the degree of laxity. Usually, only those injuries with valgus laxity in full extension are considered for operative intervention. Complete MCL avulsions of the tibial insertion can be treated acutely with direct surgical repair (**Fig. 4**), whereas most midsubstance and femoral avulsions are initially managed nonoperatively and undergo delayed reconstruction if necessary.

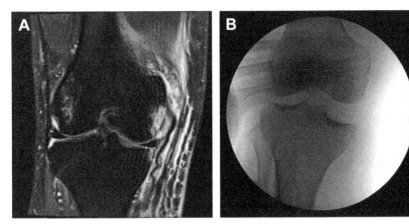

Fig. 4. Most MCL injuries are treated with a trial of nonoperative management. However, complete tibial-sided avulsions (*A*), especially those with significant medial gapping with stress (*B*), are often treated with early direct repair.

Bracing is considered long-term in groups that are at high risk for sustaining valgus-type injuries (eg, football linemen). There is evidence that supports prophylactically bracing this population to prevent MCL injury.[42]

Knee Dislocations and Multiple Ligament Injuries

Knee dislocations are an emergency and require immediate relocation to prevent catastrophic damage to the affected limb. Although fixed dislocation is obvious on physical examination, subluxations (**Fig. 5**) and dislocations with spontaneous reductions can be subtle but equally devastating. Therefore, a high level of vigilance is required for those with a PCL injury and suspected multiligamentous knee injury. A thorough vascular examination, including pulses, capillary refill, and ankle-brachial indices (ABIs), is important in identifying potential vascular injuries. In particular, ABIs are highly predictive of vascular injury following knee dislocations and ABIs less than 0.9 are associated with increased risk of vascular injury and should prompt formal vascular imaging.[43]

Knee dislocations typically occur in 3 groups: athletes, those involved in a motor vehicle accident, and the morbidly obese. Of those, the morbidly obese carry a higher risk of neurovascular injury[44] and should warrant even more thorough monitoring and aggressive imaging, especially given the limitations of physical examination in this population.

Treatment is directed largely on injury pattern and patient characteristics. Younger, physically demanding patients typically opt for surgical intervention to optimize their outcome. Initial treatment includes immobilization in a brace versus surgical application of a spanning external fixator in cases wherein a concentric reduction cannot be maintained (**Fig. 6**). If further surgical intervention is indicated and no other injuries prohibit surgery, most surgeons prefer to operate once the capsule has healed (ie, roughly 3–4 weeks).[45] Although ACL and PCL ruptures are often reconstructed, collateral ligaments can be reconstructed or repaired depending on the degree of injury, location of injury, and time from injury to surgery. Allografts are the generally preferred graft choice in the setting of multiligamentous injuries due to donor-site morbidity in the already severely injured knee. Postoperative rehabilitation proceeds slowly in this population, and full recovery takes in excess of 1 year.

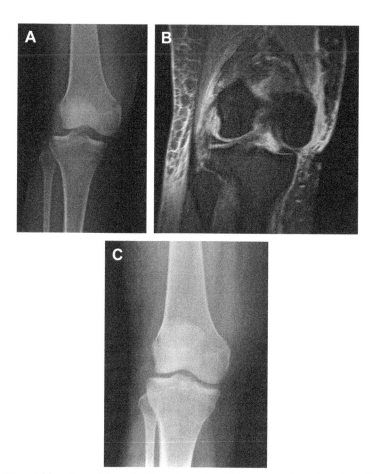

Fig. 5. Knee subluxations (*A*) and dislocations should be promptly reduced. Inability to reduce the knee closed should raise concerns over entrapped MCL and medial structures (*B*). In these cases, open reduction may be necessary to achieve an anatomic reduction (*C*).

Meniscal Tears

Meniscal tears vary greatly in their morphology and resultant limitation. Although most meniscal tears can be managed conservatively for weeks, months, or even years, bucket-handle tears and others causing restrictions in knee range of motion require prompt treatment to prevent long-term stiffness. Bucket-handle tears are long vertical tears that involve a large segment of the meniscus. The large fragment, usually the posterior horn and body of the meniscus, can flip and lodge within the notch and anterior to the femoral condyle (**Fig. 7**). This "locked" position of the meniscus limits knee extension and often requires surgical manipulation to reduce the meniscus.

Meniscal tears are relatively common in asymptomatic adults and, unless causing mechanical symptoms or associated with a ligamentous injury, can often be treated by a trial of nonoperative management. In one study, meniscal tears were detected in 36% of asymptomatic adult knees.[46] Furthermore, meniscal tears are often associated with osteoarthritis and may not be the source of pain. Studies have demonstrated only two-thirds of patients with severe osteoarthritis who underwent arthroscopic partial meniscectomy had pain relief initially and, within 5 years, only 40% reported

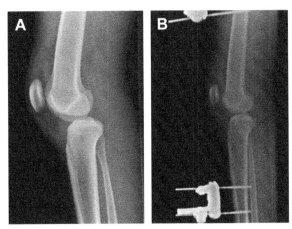

Fig. 6. Nonconcentric reductions, especially with posterior sag on lateral radiographs (A), should be treated with closed reduction and external fixation (B) to prevent compression of posterior neurovascular structures.

improved symptoms and 32% required total joint replacement or unloading osteotomy.[47] Therefore, surgical intervention in older adults should be reserved for those with a meniscal tear and relatively well-preserved articular cartilage that have mechanical symptoms and/or have failed an initial trial of nonoperative management, including physical therapy, NSAIDs, and/or injections.

Preservation of the meniscus is important to limit the progression of degenerative arthritis. Although preferable biomechanically, meniscal repair is often not possible due to the configuration of the tear and the poor blood supply of the meniscal tissue. Furthermore, recovery from a meniscal repair is lengthy compared with partial meniscectomy, in which weight-bearing as tolerated is allowed immediately following surgery. Location of the tear within 2 mm of the capsule, vertical tears less than 4 cm in length, and an associated ACL tear and concomitant reconstruction are factors most favorable for successful repair.[48,49] If a favorable milieu is present and repair is possible, especially in a young patient, early referral to an orthopedic surgeon is recommended to prevent progression of the tear.

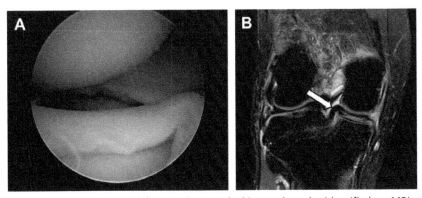

Fig. 7. Bucket-handle tears (A) frequently cause locking and can be identified on MRI as a fragment within the notch adjacent to the PCL (B). *Arrow* indicates Bucket-handle meniscus tear displaced into notch.

Patellar Dislocations

Patellar dislocations have a broad spectrum of injury. Although patellar instability can occur with minimal provocation in those with increased ligamentous laxity, dislocations in those with normal ligamentous laxity are typically more violent, can result in significant cartilaginous sheer injuries, and therefore, should be considered for MRI after initial injury. Unless imaging studies demonstrate a traumatic osteochondral body or bony avulsion, physical therapy focusing on quadriceps and core strengthening and J-bracing is the preferred initial management of most patellar dislocations.

The historical surgical treatment of recurrent patella dislocation has varied widely from tibial tubercle transfer to lateral retinacular release to medial capsular plication. The understanding that the medial patellofemoral ligament (MFPL) is the primary stabilizer of lateral patellar translation has revolutionized the treatment of patellar dislocations (**Fig. 8**). Most current surgical strategies for patellar dislocation are based on repair or reconstruction of the MPFL. Although delayed MPFL reconstructions using either hamstring autograft or allograft have produced excellent functional outcomes,[50,51] acute repair of the torn MPFL within adolescents does not confer any clinical benefit when compared with nonoperative management with physical therapy.[52]

Extensor Mechanism Injuries

Prompt recognition and referral of injuries to extensor mechanism, including quadriceps tendon, patella, and patellar tendon, are important to attain optimal clinical outcomes. Because of the unopposed proximal pull of the quadriceps musculature, disruptions of the extensor mechanism can be difficult to repair if surgery is delayed for greater than 2 to 3 weeks. In cases of acute disruption, the tendons can be directly repaired, whereas, in chronic cases, more extensive procedures such as interpositional grafts or advancement flaps may be required.

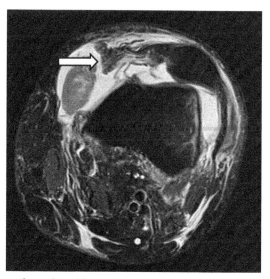

Fig. 8. The MPFL runs from the adductor tubercle of the medial femoral condyle to the superior two-thirds of the medial patella and can be compromised mid substance or at its patellar or femoral attachment (as shown here) during an acute traumatic patellar dislocation. *Arrow* indicates Torn edge of medial patellofemoral ligament.

Inability to perform a straight leg raise and a palpable defect are hallmarks of extensor mechanism and should prompt further investigation. Radiographs readily detect patellar fractures and patellar tendon disruptions where the patella is elevated (ie, patella alta) compared with the contralateral limb (**Fig. 9**). Because physical examination and radiographs can diagnose most of these injuries, MRI is often unnecessary and can delay definitive treatment. For comfort and to prevent distraction of the proximal and distal segments, the knee should be immobilized in extension before referral to an orthopedic surgeon.

Tibial Plateau Fractures

Tibial plateau fractures occur in 2 distinct subsets: in elderly patients, tibial plateau fractures are often caused by low-energy falls, whereas in younger populations, these injuries result from high-energy trauma, such as motor vehicle accidents. Vascular injuries and compartment syndrome are not uncommon among those sustaining high-energy injuries. In addition to this population, elderly with seemingly low-energy fractures but who are consuming antiplatelet agents and/or anticoagulants should be closely monitored for potential compartment syndrome.

Treatment of tibial plateau fractures is based on number, location, and amount of displacement of the fracture fragments. Nondisplaced fractures are often treated with a period of immobilization and non-weight-bearing. Although the precise amount of acceptable displacement remains controversial, unstable fractures with significant joint incongruity benefit from open reduction and internal fixation once soft tissue swelling subsides.[53]

Chondral and Osteochondral Injuries

Most chondral and osteochondral injuries are likely subclinical and occur insidiously. When symptomatic, these injuries are often associated with mechanical symptoms,

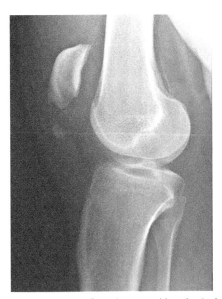

Fig. 9. Extensor mechanism injuries are often diagnosed by physical examination alone. Radiographs can be useful, especially in patellar tendon ruptures in which the patella migrates superiorly because of the unopposed action of the quadriceps.

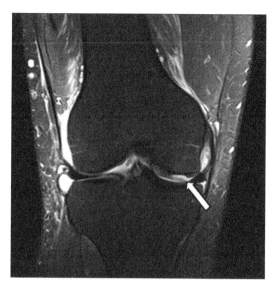

Fig. 10. Delamination injuries of the articular cartilage can cause the unstable fragment to flip and cause locking and catching sensations. *Arrow* indicates delaminated edge of articular cartilage.

such as locking and catching (**Fig. 10**). Usually, acute lesions with mechanical symptoms benefit from surgical intervention to prevent locking and potentially restore native anatomy. Osteochondral fragments are typically more amenable to surgical fixation than chondral lesions because of thickness and purchase of the osseous portion. If repair is not possible, the fragment is often removed from the joint. Delayed cartilage restoration can be considered if the patient remains in pain.

REFERENCES

1. Månsson J, Nilsson G, Strender LE, et al. Reasons for encounters, investigations, referrals, diagnoses and treatments in general practice in Sweden–a multicentre pilot study using electronic patient records. Eur J Gen Pract 2011;17(2):87–94.
2. McCaig LF, Nawar EW. National Hospital Ambulatory Medical Care Survey: 2004 emergency department summary. Adv Data 2006;372:1–29.
3. Schappert SM, Burt CW. Ambulatory care visits to physician offices, hospital outpatient departments, and emergency departments: United States, 2001-02. Vital Health Stat 13 2006;(159):1–66.
4. Solomon DH, Simel DL, Bates DW, et al. The rational clinical examination. Does this patient have a torn meniscus or ligament of the knee? Value of the physical examination. JAMA 2001;286(13):1610–20.
5. Beasley LS, Vidal AF. Traumatic patellar dislocation in children and adolescents: treatment update and literature review. Curr Opin Pediatr 2004;16(1):29–36.
6. DeHaven KE. Diagnosis of acute knee injuries with hemarthrosis. Am J Sports Med 1980;8(1):9–14.
7. Konan S, Rayan F, Haddad FS. Do physical diagnostic tests accurately detect meniscal tears? Knee Surg Sports Traumatol Arthrosc 2009;17(7):806–11.
8. Stiell IG, Greenberg GH, Wells GA, et al. Derivation of a decision rule for the use of radiography in acute knee injuries. Ann Emerg Med 1995;26(4):405–13.

9. Oei EH, Nikken JJ, Ginai AZ, et al. Costs and effectiveness of a brief MRI examination of patients with acute knee injury. Eur Radiol 2009;19(2):409–18. http://dx.doi.org/10.1007/s00330-008-1162-z.

10. Nikken JJ, Oei EH, Ginai AZ, et al. Acute peripheral joint injury: cost and effectiveness of low-field-strength MR imaging–results of randomized controlled trial. Radiology 2005;236(3):958–67.

11. Van Dyck P, Vanhoenacker FM, Lambrecht V, et al. Prospective comparison of 1.5 and 3.0-T MRI for evaluating the knee menisci and ACL. J Bone Joint Surg Am 2013;95(10):916–24. http://dx.doi.org/10.2106/JBJS.L.01195.

12. Laoruengthana A, Jarusriwanna A. Sensitivity and specificity of magnetic resonance imaging for knee injury and clinical application for the Naresuan University Hospital. J Med Assoc Thai 2012;95(Suppl 10):S151–7.

13. Crawford R, Walley G, Bridgman S, et al. Magnetic resonance imaging versus arthroscopy in the diagnosis of knee pathology, concentrating on meniscal lesions and ACL tears: a systematic review. Br Med Bull 2007;84:5–23.

14. Mathieu L, Bouchard A, Marchaland JP, et al. Knee MR-arthrography in assessment of meniscal and chondral lesions. Orthop Traumatol Surg Res 2009;95(1): 40–7. http://dx.doi.org/10.1016/j.otsr.2008.09.005.

15. Wicky S, Blaser PF, Blanc CH, et al. Comparison between standard radiography and spiral CT with 3D reconstruction in the evaluation, classification and management of tibial plateau fractures. Eur Radiol 2000;10(8):1227–32.

16. Macarini L, Murrone M, Marini S, et al. Tibial plateau fractures: evaluation with multidetector-CT. Radiol Med 2004;108(5–6):503–14.

17. Sladjan T, Zoran V, Zoran B. Correlation of clinical examination, ultrasound sonography, and magnetic resonance imaging findings with arthroscopic findings in relation to acute and chronic lateral meniscus injuries. J Orthop Sci 2014; 19(1):71–6.

18. Abbasi D, May MM, Wall EJ, et al. MRI findings in adolescent patients with acute traumatic knee hemarthrosis. J Pediatr Orthop 2012;32(8):760–4. http://dx.doi.org/10.1097/BPO.0b013e3182648d45.

19. Leivo I, Kauhanen S, Michelsson JE. Abnormal mitochondria and sarcoplasmic changes in rabbit skeletal muscle induced by immobilization. APMIS 1998; 106(12):1113–23.

20. Walsh S, Frank C, Shrive N, et al. Knee immobilization inhibits biomechanical maturation of the rabbit medial collateral ligament. Clin Orthop Relat Res 1993;(297):253–61.

21. Padgett LR, Dahners LE. Rigid immobilization alters matrix organization in the injured rat medial collateral ligament. J Orthop Res 1992;10(6):895–900.

22. Wall BT, Dirks ML, Snijders T, et al. Substantial skeletal muscle loss occurs during only 5 days of disuse. Acta Physiol (Oxf) 2014;210(3):600–11.

23. Long BC, Knight KL, Hopkins T, et al. Production of consistent pain by intermittent infusion of sterile 5% hypertonic saline, followed by decrease of pain with cryotherapy. J Sport Rehabil 2012;21(3):225–30.

24. Hubbard TJ, Denegar CR. Does cryotherapy improve outcomes with soft tissue injury? J Athl Train 2004;39(3):278–9.

25. Lee CK, Pardun J, Buntic R, et al. Severe frostbite of the knees after cryotherapy. Orthopedics 2007;30(1):63–4.

26. Keskin M, Tosun Z, Duymaz A, et al. Frostbite injury due to improper usage of an ice pack. Ann Plast Surg 2005;55(4):437–8.

27. Maffulli N, Binfield PM, King JB, et al. Acute haemarthrosis of the knee in athletes. A prospective study of 106 cases. J Bone Joint Surg Br 1993;75(6):945–9.

28. Wallman P, Carley S. Aspiration of acute traumatic knee haemarthrosis. Emerg Med J 2002;19(1):50.

29. Shaarani SR, O'Hare C, Quinn A, et al. Effect of prehabilitation on the outcome of anterior cruciate ligament reconstruction. Am J Sports Med 2013;41(9): 2117–27.

30. Hurd WJ, Axe MJ, Snyder-Mackler L. A 10-year prospective trial of a patient management algorithm and screening examination for highly active individuals with anterior cruciate ligament injury: part 2, determinants of dynamic knee stability. Am J Sports Med 2008;36(1):48–56.

31. Dumont GD, Hogue GD, Padalecki JR, et al. Meniscal and chondral injuries associated with pediatric anterior cruciate ligament tears: relationship of treatment time and patient-specific factors. Am J Sports Med 2012;40(9): 2128–33.

32. Lawrence JT, Argawal N, Ganley TJ. Degeneration of the knee joint in skeletally immature patients with a diagnosis of an anterior cruciate ligament tear: is there harm in delay of treatment? Am J Sports Med 2011;39(12):2582–7.

33. Neuman P, Englund M, Kostogiannis I, et al. Prevalence of tibiofemoral osteoarthritis 15 years after nonoperative treatment of anterior cruciate ligament injury: a prospective cohort study. Am J Sports Med 2008;36(9):1717–25.

34. Taylor DC, Posner M, Curl WW, et al. Isolated tears of the anterior cruciate ligament: over 30-year follow-up of patients treated with arthrotomy and primary repair. Am J Sports Med 2009;37(1):65–71.

35. Kaeding CC, Aros B, Pedroza A, et al. Allograft versus autograft anterior cruciate ligament reconstruction: predictors of failure from a MOON prospective longitudinal cohort. Sports Health 2011;3:73–81.

36. Macaulay AA, Perfetti DC, Levine WN. Anterior cruciate ligament graft choices. Sports Health 2012;4:63–8.

37. Shelbourne KD, Wilckens JH, Mollabashy A, et al. Arthrofibrosis in acute anterior cruciate ligament reconstruction. The effect of timing of reconstruction and rehabilitation. Am J Sports Med 1991;19(4):332–6.

38. Decarlo MS, Shelbourne KD, McCarroll JR, et al. Traditional versus accelerated rehabilitation following ACL reconstruction: a one-year follow-up. J Orthop Sports Phys Ther 1992;15(6):309–16.

39. Shelbourne KD, Clark M, Gray T. Minimum 10-year follow-up of patients after an acute, isolated posterior cruciate ligament injury treated nonoperatively. Am J Sports Med 2013;41(7):1526–33.

40. Torg JS, Barton TM, Pavlov H, et al. Natural history of the posterior cruciate ligament-deficient knee. Clin Orthop Relat Res 1989;(246):208–16.

41. Matava MJ, Ellis E, Gruber B. Surgical treatment of posterior cruciate ligament tears: an evolving technique. J Am Acad Orthop Surg 2009;17:435–46.

42. Albright JP, Powell JW, Smith W, et al. Medial collateral ligament knee sprains in college football. Effectiveness of preventive braces. Am J Sports Med 1994; 22(1):12–8.

43. Mills WJ, Barei DP, McNair P. The value of the ankle-brachial index for diagnosing arterial injury after knee dislocation: a prospective study. J Trauma 2004;56:1261–5.

44. Werner BC, Gwathmey FW Jr, Higgins ST, et al. Ultra-low velocity knee dislocations: patient characteristics, complications, and outcomes. Am J Sports Med 2014;42(2):358–63.

45. Harner CD, Waltrip RL, Bennett CH, et al. Surgical management of knee dislocations. J Bone Joint Surg Am 2004;86:262–73.

46. Zanetti M, Pfirrmann CW, Schmid MR, et al. Patients with suspected meniscal tears: prevalence of abnormalities seen on MRI of 100 symptomatic and 100 contralateral asymptomatic knees. AJR Am J Roentgenol 2003;181(3):635–41.

47. Pearse EO, Craig DM. Partial meniscectomy in the presence of severe osteoarthritis does not hasten the symptomatic progression of osteoarthritis. Arthroscopy 2003;19(9):963–8.

48. Laible C, Stein DA, Kiridly DN. Meniscal repair. J Am Acad Orthop Surg 2013; 21(4):204–13.

49. Cannon WD Jr, Vittori JM. The incidence of healing in arthroscopic meniscal repairs in anterior cruciate ligament-reconstructed knees versus stable knees. Am J Sports Med 1992;20(2):176–81.

50. Csintalan RP, Latt LD, Fornalski S, et al. Medial patellofemoral ligament (MPFL) reconstruction for the treatment of patellofemoral instability. J Knee Surg 2014; 27(2):139–46.

51. Howells NR, Barnett AJ, Ahearn N, et al. Medial patellofemoral ligament reconstruction: a prospective outcome assessment of a large single centre series. J Bone Joint Surg Br 2012;94(9):1202–8.

52. Palmu S, Kallio PE, Donell ST, et al. Acute patellar dislocation in children and adolescents: a randomized clinical trial. J Bone Joint Surg Am 2008;90(3):463–70.

53. Koval KJ, Helfet DL. Tibial plateau fractures: evaluation and treatment. J Am Acad Orthop Surg 1995;3(2):86–94.

Practical Approach to Hip Pain

 CrossMark

Christopher Karrasch, MD, Scott Lynch, MD*

KEYWORDS

- Hip pain • Labral tear • FAI • Osteoarthritis

KEY POINTS

- Detailed history including age, onset of symptoms, location of pain, history of trauma or overuse, duration of symptoms, rheumatologic conditions, and previous therapy is important in narrowing the differential diagnosis.
- Owing to the high sensitivity and specificity of magnetic resonance imaging (MRI) in detecting common injuries, it has become the modality of choice in diagnosing soft tissue abnormality of the hip, but it must be used with prudence because it may reveal pathologic condition that are asymptomatic and could lead to overtreatment.
- Initial treatment centers on analgesia, nonsteroidal antiinflammatory drugs (NSAIDs), cryotherapy, physical therapy, and, if necessary, a brief period of immobilization.
- Intra-articular anesthetic/cortisone injections can be both diagnostic and therapeutic.
- Timely diagnosis is important because time to operative intervention can have a significant effect on surgical outcomes, patient recovery, and satisfaction.

INTRODUCTION

Musculoskeletal ailments are the presenting complaint in nearly 21.5% of visits in the primary care office[1] and 13.8% of emergency room visits.[2] Diagnosis and treatment of hip pain, especially in young patients, is an evolving field. The differential diagnosis is vast for pain about the hip and can be caused by a wide spectrum of pathologic conditions. Recently, there has been a large focus on the labrum and its associated pathologies, which are usually referred to as femoroacetabular impingement (FAI). Like any new diagnosis, there becomes a rush to attribute any and all unexplained pain to the newly discovered pathologic condition. This rush causes a loss of focus on other potential causes of pain, often to the detriment of the patient. Such has been the case with labral tears and FAI. One must resist this temptation and continue to adhere to the fact that a good history and examination are the cornerstones of diagnosis and thus

Department of Orthopaedic Surgery, Penn State Milton S. Hershey Medical Center, Pennsylvania State University College of Medicine, 30 Hope Drive, Hershey, PA 17033, USA
* Corresponding author. Penn State Hershey Medical Center, Bone and Joint Institute, Pennsylvania State University College of Medicine, 30 Hope Drive, PO Box 859, Hershey, PA 17033.
E-mail address: slynch@hmc.psu.edu

Med Clin N Am 98 (2014) 737–754
http://dx.doi.org/10.1016/j.mcna.2014.03.003
0025-7125/14/$ – see front matter © 2014 Elsevier Inc. All rights reserved.
medical.theclinics.com

start from the perspective of a large differential diagnosis. A general diagnostic knowledge of the pathologic condition and overall treatment strategies is paramount to avoid long-term disability and progression of disease caused by a delay in appropriate treatment.

HISTORY

A comprehensive history helps narrow the differential diagnosis. A detailed history should include the following aspects: patient age; onset, nature, and location of pain; referred pain; precipitating or provoking causes; mechanical symptoms (ie, snapping, popping, locking, reduced range of motion); ability to bear weight; history of a traumatic event; congenital or childhood hip deformities; recent alterations in activity level; previous musculoskeletal injuries and/or surgeries; underlying rheumatologic conditions; and systemic symptoms.

Differentiating intra-articular from extra-articular causes of pain is important. Many extra-articular pathologies can be mimickers of hip pain but may not be directly associated with the hip joint itself.[3] Categorizing hip pain makes synthesizing a differential diagnosis more systematic, objective, and accurate. Simply asking a patient to point with 1 finger where the pain is can help guide a differential diagnosis. **Box 1** presents various pathologic conditions categorized into intra-articular, extra-articular, and mimickers that can be presenting causes of hip pain at the clinic.

Patients with intra-articular pathology typically complain of pain in the groin and may have mechanical symptoms such as catching, popping, or clicking.[4] Such patients often have difficulty with torsional or twisting activities, prolonged sitting, and rising from a seated position and greater difficulty on inclined surfaces when compared with level ones.[5–7] An acute change in pain and inability to bear weight should raise concern for more serious hip pathology and prompt an urgent referral to an orthopedist or the emergency room.

PHYSICAL EXAMINATION

Examination of the painful hip can be challenging. Although the literature focuses on many provocative maneuvers for specific pathology, the physical examination should begin with the basics of any musculoskeletal evaluation: observation, palpation, range of motion, motor strength, sensation, vascularity, stability, and provocative maneuvers. As with any musculoskeletal examination, the affected limb should be compared with the unaffected limb.

A systematic approach to the physical examination helps limit undiagnosed pathologic condition.[8] A positional approach in which specific examinations are performed with the patient in standing, seated, supine, lateral, and prone positions has been described by Martin.[9] This approach allows good flow through the examination with less patient discomfort and repetitive positional changes.[10] During an examination, many provocative maneuvers can be performed to assess for intra-articular joint pathology. A single test on its own is not diagnostic, but multiple maneuvers in combination with a thorough history increase the accuracy of a clinical diagnosis.[11]

Standing Position

General overall ligamentous laxity should be assessed. The ability to touch thumbs to the forearm and hyperextend the elbow and knee recurvatum are signs of increased laxity, which predisposes affected individuals to hip instability and pain. The patient's gait should be evaluated and any abnormalities as well as the patient's overall mechanical alignment (varus/valgus) should be documented. A limp can be caused by

---

Box 1
Common causes of pain around the hip

Intra-articular

Osteoarthritis

Labral tears

Femoroacetabular impingement

Loose bodies

Chondral lesions

Avascular necrosis

Septic arthritis

Fracture

Ligamentum teres tears

Extra-articular

Trochanteric bursitis

Iliotibial band snapping

Iliopsoas tendonitis/snapping

Piriformis syndrome

Stress fracture

Other non-hip-related causes

Sports hernia

Osteitis pubis

Adductor strain

Abdominal/pelvic viscera

Lumbar radiculopathy

Adapted from Tibor LM, Sekiya JK. Differential diagnosis of pain around the hip joint. Arthroscopy 2008;24:1407–21.

---

pain, limb length discrepancy, or weakness. A Trendelenburg gait is seen when the patient has weak abductor musculature. The patient compensates by laterally leaning his or her thorax over the affected hip to keep the center of gravity over the stance leg. The Trendelenburg test is performed by asking patients to stand on their affected leg. If the abductors are weak, the pelvis droops to the contralateral side.[12] Patients' pelvis should be assessed for obliquity by placing hands on the iliac crests. The iliac crests should be parallel to the floor, and if not, a block should be placed under the foot of the lower crest to evaluate for limb length discrepancy as the cause for the obliquity. The spine should be assessed and any excessive scoliosis, lordosis, kyphosis, or stiffness should be documented. The sacroiliac joints should be palpated for tenderness.

Seated Position

With the patient in sitting position, the neurologic status, including sensory, motor, and reflexes (**Table 1**); skin; and circulation, should be evaluated.

Table 1
Motor and sensory testing for major peripheral nerves of lower extremity

Nerve	Motor	Sensory
Genitofemoral (L1–L2)	None	Proximal anteromedial thigh
Lateral femoral cutaneous (L2–L3)	None	Lateral thigh (meralgia paresthetica)
Obturator (L2–L4)	Thigh/hip adduction	Inferomedial thigh
Superior gluteal (L5)	Thigh abduction	None
Inferior gluteal (L5–S2)	Hip extension	None
Posterior femoral cutaneous (S1–S3)	None	Posterior part of the thigh
Femoral (L2–L4)	Hip flexion/knee extension	Anteromedial thigh, medial leg and foot (saphenous)
Deep peroneal	Ankle and great toe dorsiflexion	Dorsal first web space
Superficial peroneal	Hindfoot eversion	Dorsal lateral foot
Tibial nerve (L4–S3)	Ankle plantarflexion	Plantar surface foot

Supine Position

An abdominal examination including palpation of all 4 quadrants should be performed to screen for acute visceral pathology that can mimic hip pain such as splenic or liver laceration, appendicitis, pelvic inflammatory disease, hernias, and so forth. Palpation should be done laterally over the greater trochanter, the anterior part of the hip, along the inguinal ligament, and pubis for tenderness as well as warmth and any enlarged lymph nodes. Generally, intra-articular hip pathology is not tender to palpation. Muscular strains, tendinitis, and bursitis are tender. Range of motion, both passive and active, should be assessed (**Table 2**).

The Thomas test assesses for hip flexion contractures and is performed by flexing both hips and allowing the affected lower extremity to extend to lay flat on the table.[13] Normal range of motion allows a patient to lay the leg flat on the table with the other hip flexed. Inability to lay the affected leg flat on the table is a positive result of examination and suggests a hip flexion contracture. A straight leg raise against resistance (Stinchfield test) loads the anterolateral joint and produces intra-articular joint pain. The impingement test is performed by flexing, adducting, and internally rotating the hip. Pain can indicate FAI and labral pathology and has been shown to be sensitive in up to 95% of patients with labral tears.[14] However, it is not very specific, because many other disorders also have pain with this maneuver. The flexion, abduction, and external rotation (FABER) test can elicit pain stemming from the sacroiliac and hip joints. Once in the FABER position, extending, adducting, and internally rotating the leg while palpating the anterior part of the hip may elicit a palpable snap that suggests iliopsoas snapping syndrome.[15]

Table 2
Normal hip range of motion

Flexion (tested supine)	120°–135°
Extension (tested prone)	20°–30°
Abduction/adduction (tested supine)	45°–50°/20°–30°
Internal/external rotation (supine with hip at 90°)	30°/50°

Lateral Position

The greater trochanter should be palpated. If tender, the likely diagnosis is trochanteric bursitis or iliotibial (IT) band pathology. The Ober test is performed by flexing and abducting the hip with the knee at 90° and then extending and adducting the hip.[16] If the lower extremity stays in abduction then the IT band is tight. Snapping of the IT tendon, as it passes over the greater trochanter, may be reproduced by extending and externally rotating the hip from a flexed and internally rotated position.[17] The piriformis syndrome is assessed by adducting and internally rotating the hip putting the piriformis muscle on stretch; this can compress the sciatic nerve, reproduce the posterior part of the hip and thigh pain, and sometimes cause tingling or numbness in the sciatic distribution.[18]

Prone Position

Extension as well as internal/external rotation of the hip should be tested. Ely test is performed by passively flexing the knee. Flexing of the hip suggests a tight rectus femoris muscle.[9]

DIAGNOSTIC TEST/IMAGING

Orthogonal radiographs including anterior/posterior (A/P) radiograph of the pelvis and a cross-table lateral view of the proximal femur are the essential initial imaging studies to evaluate the hip. Radiographs are relatively inexpensive, widely available, and can quickly triage hip complaints that may require immediate treatment by an orthopedic surgeon such as a gross fracture or chronic conditions such as osteoarthritis (OA). The A/P radiograph of the pelvis must be critically evaluated to ensure that it is an appropriate examination. On an appropriately performed pelvic A/P radiograph the coccyx should be in line with and 1 to 2 cm above the pubic symphysis to ensure that there is no inletization or rotation. Radiographs can also screen for FAI. Acetabular retroversion makes the hip prone to acetabular overcoverage (pincer deformity) that can cause impingement and pain.[19] This condition can be seen on the A/P pelvic radiograph as the described crossover or posterior wall sign (**Fig. 1**). However, the A/P radiograph must be appropriate because the crossover or posterior wall sign can be overcalled on a pelvic film that is inletized (**Fig. 2**). Obtaining a false profile view may help to delineate acetabular overcoverage further.[20,21] On the cross-table lateral view, the sphericity of the femoral head can be quantified using the described α-angle (**Fig. 3**).[22] An increased α-angle is seen with an aspherical femoral head (cam lesion), which can predispose patients to impingement, labral tears, and early OA.[6,7,23] Plain radiographs can also evaluate for hip deformities such as hip dysplasia (**Fig. 4**) and slipped capital femoral epiphysis as well as other pathologic conditions such as osteitis pubis (**Fig. 5**), which may be causes of pain around the hip.

Ultrasonography is becoming more readily available and can evaluate both intra- and extra-articular ailments. This modality can be used in real time dynamically to evaluate pathologic conditions such as bursitis, snapping hip, hematoma, hip effusions, paralabral cyst formation, as well as nonhip pathology such as hernias, abscess, tumor, and lymphadenopathy.[24] Ultrasonography predictably provides anatomic verification for injections and/or aspirations and improves accuracy of placement for both intra-articular and extra-articular pathologies.[25–28]

Computed tomographic (CT) scans can be helpful in evaluating the anatomic position and orientation of the acetabulum, and to assess for excess femoral anteversion. Three-dimensional reconstructions can be helpful in surgical planning and in further characterizing acetabular retroversion, but, in general, these are not necessary in

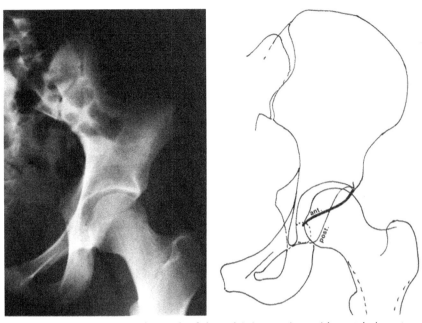

Fig. 1. This is a cropped A/P radiograph of the pelvis in a patient with acetabular retroversion. The crossover or posterior wall sign is outlined.

the primary workup of hip pain. These reconstructions can aid in the diagnosis of occult fractures when a patient is unable to obtain an MRI secondary to a pacemaker, certain cardiac stents, or other pathologic condition that excludes them from the study. MRI has been shown to be superior to CT scans in defining occult and stress fractures about the hip.[29]

MRI of the hip is the most sensitive and specific imaging modality for pathology about the hip. MRI is expensive and should be used with prudence because it can uncover presumed pathologic condition that may be asymptomatic.[30] When prescribing

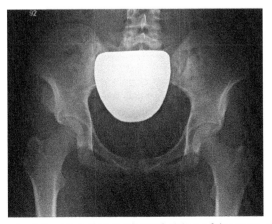

Fig. 2. A/P radiograph of the pelvis that is inletized giving a false sense of a crossover sign, although there is no true acetabular retroversion.

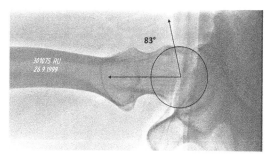

Fig. 3. Cross-table lateral view with a labeled increased α-angle indicating a significant cam lesion and asphericity of the femoral head. Normal α-angle is less than 50° to 55°. MRI of the same hip with concomitant labral tear.

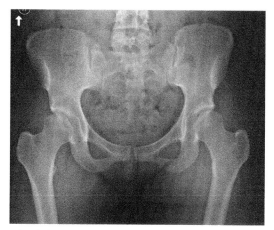

Fig. 4. A/P radiograph of the pelvis demonstrating bilateral hip dysplasia.

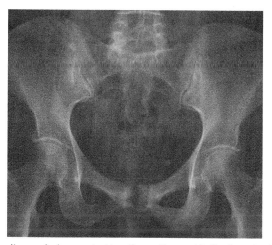

Fig. 5. A/P pelvic radiograph demonstrating the radiographic findings in chronic osteitis pubis with sclerosis and bone remodeling of the pubic symphysis.

an MRI of the hip, it should be ensured that it is an isolated hip MRI and not an MRI of the pelvis because they are vastly different and this mistake can lead to delayed diagnosis as well as increased cost. However, if the clinical diagnosis is more suggestive of adductor strain, osteitis pubis, or sports hernia, an MRI of the pelvis is indicated because an isolated hip MRI may not fully evaluate these pathologic conditions. To rule out intra-articular hip pathology, an MRI with an arthrogram (MRA) can be a powerful tool. When ordering the MRA, patients must be prescribed an intra-articular injection of anesthetic such as bupivacaine and asked to pay particular attention to their pain immediately after the study. Pain relief from the anesthetic has been shown to have a 90% predictability of an intra-articular abnormality.[31]

DIFFERENTIAL DIAGNOSIS/TREATMENT
OA

Of all joint diseases, OA is the leading cause of impaired quality of life, disability, and lost work days in the United States.[32,33] Symptoms are insidious, but may wax and wane in severity, and are felt predominantly in the groin. This condition is the first on the differential for an elderly patient with chronic hip pain. Generally, the pain is exacerbated with activity and improves with rest. Risk factors include female gender, obesity, history of high-demand work (such as farming), high-impact competitive athletics, higher bone density, developmental abnormalities (dysplasia, Legg-Calvé-Perthes disease, slipped capital femoral epiphysis, and FAI), and a family history.[34–40]

The hallmarks on physical examination are decreased passive and active range of motion that is associated with pain. Patients generally lose internal rotation range of motion first. Radiographically, there is joint space narrowing, subchondral sclerosis, and in later disease, bone cysts. Radiographs include weight-bearing A/P pelvic and cross-table lateral views of the proximal femur. These radiographs are to be an adjunct to the history and physical examination while ruling out other conditions. Radiographs should not be relied on independently because radiographic severity does not necessarily correlate with functional disability.[41]

Treatment of OA is based on symptoms, with the goal of pain relief and improved physical function. At present, neither is there any cure for OA nor is there any cartilage regeneration pharmacologics or procedure.[42] Antiinflammatories (NSAIDs) are currently the mainstay of nonoperative management. Patients should be encouraged to stay as active as they can be as well as initiate an exercise program. In a recent meta-analysis of the literature, an approach combining exercises to increase strength, flexibility, and aerobic capacity was significantly more effective in improving limitation in function than a program having no regimented exercise.[43] Intra-articular cortisone injections are effective both therapeutically and diagnostically for those who fail NSAIDs alone. These injections can be administered every 3 to 4 months without a significant increase in cartilage compromise. In the setting of OA once patients have exhausted NSAIDs, physical therapy, and intra-articular cortisone injections, the next step in treatment is a total hip arthroplasty. To obtain the most reliable outcomes, patients should be referred to high-volume surgeons and centers specializing in joint replacement.[44]

Labral Tears

The labrum of the hip is a fibrocartilagenous ring that forms a rim around the articular surface of the acetabulum. Although it has minimal mechanical properties for distributing forces over the articular surface of the acetabulum, it acts as a gasket and creates an important hydraulic seal in the hip joint to provide stability via negative pressure.[45,46] The labrum has neuroreceptors and may have a functional role in proprioception.[47] The blood supply of the labrum is limited to the peripheral ring nearest the acetabulum where healing of repairs can occur.[48] Tears of the labrum can become symptomatic and present with a combination of dull and sharp pain in the groin that is often made worse with activity and prolonged sitting.[14] Activities that cause repetitive loading of the joint, specifically pivoting and hip flexion, increase the risk of labral tears predisposing individuals such as athletes to pathologic condition.[14] Acute subluxations, dislocations, or trauma can cause a tear in the labrum and must be differentiated from labral tears secondary to associated chronic conditions such as dysplasia, FAI, iliopsoas impingement, OA, or acetabular anteversion/retroversion.[49] These secondary tears are thought to be much more common.

On physical examination, maneuvers that assess intra-articular pathology such as log roll, hip range of motion, flexion adduction, and internal rotation reproduce pain in the groin. A/P radiograph of the pelvis and cross-table lateral radiograph are indicated and can help to delineate other pathologies as described above. A hip MRA (**Fig. 6**) is the most sensitive and specific test to diagnose labral tears, approaching 90% and 100%, respectively.[50,51] Patients with a labral tear on MRI who report significant pain relief from the intra-articular anesthetic administered during the test have a significantly increased probability that the labral tear is symptomatic. Hip MRI results must be critically analyzed in conjunction with a clinical history and examination because most labral tears, including those in athletes, are asymptomatic.[30] Nearly all patients older than 70 years have MRI-positive labral pathology that is degenerative in nature and related to degenerative arthritis and age.[52]

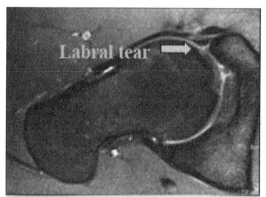

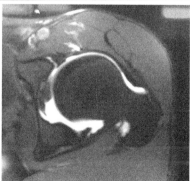

Fig. 6. MRI with intra-articular gadolinium of the hip depicting an anterior labral tear.

Treatment begins with conservative measures including NSAIDs, activity modification, physical therapy, and intra-articular cortisone injections. Once conservative therapy has failed, open versus arthroscopic surgical intervention may be indicated, including labral repair or debridement (**Fig. 7**). Clinical improvement in hip symptoms after surgery has been reported from 68% to 82% in the literature.[5,53,54]

FAI

In normal hip anatomy, the acetabulum and proximal femur articulate without abutment or impingement through a physiologic range of motion. FAI occurs when there is abnormal anatomy of the acetabulum and/or femoral head-neck junction that results in abnormal contact between the two. On the acetabular side, this abnormal contact is a result of acetabular overcoverage of the proximal femur and is termed pincer impingement. This impingement can be caused by a deep acetabulum (coxa profunda), or anterior overcoverage due to acetabular retroversion. A normal femoral head-neck junction is spherical. An aspherical femoral head-neck junction can lead to abutment at the end ranges of hip motion and is termed cam impingement. An aspherical femoral head-neck junction can be caused by various pathologic conditions including slipped capital femoral epiphysis, malunion or malreduced femoral neck fractures, femoral retroversion, and coxa vara. Most frequently, the aspherical portion of the femur is the anterolateral head-neck junction.[55] Although these 2 types of FAI have been described as separate entities, often patients have a combination of both. These nonanatomic relationships leading to impingement can cause pain, decreased range of motion, labral tears, chondral defects of the acetabulum, and eventual OA.[6,7]

Patients are generally young to middle aged and present with pain in the groin provoked by activity. Pain comes on insidiously and often is present for months to years. Prolonged sitting, movements requiring flexion and internal rotation such as getting in and out of cars, and getting up from seated positions often cause pain.[55]

On physical examination, a straight leg raise against resistance loads the anterolateral joint and produces intra-articular joint pain. Pain with the impingement test (flexion, adduction, and internal rotation) can indicate FAI.

Radiographic evaluation to assess for FAI includes an A/P view, a cross-table lateral view with the hip internally rotated 15° (see **Fig. 3**), and in some cases, a false profile

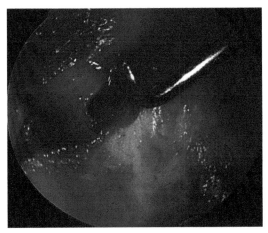

Fig. 7. Arthroscopic hip procedure demonstrating a labral tear.

view (**Fig. 8**).[56] The A/P view evaluates for acetabular overcoverage (pincer), and the cross-table lateral view evaluates for asphericity of the femoral head-neck junction (cam). The α-angle is measured off the lateral view by fitting a best fit circle to the femoral head. Then a point in the circle is centered and an angle is created from the femoral shaft to the leading edge of asphericity that deviates from the best fit circle (see **Fig. 3**). A normal α-angle is less than 50° to 55°, and an angle greater than this is considered a cam lesion. An α-angle greater than 65° is associated with a higher incidence of chondral defects.[57] On the A/P film, a crossover or posterior wall sign can be seen when the acetabulum is retroverted (see **Fig. 1**). Normally the shadows of the posterior and anterior acetabular walls do not cross. A crossover or posterior wall sign indicates anterosuperior acetabular overcoverage.[19] An MRI can further delineate FAI as well as evaluate for concomitant chondral lesions, labral tears, or other intra-articular pathology.

Treatment of FAI includes NSAIDs, activity modification, physical therapy, and, if necessary, intra-articular cortisone injections. When conservative measures fail, surgical intervention may be warranted, which can be done through an open procedure (**Fig. 9**) or an arthroscopic procedure, with both yielding good results. With recent arthroscopic technology and technique advancements, arthroscopic acetabular osteoplasty and femoral head-neck resection has become the treatment of choice in most cases.

Snapping Hip

The painful snapping hip (coxa saltans) can be difficult to diagnose and treat.[58] The condition can be systematically categorized into intra-articular (labral tears, loose bodies, chondral defects, etc), internal (iliopsoas snapping), and external (IT band snapping). Differentiating the location of the condition is predicated on a thorough history, physical examination, and diagnostic imaging.

External snapping is caused by a thickened or tight IT band snapping over the greater trochanter of the proximal femur. More often than not, the snapping is

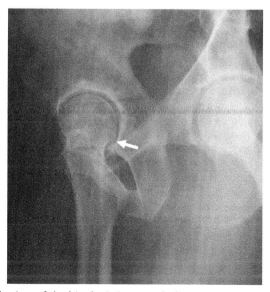

Fig. 8. False profile view of the hip depicting acetabular overcoverage or pincer deformity. Arrow pointing to associated posterior inferior joint space narrowing.

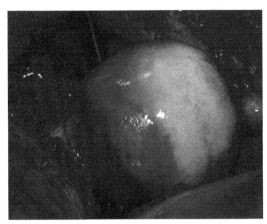

Fig. 9. Open surgical dislocation of the hip demonstrating an aspherical femoral head or cam deformity. The femoral head is more mushroom shaped compared to the normal, which is spherical.

nonpainful. In symptomatic cases, it is often associated with trochanteric bursitis.[59] Most often it is found in middle-aged women or running athletes. The thickened posterior portion of the IT band snaps over the greater trochanter from posterior to anterior when the hip goes from an extended to a flexed position. This snapping can be painful when the bursa is inflamed. Patients often have pain over the greater trochanter that radiates down the lateral thigh and have difficulty sleeping on the affected side. Patients often complain of the feeling that their hip is giving out.

On examination the patient may be able to reproduce the snapping actively, and this may be palpated or observed grossly. The patient has pain with palpation of the greater trochanter if the bursa is inflamed. If the patient is unable to reproduce the snapping, the IT tendon may be palpated as it passes over the greater trochanter during active hip motion. This palpation is done by starting the hip flexed and internally rotated, and then extending and externally rotating the leg.[17] IT band tightness should be assessed with the Ober test by flexing and abducting the hip with the knee at 90° and then extending and adducting the hip.[16] If the lower extremity stays in abduction then the IT band is tight.

Newer advances in ultrasonographic techniques have made it the imaging modality of choice if the clinical examination is unclear. Sometimes IT band snapping can be seen dynamically during an ultrasonography, providing a definitive diagnosis.

The mainstay of treatment is antiinflammatory medications, physical therapy for stretching of the IT band, and if necessary, corticosteroid injections. This treatment resolves symptoms in most cases, but for those who fail conservative treatment referral to an orthopedic surgeon is warranted. Historically, an open surgery has been performed to create tendon relaxing incisions in the IT band over the greater trochanter. It is important that surgery maintains the structural integrity of the abductor mechanism or patients can have abductor weakness that can affect their gait.[60] More recently, endoscopic techniques have been developed with similar good results in eliminating external snapping in most cases.[61]

Internal snapping of the hip is caused by the iliopsoas tendon snapping over the femoral/acetabular capsule or more commonly over the pectineal eminence of the pelvis. The iliopsoas is a powerful hip flexor formed by the confluence of the iliacus and psoas muscles that inserts on the lesser trochanter of the femur. Approximately

10% of the active population has asymptomatic snapping of the iliopsoas tendon. Painful snapping is a sign of either acute iliopsoas tendonitis or more chronic tendinopathy. Such snapping may be caused by repetitive microtrauma, and is seen with a higher incidence in runners, athletes, and elite ballet dancers.[17,62] Patients complain of clicking/popping that can be audible and is felt in the anterior region of the groin. Because the psoas muscle originates from the back, patients often concomitantly complain of low-back pain.[63]

On physical examination, the patient may be able to actively re-create the snapping. Passively the snapping is best evaluated in the supine position by taking the hip from a flexed, abducted, and externally rotated position down to an extended and internally rotated position while palpating over the anterior part of the groin. The snap of the iliopsoas tendon may be grossly palpable, very subtle, or not felt at all with the patient simply feeling an internal snap.

Dynamic ultrasonography is the imaging modality of choice and can be both diagnostic and a means for a therapeutic/diagnostic injection.

Treatment consists of NSAIDs, physical therapy, and if needed, corticosteroid injections. Response to an injection provides improved predictability that surgical intervention will be successful in patients who fail conservative measures.[64] Arthroscopic iliopsoas tendon release has become the surgical treatment of choice secondary to the minimally invasive approach and addresses associated intra-articular pathology.

Pubalgia

A wide spectrum of conditions can lead to pubic pain, including orthopedic (sports hernia, osteitis pubis, adductor strains, etc) as well as nonorthopedic (true hernias, genitourinary pathology, endometriosis, pelvic inflammatory disease, abdominal strains, etc) pathologies. A thorough knowledge of the pelvic anatomy is important in making the diagnosis.

Sports hernia is caused by a tear in the inguinal floor that does not result in a clinically obvious hernia but results in chronic groin pain.[65] Various injury mechanisms have been described, from simultaneous trunk hyperextension and thigh hyperabduction, which causes shearing forces, to muscular imbalances between strong thigh muscles and a concomitantly week abdominal core.[3] Athletes who participate in sports requiring repetitive twisting and torque of the proximal thigh and lower abdominal musculature (hockey, soccer, rugby, etc) are at a higher risk of occurrence.[65] The pain comes on insidiously and often radiates into the adductors, perineum, inguinal ligament, or testicular area and can be provoked by sudden movements such as sprints, quick cuts, sit-ups, or even coughing and sneezing.[3] Periods of rest typically improve symptoms.

On examination there is no appreciable hernia, but tenderness may be elicited around the conjoined tendon, pubic tubercle, external inguinal ring, or posterior inguinal canal. Having the patient perform a Valsalva maneuver may reproduce the pain.

Osteitis pubis is on a continuum with sports hernia and develops when there are increased forces on the symphysis pubis, which can be from repetitive stresses and/or the pull of pelvic musculature. Patients have specific pain located over the pubic symphysis and are generally tender over the symphysis on examination.

Adductor strains/sprains are the most common traumatic causes of groin pain in athletes, with a higher incidence in soccer and ice hockey players.[66] The pain is usually acute, in the groin, and patients can often recall a specific time or incident when the pain started. The acuity may help to differentiate this from a sports hernia and osteitis pubis, which have a more insidious onset. On examination, patients report tenderness to palpation along the adductor complex and have pain with resisted adduction.

Radiographic evaluation in pubalgia can be helpful to rule out fractures or avulsions and can establish a diagnosis of chronic osteitis pubis when the classic bone resorption, irregular contour, and widening of the pubic symphysis is seen (see **Fig. 5**). If there is doubt in diagnosis, an MRI of the pelvis is the most sensitive and specific imaging modality. Patients with athletic pubalgia (sports hernia) often have a secondary cleft sign near the pubic symphysis on MRI (**Fig. 10**).

Treatment of all pubalgia starts with activity modification, NSAIDs, and physical therapy. Treatment of acute adductor strains begins with rest, ice, and compression until the pain is improved. The second step is a regimen focused on range of motion. Once pain-free range of motion is obtained, the patient is advanced to regaining strength, flexibility, and endurance. Osteitis pubis is generally self-limiting, and its treatment should be done following the same protocol as for an adductor strain. True sports hernias may not respond to nonoperative treatment. Surgical intervention for unresolved sports hernias includes repair of the abdominal musculature, inguinal ligament, and its attachments. Historically this has been done either in an open manner or laproscopically using the patient's native tissue. Advances in synthetic materials and technology have produced light-weight mesh that allows both anterior and posterior repairs that allow normalization of the torn anatomy. This technique has been studied and yields excellent results in pain improvement, mobility, and return to previous activities.[67]

Stress Fractures

Stress fractures that can cause hip pain are relatively common in runners and highly competitive athletes. The treatment of stress fractures depends on their location. Most can be treated nonoperatively with activity modification and protected weight bearing. Some specific fractures with a history of poor healing may require surgery. Many patients have a history of a recent increase in activity such as a long run, competition, starting a new season of sport, increase in training, etc. The pain is worse with weight bearing and improves with rest and time.

On examination, the only positive feature may be pain with weight bearing and an altered gait. Patients may have tenderness to palpation over the area, but this may be unreliable.

Radiographs can show evidence of a fracture if it has been chronic with associated sclerosis or bone remodeling in the area of the stress fracture. However, in the early stages of stress fractures, radiographs may have only a 10% sensitivity and are often

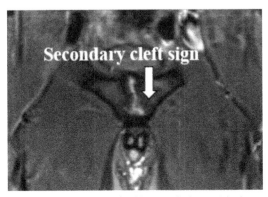

Fig. 10. MRI of the pelvis in the setting of athletic pubalgia with the arrow indicating the secondary cleft sign often seen in the chronic setting.

read as normal.[3,68,69] MRI has been shown to be more reliable than CT scans and is the most sensitive and specific for stress fractures.[29]

Stress fractures of the pubic bones can be treated with activity modification and weight bearing as tolerated. Fractures of the femoral neck are treated with protected weight bearing or surgery depending on their location. If the fracture is on the compression side of the femur during weight bearing (inferior neck), it can be treated with protected weight bearing and has a low incidence of displacement. If the fracture is on the tension side of the femoral neck during weight bearing (superior neck), it has a high incidence of displacement and requires surgical fixation. Displaced femoral neck fractures have a significant incidence of going on to develop avascular necrosis of the femoral head with eventual collapse, arthritis, and probable need for a total hip arthroplasty.

SUMMARY

Hip pain is a common complaint among patients presenting to outpatient clinics. Stratifying patients based on age, acuity, and location (extra-articular vs intra-articular) can help to aid in appropriate imaging and timely referral to an orthopedic surgeon. A thorough history and an organized physical examination combined with radiographs are usually sufficient to diagnose most hip complaints. If the diagnosis remains uncertain, MRI, usually with intra-articular gadolinium, is the imaging modality of choice in diagnosing both intra-articular and extra-articular pathologies.

REFERENCES

1. Månsson J, Nilsson G, Strender LE, et al. Reasons for encounters, investigations, referrals, diagnoses and treatments in general practice in Sweden–a multicentre pilot study using electronic patient records. Eur J Gen Pract 2011;17(2): 87–94.
2. McCaig LF, Nawar EW. National Hospital Ambulatory Medical Care Survey: 2004 emergency department summary. Adv Data 2006;(372):1–29.
3. Tibor LM, Sekiya JK. Differential diagnosis of pain around the hip joint. Arthroscopy 2008;24:1407–21.
4. Carreira D, Bush-Joseph CA. Hip arthroscopy. Orthopedics 2006;29:517–23.
5. Byrd JW, Jones KS. Prospective analysis of hip arthroscopy with two year follow up. Arthroscopy 2000;16:578–87.
6. Beck M, Kalhor M, Leunig M, et al. Hip morphology influences the pattern of damage to the acetabular cartilage: femoracetabular impingement as a cause of early osteoarthritis of the hip. J Bone Joint Surg Br 2005;87:1012–8.
7. Ganz R, Parvizi J, Beck M, et al. Femoroacetabular impingement: a cause for osteoarthritis of the hip. Clin Orthop Relat Res 2003;(417):112–20.
8. Shindle M, Voos J, Nho S, et al. Arthroscopic management of labral tears in the hip. J Bone Joint Surg Am 2008;90:2–19.
9. Martin HD. Clinical examination of the hip. Oper Tech Orthop 2005;15:177–81.
10. Braly BA, Beall DP, Martin HD. Clinical examination of the athletic hip. Clin Sports Med 2006;25:199–210.
11. Maslowski E, Sullivan W, Forster-Harwood J, et al. The diagnostic validity of hip provocation maneuvers to detect intra-articular hip pathology. PM R 2010;2: 174–81.
12. Hardcastle P, Nade S. The significance of the Trendelenburg test. J Bone Joint Surg Br 1985;67:741–6.

13. Hoppenfeld S. Physical examination of the spine and extremities. New York: Appleton-Century-Crofts; 1976. p. 143 Physical examination of the hip and pelvis.

14. Burnett RS, Della Rocca GJ, Prather H, et al. Clinical presentation of patients with tears of the acetabular labrum. J Bone Joint Surg Am 2006;88:1448–57.

15. Ilizaliturri V, Villalobos F, Chaidez P, et al. Internal snapping hip syndrome: treatment by endoscopic release of the iliopsoas tendon. Arthroscopy 2005;21: 1375–80.

16. Farr D, Selesnick H, Janecki C, et al. Arthroscopic bursectomy with concomitant iliotibial band release for the treatment of recalcitrant trochanteric bursitis. Arthroscopy 2007;23:905.

17. Winston P, Awan R, Cassidy J, et al. Clinical examination and ultrasound of self-reported snapping hip syndrome in elite ballet dancers. Am J Sports Med 2007; 35:118–26.

18. Windisch G, Braun EM, Anderhuber F. Piriformis muscle: clinical anatomy and consideration of the piriformis syndrome. Surg Radiol Anat 2007;29:37–45.

19. Reynolds D, Lucac J, Klaue K. Retroversion of the acetabulum. A cause of hip pain. J Bone Joint Surg Br 1999;81:281–8.

20. Lequesne M, De Seze S. False profile of the pelvis, a new radiographic incidence for the study of the hip. Its use in dysplasias and different coxopathies. Rev Rhum Mal Osteoartic 1961;28:643–52.

21. Chosa E, Tajima N. Anterior acetabular head index of the hip on false-profile views. New index of anterior acetabular cover. J Bone Joint Surg Br 2003;85: 826–9.

22. Nötzli H, Wyss T, Stöcklin C, et al. The contour of the femoral head-neck-junction as a predictor for the risk of anterior impingement. J Bone Joint Surg Br 2002;84: 556–60.

23. Eijer H, Leunig M, Mahomed M, et al. Crosstable lateral radiograph for screening of anterior femoral head-neck offset in patients with femoro-acetabular impingement. Hip Int 2001;11:37–41.

24. Cho K, Park B, Yeon K. Ultrasound of the adult hip. Semin Ultrasound CT MR 2000;21:214–30.

25. Micu MC, Bogdan GD, Fodor D. Steroid injection for hip osteoarthritis: efficacy under ultrasound guidance. Rheumatology 2010;49:1490–4.

26. Sofka CM, Collins AJ, Adler RS. Use of ultrasonographic guidance in interventional musculoskeletal procedures: a review from a single institution. J Ultrasound Med 2001;20:21–6.

27. Rowbotham E, Grainger A. Ultrasound-guided intervention around the hip joint. AJR Am J Roentgenol 2011;197:122–7.

28. Gilliland CA, Salazar LD, Borchers JR. Ultrasound versus anatomic guidance for intra-articular and periarticular injection: a systematic review. Phys Sportsmed 2011;39:121–31.

29. Chatha H, Ullah S, Cheema Z. Review article: magnetic resonance imaging and computed tomography in the diagnosis of occult proximal femur fractures. J Orthop Surg (Hong Kong) 2011;19:99–103.

30. Silvis M, Mosher T, Smetana B, et al. High prevalence of pelvic and hip magnetic resonance imaging findings in asymptomatic collegiate and professional hockey players. Am J Sports Med 2011;39:715–21.

31. Byrd JW, Jones KS. Diagnostic accuracy of clinical assessment, magnetic resonance imaging, magnetic resonance arthrography, and intra-articular injection in hip arthroscopy patients. Am J Sports Med 2004;32:1668–74.

32. Centers for Disease Control and Prevention (CDC). Prevalence of disabilities and associated health conditions among adults: United States, 1999. MMWR Morb Mortal Wkly Rep 2001;50:120–5.

33. Hootman J, Bolen J, Helmick C, et al. Prevalence of doctor-diagnosed arthritis and arthritis attributable activity limitation-United States, 2003-2005. MMWR Morb Mortal Wkly Rep 2006;55:1089–92.

34. Ganz R, Leunig M, Leunig-Ganz K, et al. The etiology of osteoarthritis of the hip: an integrated mechanical concept. Clin Orthop Relat Res 2008;466:264–72.

35. Gabay O, Hall D, Berenbaum F, et al. Osteoarthritis and obesity. Experimental models. Joint Bone Spine 2008;75:675–9.

36. Spector R, Harris P, Hart D, et al. Risk of osteoarthritis associated with long-term weight-bearing sports: a radiologic survey of the hips and knees in female ex-athletes and population controls. Arthritis Rheum 1996;39:988–95.

37. Cheng Y, Macera C, Davis D, et al. Physical activity and self-reported, physician-diagnosed osteoarthritis: is physical activity a risk factor. J Clin Epidemiol 2000;53:315–22.

38. Hochber M, Lethbridge-Cejku M, Tobin J. Bone mineral density and osteoarthritis: data from the Baltimore longitudinal study of aging. Osteoarthritis Cartilage 2004;12:S45–8.

39. Bos S, Slagboom P, Meulenbelt I. New Insights into osteoarthritis: early developmental features of an ageing-related disease. Curr Opin Rheumatol 2008;20:553–9.

40. Baldes A, Spector T. The contribution of genes to osteoarthritis. Rheum Dis Clin North Am 2008;34:581–603.

41. Hunter D, McDougall J, Keefe F. The symptoms of osteoarthritis and the genesis of pain. Rheum Dis Clin North Am 2008;34:623–43.

42. Steinert A, Nöth U, Tuan R. Concepts in gene therapy for cartilage repair. Injury 2008;39:97–113.

43. Uthman OA, van der Windt DA, Jordan JL, et al. Exercise for lower limb osteoarthritis: systematic review incorporating trial sequential analysis and network meta-analysis. BMJ 2013;347:5555.

44. Katz J, Losina E, Barrett J, et al. Association between hospital and surgeon procedure volume and outcomes of total hip replacement in the United States medicare population. J Bone Joint Surg Am 2001;83:1622–9.

45. Konrath F, Hamel A, Olson S, et al. The role of the acetabular labrum and the transverse acetabular ligament in load transmission in the hip. J Bone Joint Surg Am 1998;80:1781–8.

46. Ferguson S, Bryant J, Ganz R, et al. The acetabular labrum seal: poroelastic finite element model. Clin Biomech 2000;15:463–8.

47. Kim YT, Azuma H. The nerve endings of the acetabular labrum. Clin Orthop Relat Res 1995;(320):176–81.

48. Kelly BT, Shapiro GS, Digiovanni CW, et al. Vascularity of the hip labrum: a cadaveric investigation. Arthroscopy 2005;21:3–11.

49. Robertson WJ, Kadrmas WR, Kelly BT. Arthroscopic management of labral tears in the hip: a systematic review. Clin Orthop Relat Res 2006;455:88–92.

50. Toomayan GA, Holman WR, Major NM, et al. Sensitivity of MR arthrography in the evaluation of acetabular labral tears. AJR Am J Roentgenol 2006;186:449–53.

51. Freedman BA, Potter BK, Dinauer PA, et al. Prognostic value of magnetic resonance arthrography for Czerny stage II and III acetabular labral tears. Arthroscopy 2006;22:742–7.

52. McCarthy J, Noble P, Schuck M, et al. The watershed labral lesion: its relationship to early arthritis of the hip. J Arthroplasty 2001;16:81–7.
53. Farjo LA, Glick JM, Sampson TG. Hip arthroscopy for acetabular labrum tears. Arthroscopy 1999;15:132–7.
54. Santori N, Villar RN. Acetabular labral tears: results of arthroscopic partial limbectomy. Arthroscopy 2000;16:11–5.
55. Larson CM, Stone RM. Arthroscopic Management of Femoroacetabular Impingement. In: Wiesel S. Operative Techniques in Orthopaedic Surgery. Philadelphia: Lippincott Williams & Wilkins; 2011:1(26):213–21.
56. Tannast M, Siebenrock KA. Conventional radiographs to assess femoroacetabular impingement. Instr Course Lect 2009;58:203–12.
57. Beaulé PE, Hynes K, Parker G, et al. Can the alpha angle assessment of cam impingement predict acetabular cartilage delamination? Clin Orthop Relat Res 2012;470:3361–7.
58. Allen WC, Cope R. Coxa saltans: the snapping hip revisited. J Am Acad Orthop Surg 1995;3:303–8.
59. Baker CL, Massie V, Hurt WG, et al. Arthroscopic bursectomy for recalcitrant trochanteric bursitis. Arthroscopy 2007;23:827–32.
60. Byrd JW. Snapping hip. Oper Tech Sports Med 2005;13:46–54.
61. Ilizaliturri VM Jr, Villalobos FE Jr, Chaidez PA, et al. Endoscopic iliotibial band release for external snapping hip syndrome. Arthroscopy 2006;22:505–10.
62. Hölmich P. Long-standing groin pain in sportspeople falls into three primary patterns, a "clinical entity" approach: a prospective study of 207 patients. Br J Sports Med 2007;41:247–52.
63. Little TL, Mansoor J. Low back pain associated with internal snapping hip syndrome in a competitive cyclist. Br J Sports Med 2008;42:308–9.
64. Flanum ME, Keene JS, Blankenbaker DG, et al. Arthroscopic treatment of the painful "internal" snapping hip: results of a new endoscopic technique and imaging protocol. Am J Sports Med 2007;35:770–9.
65. Farber AJ, Wilckens JH. Sports hernia: diagnosis and therapeutic approach. J Am Acad Orthop Surg 2007;15:507–14.
66. Schilders E, Bismil Q, Robinson P, et al. Adductor-related groin pain in competitive athletes. J Bone Joint Surg Am 2007;89:2173–8.
67. Meyers WC, Foley DP, Garrett WE, et al. Management of severe lower abdominal or inguinal pain in high-performance athletes. Am J Sports Med 2000;28: 2–8.
68. Mattila VM, Niva M, Kiuru M, et al. Risk factors for bone stress injuries: a follow-up study of 102,515 person years. Med Sci Sports Exerc 2007;39:1061–6.
69. Niva MH, Kiuru MJ, Haataja R, et al. Fatigue injuries of the femur. J Bone Joint Surg Br 2005;87:1385–90.

Evaluation and Management of Adult Shoulder Pain
A Focus on Rotator Cuff Disorders, Acromioclavicular Joint Arthritis, and Glenohumeral Arthritis

April Armstrong, BSc(PT), MD, MSc, FRCSC

KEYWORDS

- Shoulder • Rotator cuff disorders • Rotator cuff tears
- Acromioclavicular joint arthritis • Glenohumeral joint arthritis • Examination
- Evaluation • Treatment

KEY POINTS

- Limited passive external rotation is a salient feature of glenohumeral joint arthritis but not for rotator cuff disease or acromioclavicular (AC) joint disease.
- Plain radiographs may show AC joint arthritis, but unless they are tender on palpation in this region, this is a clinically insignificant radiographic finding.
- Rotator cuff disease is best categorized into 3 different groups to help guide treatment. Group 1 and Group 3 are best treated nonoperatively, whereas group 2 should be given consideration for earlier surgical treatment.
- There are risks of nonoperative treatment of rotator cuff tears, which include tear progression, muscle fatty degeneration, tendon retraction increasing difficulty with tendon mobilization and repair, and potential for future arthritis.
- Initial treatment of most nontraumatic shoulder problems involves a physical therapy program, medication such as nonsteroidal antiinflammatory drugs, and joint injections. However, early surgical repair is considered for rotator cuff tears in a physiologically younger individual with an acute tear or who has a chronic rotator cuff tear with minimal irreversible changes on magnetic resonance imaging.

Disclosure: consultant for Zimmer, not related to this work.
Department of Orthopaedics and Rehabilitation, Bone and Joint Institute, Penn State Milton S. Hershey Medical Center, 30 Hope Drive, Building A, Hershey, PA 17033, USA
E-mail address: aarmstrong@hmc.psu.edu

Med Clin N Am 98 (2014) 755–775
http://dx.doi.org/10.1016/j.mcna.2014.03.004
0025-7125/14/$ – see front matter © 2014 Elsevier Inc. All rights reserved.

medical.theclinics.com

INTRODUCTION

Shoulder pain is a common reason for an office visit with a primary care physician, in some reports as high as 30% of referrals.[1–3] The focus of this article is on the evaluation and management of adult shoulder pain with a specific focus on rotator cuff disorders, acromioclavicular (AC) joint arthritis, and glenohumeral arthritis. Typically, these shoulder conditions are seen in individuals older than 40 years. Under extenuating circumstances, these entities may be seen in younger individuals, but there is usually a special circumstance, such as a history of trauma or previous surgery.

PATIENT HISTORY AND PHYSICAL EXAMINATION

Patients with a rotator cuff problem usually present with 1 of 2 typical histories. The first is a history of an abrupt onset of shoulder pain associated with a traumatic event, such as a fall on an outstretched arm or something as trivial as reaching above shoulder height and suddenly feeling a sharp pain. The patient may describe, "something tore in the shoulder." The second is a history of a gradual onset of aching shoulder pain that has not improved over time and the patient cannot recall any specific event or reason for the shoulder pain. Patients with shoulder arthritis, adhesive capsulitis, and AC joint arthritis tend to have more of a gradual onset of pain. Identifying aggravating and alleviating factors for the pain can also help to characterize the shoulder problem. Rotator cuff disease typically hurts more with elevation above the shoulder and is less painful at waist level. Adhesive capsulitis and arthritis tend to be painful with any shoulder motion. AC joint arthritis is often painful when reaching across the body (**Table 1**).

Often with rotator cuff disease, the patient describes the pain near the insertion of the deltoid in the lateral upper third of the arm rather than specifically at the shoulder. The patient may grab the whole side of the shoulder and describe pain in this region. The patient may describe the pain as less intense at rest during the day with worsening of their symptoms with movement of the shoulder, particularly with activities requiring reaching overhead, and at night, when they have fewer distractions for their pain. The pain experienced with adhesive capsulitis is intense, particularly at night, and also during the day, and is not relieved with rest, which differentiates it from a rotator cuff problem. Patients with glenohumeral arthritis or adhesive capsulitis are less specific about the location of the pain, but they focus usually on the fact that motion of the shoulder worsens their pain. Patients with AC joint arthritis are typically specific about the location of the pain and localize the pain right at the AC joint, on top of the shoulder. Patients may also show a positive cross-body test.[4] The examiner passively forward flexes the shoulder to 90° and horizontally adducts the arm as far as possible, which provokes the AC joint pain. Palpable pain localized over the AC joint is common. An injection of local anesthetic and corticosteroid into the AC joint can confirm whether this joint is a significant reason for their pain if it relieves the pain they are experiencing.

Table 1
Distinguishing features of pain

	Distinguishing Features of Pain	
	Onset	Aggravating Factors
Rotator cuff disease	Sudden or gradual	Overhead elevation
AC joint arthritis	Gradual	Reaching across the body
Glenohumeral arthritis	Gradual	Any shoulder motion

Often, the injection takes away 90% of their pain and confirms the diagnosis. It is not uncommon for AC joint arthritic changes to be seen on plain radiographs, but this is frequently an incidental finding. Unless the patient is symptomatic in this region on examination, this radiographic finding is not clinically significant. Pain related to the shoulder does not usually refer below the elbow; if you see this pattern, you must distinguish this from referred pain from the cervical spine.

The physical examination of the shoulder focuses on observation, palpation, range of motion, and strength testing (**Table 2**). Examination of the shoulder requires that the shoulder be exposed for observation of the entire shoulder, allowing for comparison with the opposite shoulder. Health care providers need to look for asymmetries and any evidence of atrophy of the rotator cuff musculature. Typically, this condition is most evident when looking at the infraspinatus, because chronic atrophic changes of this muscle belly are easy to identify, with prominence of the scapular spine and a scalloped appearance of the infraspinatus fossa. Atrophic changes of the supraspinatus may not be so readily appreciated, because the trapezius muscle lies above this muscle belly and can hide these changes. One should observe for other atrophic changes, such as with the deltoid, which would suggest possibly a neurologic reason, axillary neuropathy, for the shoulder problem.

It is important to observe the patient's willingness to move the shoulder and to assess the flow of movement of the shoulder, which allows you to assess their degree of pain, active weakness, and also the scapulohumeral rhythm.[5] If there is significant scapular winging, you need to distinguish this from a neurologic reason versus a scapular dyskinesis from poor mechanics.[6] Range of motion testing includes forward elevation, external rotation at their side, and internal rotation behind their back, both with active (patient uses their own muscle to generate the movement) and passive (motion generated by someone else moving the extremity and patient does not use their own muscles) motion. In patients with isolated rotator cuff disease, shoulder motion is not limited passively but may be limited actively. If active and passive motion is limited, diagnoses such as adhesive capsulitis and glenohumeral arthritis should be higher on the differential. Loss of passive motion in 3 planes of motion such as forward elevation, external rotation, and internal rotation suggests an articular problem or joint contracture. Loss of passive external rotation at the side is one of the first classic findings for glenohumeral arthritis and adhesive capsulitis. Some patients with massive rotator cuff tears develop glenohumeral joint arthritis, and once this develops, the

Table 2
Distinguishing features on physical examination

| | Distinguishing Features on Physical Examination | | | |
	Range of Motion	Strength of Rotator Cuff	Palpation	Special Tests
Rotator cuff disease	Full passive Full or limited active	Weakness	Occasionally, pain at greater tuberosity	Neer and Hawkins impingement tests
AC joint arthritis	Full passive Full active	No weakness	Localized pain at AC joint	Cross-body test
Glenohumeral Arthritis	Limited passive Limited active Limited external rotation salient feature	No weakness	No localized pain	None

treatment typically becomes focused on managing the arthritis and not the rotator cuff tear.

The Neer and Hawkins impingement tests may be used to identify rotator cuff irritability.[7] However, there is significant clinical diversity regarding the usefulness of these tests, and it is difficult to assess the relative sensitivity and specificity of shoulder diagnostic tests.[8,9] Therefore, the clinician should consider the components of the history and physical examination as adjunctive tools to gain more insight into the clinical picture of the problem. The Neer impingement sign passively elevates the shoulder above the patient's head, and stabilizes the scapula superiorly, to impinge the rotator cuff under the acromion (**Fig. 1**). The Hawkins impingement sign forward elevates the shoulder to 90° in neutral rotation and then internally rotates the shoulder, stabilizing the scapula, to impinge the rotator cuff under the acromion (**Fig. 2**).

When observing the patient reach behind the back, it is also important to watch for scapular winging, which suggests that the observed motion is occurring at the scapulothoracic joint rather than the glenohumeral joint. If scapular winging or loss of internal rotation motion is recognized, it is important to assess further for posterior shoulder capsular tightness.[10] The sleeper stretch is an effective way to assess for this posterior capsular tightness, because the patient lying on their side limits the scapulothoracic joint contribution to the motion (**Fig. 3**).[11] The patient lies on their side with the dependent arm flexed to 90°. The patient then pushes on the wrist of the dependent arm into internal rotation toward the bed, with the opposite arm, to show restricted internal rotation range of motion. This limited motion can be identified with rotator cuff disease, AC joint arthritis, and glenohumeral joint arthritis. The difference is found when using this stretch as a treatment. Patients with rotator cuff disease and AC joint arthritis are more likely to stretch and improve their posterior capsule tightness and thus improve their pain symptoms, whereas in patients with glenohumeral arthritis, this tightness is likely permanent.

Strength testing is important for any shoulder examination, but especially for patients with suspected rotator cuff tears. The rotator cuff is made up of 4 distinct tendons: (1) supraspinatus, (2) infraspinatus, (3) subscapularis, and (4) teres minor. Each of these tendons can be specifically tested for strength and integrity. The supraspinatus tendon is evaluated using the Jobe test (**Fig. 4**). The patient is asked to elevate their arm in the plane of the scapula on the chest wall until they are just short of 90° of forward elevation. They are then asked to turn their thumb down toward the floor to theoretically bring the supraspinatus tendon on top of the shoulder joint, and the examiner

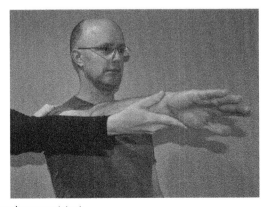

Fig. 1. The Neer impingement test.

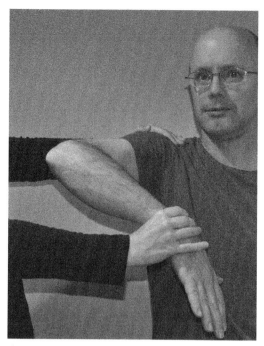

Fig. 2. The Hawkins impingement test.

then tries to push their arm to the floor, comparing at the same time with the opposite shoulder. Weakness or giving way could suggest a rotator cuff weakness involving the supraspinatus. More recently, a modified lateral Jobe test has been reported as effective in diagnosing supraspinatus tears.[12] Instead of the patient's arm held straight, the arm is bent 90° at the elbow. Infraspinatus weakness is tested with the arm at their side, elbow flexed to 90°, and neutral shoulder rotation, with their forearm pointing directly forward (**Fig. 5**). The examiner then attempts to rotate the arm internally while the patient resists with external rotation strength. This test has been described as one of the more effective tests to detect a rotator cuff tear.[13] A positive external lag test is

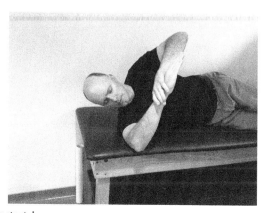

Fig. 3. The sleeper stretch.

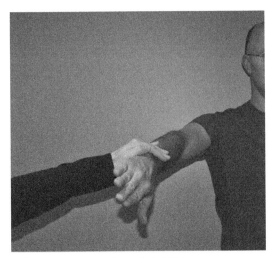

Fig. 4. The Jobe test for supraspinatus strength testing.

one in which a patient is positioned in full external rotation at their side and is unable to hold this position because of significant external rotation weakness.[14] A positive external lag test suggests a large tear of the rotator cuff, and associated atrophy of the infraspinatus muscle belly on observation supports this finding. Subscapularis function is assessed using the belly press test (**Fig. 6**) or the liftoff test (**Fig. 7**).[15,16] The belly press test requires that the patient place both hands on their belly with neutral wrist alignment, and the patient is asked to bring their elbows forward to simulate internal rotation of the shoulder. Weakness is detected when the elbow lags behind and the patient cannot bring it forward. This test is useful for patients who are in too much pain to reach behind their back. The liftoff test requires that the patient reach behind their low back and then lift their hand off their back. This test requires patient to have enough internal rotation to perform the movement. The health care provider must ensure that the patient is truly activating the subscapularis and not the triceps muscle, which extends the elbow rather than lifting the arm off the low back. The

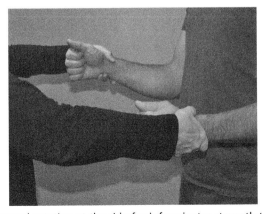

Fig. 5. Resisted external rotation at the side for infraspinatus strength testing.

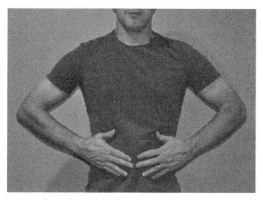

Fig. 6. The belly press test for subscapularis strength testing.

last tendon to assess is the teres minor, and this is typically not involved unless there is a massive rotator cuff tear or an axillary nerve palsy. The hornblower test was described to test this muscle belly (**Fig. 8**).[17] The teres minor is most active when the shoulder is externally rotated in the abducted position, so the patient is asked to bring their arm overhead, with the shoulder abducted to 90° and elbow flexed to 90°. The patient is then asked to rotate their arm from 90° of shoulder elevation to full external rotation like a hitch-hiking motion. Inability of the arm to perform this movement results in the arm dropping to the face and overactivity of the deltoid muscle with increased abduction of the shoulder, looking like you are blowing on a horn, or the hornblower sign (**Fig. 9**). Patients with glenohumeral arthritis, adhesive capsulitis, and AC joint arthritis do not show significant rotator cuff weakness. However, if they are in too much pain, this may inhibit their ability to generate a forceful contraction and good strength on their examination.

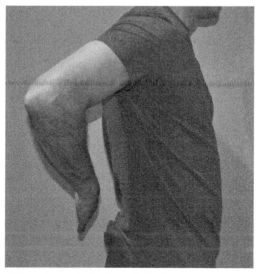

Fig. 7. The liftoff test for subscapularis strength testing.

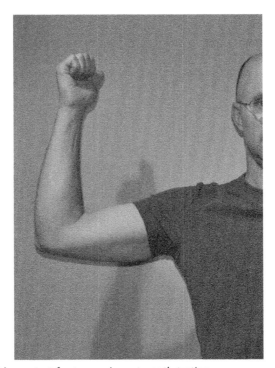

Fig. 8. The hornblower test for teres minor strength testing.

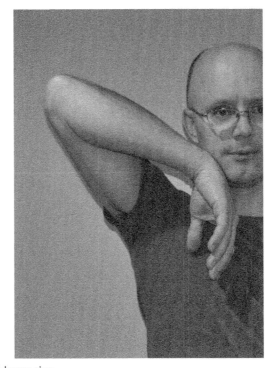

Fig. 9. The hornblower sign.

IMAGING

A standard anteroposterior (AP), true AP, outlet, and axillary shoulder radiographic series is recommended (**Fig. 10**). In patients with rotator cuff disorders, the radiographs are often normal (see **Fig. 10**). There may be some spurring of the anterior or lateral acromion and possibly a traction osteophyte at the location of the coracoacromial ligament traveling medially to the coracoid. It is controversial whether these spurs should be dealt with surgically, with more recent literature supporting isolated bursectomies and not resecting these bony prominences.[18] In patients with large to massive rotator cuff tears, superior migration of the humeral head and possibly arthritic signs may be observed (**Fig. 11**). The standard AP film is most useful for visualizing the AC joint in profile and better identifies joint space narrowing, osteophytosis, sclerosis, or cystic formation (**Fig. 12**). However, these radiographic findings are not uncommon in patients with no pain related to the AC joint, and so you must be careful to not overdiagnose this condition. The true AP and axillary images show the glenohumeral joint in

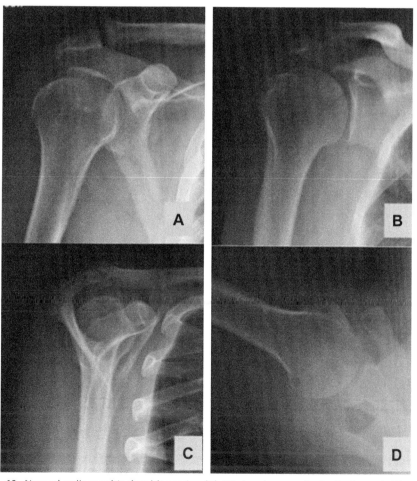

Fig. 10. Normal radiographic shoulder series. (*A*) AP view (perpendicular to thorax), (*B*) true AP view (perpendicular to glenohumeral joint), (*C*) outlet view, and (*D*) axillary view.

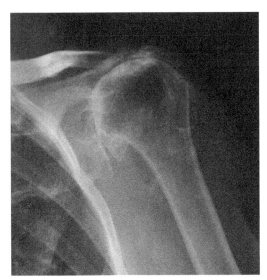

Fig. 11. True AP image of left shoulder of a patient with a chronic rotator cuff tear and superior migration of the humeral head and resultant arthritis of the glenohumeral joint.

profile and help to show joint space narrowing and arthritic changes associated with glenohumeral arthritis (**Fig. 13**). These images are important for distinguishing between shoulder arthritis and adhesive capsulitis. In patients with adhesive capsulitis, the radiographs are normal, with no evidence of arthritis.

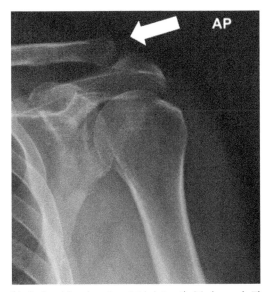

Fig. 12. AP image of left shoulder showing AC joint arthritis (*arrow*). There is narrowing of the joint space, sclerosis, and osteophyte formation.

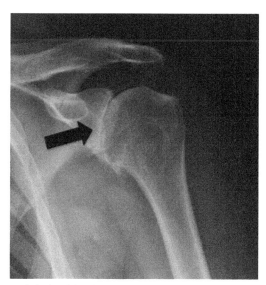

Fig. 13. True AP image left shoulder showing advanced glenohumeral joint arthritis. The *arrow* is pointing to the glenohumeral joint, which shows significant joint space narrowing, sclerosis, cystic formation, and osteophyte formation.

MANAGEMENT OF ROTATOR CUFF DISORDERS

When deciding on management of rotator cuff disorders, it is helpful to divide the patients into one of 3 groups to help guide treatment.[19] Both nonoperative and operative of treatment of rotator cuff disorders have risks (**Tables 3** and **4**). These groupings take into consideration the natural history of full and partial thickness rotator cuff tears, the reparability of the tendon tear, and the potential for healing of rotator cuff tears. The surgical risks of treatment are readily easy to understand; however, the nonoperative risks of treating rotator cuff disease may be less obvious. These nonoperative risks include tear progression, muscle fatty degeneration, tendon retraction increasing difficulty with tendon mobilization and repair, and potential for future arthritis (**Fig. 14**). Tear progression has been reported in several studies when following the natural history of asymptomatic and symptomatic rotator cuff tears.[20–25] Increased tear size and poorer muscle quality have been associated with worse surgical outcomes, and therefore, earlier consideration for surgical repair is warranted in some cases.

Table 3 Risks of treatment		
	Risks of Treatment	
Nonoperative	Tear progression Muscle fatty degeneration Tendon retraction increasing difficulty with tendon mobilization and repair Potential for future arthritis	
Operative	Anesthetic complications Infection Nerve injury Arterial injury Failure of tendon to heal	

Table 4
Three groups of rotator cuff disease

	Defining Features	Risk of Nonoperative Treatment
Group 1	Rotator cuff tendonitis, impingement, or bursitis, partial thickness tear, or maybe a small (<1 cm) full thickness rotator cuff tear	Minimal
Group 2	<65 y old (or older individuals who act physiologically younger) with a chronic full thickness rotator cuff tear (except maybe <1 cm tear), an acute full thickness rotator cuff tear (except maybe <1 cm tear), or an acute or chronic rotator cuff tear with a significant change in functional status of the arm, or >40 y old with an acute shoulder dislocation and an acute rotator cuff tear	High
Group 3	>65–70 y old or physiologically older with a chronic full thickness rotator cuff tear or individuals of any age with a massive irreparable tear with significant retraction, fatty degeneration, and humeral head superior migration, and early articular arthritic change	Minimal

The first group (group 1) of patients refers to patients who have an examination consistent with a rotator cuff tendonitis, impingement, or bursitis, partial thickness tear, or it may be a small (<1 cm) full thickness rotator cuff tear. There is minimal risk to this patient group with nonoperative treatment. The likelihood that they will develop chronic irreversible rotator cuff change, such as tendon retraction, fatty degeneration, and glenohumeral arthritis, is small. Nonoperative treatment in patients with rotator cuff tendonitis, impingement, or bursitis has a high success rate.[26–28] In 1 randomized prospective control study,[29] there was no significant difference between

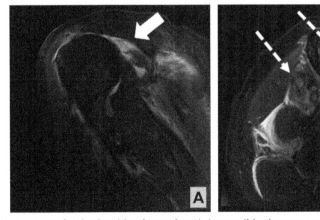

Fig. 14. MRI of right shoulder shows chronic irreversible changes to the rotator cuff. (*A*) Coronal image shows significant retraction of the rotator cuff tendon to the glenoid margin (*solid white arrow*) and superior migration of the humeral head. (*B*) Sagittal image shows significant fatty infiltration and atrophy of the supraspinatus and infraspinatus (*dotted white arrows*).

supervised physical therapy treatment and surgical treatment of arthroscopic subacromial decompression. With respect to partial thickness rotator cuff tears, there has been shown to be a slow, small risk for tear progression.[20,25] However, bursal sided partial thickness tears may not be so responsive to physical therapy treatment compared with articular partial thickness rotator cuff tears and may lead to earlier surgical intervention.[30,31] More recently, there has been some evidence that acute or chronic small (<1–1.5 cm) rotator cuff tears have a small risk of tear progression.[22] However, yearly monitoring, by the primary care provider or orthopedic surgeon, for tear progression and increased symptoms is recommended for younger individuals, who are at higher risk for irreversible changes if the tear increases in size. Nonoperative treatment options include physical therapy, antiinflammatory medications, and subacromial local and corticosteroid injections. Magnetic resonance imaging (MRI) is not indicated in this patient group.

The mainstay of treatment is physical therapy and the rehabilitation goals are to improve function for the patient and decrease pain. Patient education regarding activity modification as an effective initial treatment is important. The patient should be counseled to avoid or reduce any repetitive overhead activity or heavy lifting with the arm. Once the pain and function are improved, these aggravating activities may be reintroduced. The therapy program usually focuses on reestablishing normal range of motion, shown through normal glenohumeral and scapulohumeral kinematics. As mentioned earlier, often these patients have a tight posterior capsule, and therefore, physical therapy treatment often includes specific stretching for the posterior capsule. Strengthening exercises are gradually introduced when normal kinematics are established. Therapeutic modalities such as ultrasonography may also be included. A recent study analyzed the nonsurgical modifiable factors that contributed to pain and dysfunction in patients with symptomatic rotator cuff tears.[32] These investigators determined that scapulothoracic dyskinesis, range of motion in active abduction and forward elevation, and strength in abduction and forward elevation contributed significantly to pain or poor function.[32] They postulated that focused physical therapy treatment of these factors may provide better pain control in patients with symptomatic rotator cuff tears. Medications such as nonsteroidal antiinflammatory drugs (NSAIDs), acetaminophen, and possibly, a short-term opiate medication may be necessary to help control pain. Adequate pain control is important for the patient to be compliant with the physical therapy program.

If the patient has a poor response to the therapy and medications, a subacromial corticosteroid injection may be used as an adjunct to the treatment program. Subacromial injections can be approached from an anterior, lateral, or posterior approach. I prefer the posterior approach, with the patient sitting. The posterolateral corner of the acromion and the site of injection is typically 1 cm medial and 2 cm distal to the posterolateral corner of the acromion to avoid hitting the acromion (**Fig. 15**). The patient is asked to rest their forearm comfortably on their lap to relax the deltoid. I mix the lidocaine and corticosteroid in the same syringe for 1 injection. You must make sure that the needle is deep enough and penetrates the subacromial space to avoid complications of skin depigmentation and subcutaneous atrophy. The use of subacromial injections is controversial. A systematic review[33] concluded that there was little evidence to support the use of corticosteroid injections in managing rotator cuff disease; however, the available literature to make this conclusion was suboptimal. There was evidence that subacromial injections may help, particularly in the short-term, to improve range of motion and pain, but not in the long-term.[34–37] The decision to inject a patient should be individualized to the patient's circumstances. Injections are helpful for patients with calcific tendonitis, for patients who are acutely painful and unable to

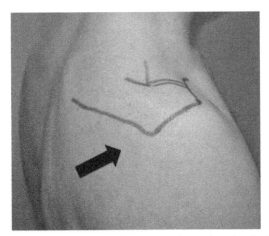

Fig. 15. Posterior approach to subacromial injection. The patient is asked to rest their forearm comfortably on their lap to relax the deltoid. The posterolateral corner of the acromion is identified, and the site of injection is typically 1 cm medial and 2 cm distal to the posterolateral corner of the acromion to avoid hitting the acromion (*arrow*).

participate in physical therapy, or for patients who have reached a plateau with the therapy program and are having difficulty progressing. The injections should be used sparingly, because there is evidence that corticosteroids can weaken the tendons and cause histologic changes.[38,39] It is recommended to wait at least 4 months between injections. If pain persists after 1 or 2 injections and physical therapy treatment has been optimized, advanced imaging, such as MRI, to better define the soft tissue disease, should be considered.

The second group (group 2) refers to patients younger than 65 years (or older individuals who act physiologically younger) who present with a chronic full thickness rotator cuff tear (except maybe <1 cm tear), an acute full thickness rotator cuff tear (except maybe <1 cm tear), or an acute or chronic rotator cuff tear with a significant change in their functional status of the arm (**Fig. 16**). This group includes the patient older than 40 years who had an acute shoulder dislocation and is therefore at a higher risk for an acute rotator cuff tear. Early surgical repair should be considered for this group of patients without significant muscle deterioration secondary to risk for chronic irreversible rotator cuff changes.[40–44] There is a high risk for tear progression, including fatty changes of the rotator cuff muscle and tendon retraction, with nonoperative treatment. Patients with a symptomatic rotator cuff tear have a 50% risk of tear progression in 2 years and tear progression, which correlates with increasing symptoms.[20,21,25] Patients presenting with a symptomatic rotator cuff tear have a 35% risk of contralateral rotator cuff tear, and this increases to 50% risk if age is greater than 80 years.[23] It is recommended that this patient group obtain MRI and a referral to a specialist for consideration of surgical repair of the rotator cuff.

The surgical literature also supports that group 2 has a higher rate of healing of the rotator cuff with surgery.[45–48] Surgical treatment options include arthroscopic and mini-open rotator cuff repair. An arthroscopic approach requires the surgeon to make approximately 3 to 6 small (<1 cm), incisions to repair the rotator cuff while watching a video camera and working through the small incisions. The mini-open approach requires an open incision through the deltoid muscle to repair the rotator cuff.

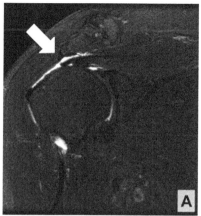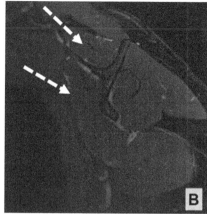

Fig. 16. MRI of right shoulder shows rotator cuff without significant chronic changes. (*A*) Coronal image shows retraction of the rotator cuff tendon half the width of the humeral head (*solid white arrow*) and no superior migration of the humeral head. (*B*) Sagittal image shows no significant fatty infiltration of the supraspinatus or infraspinatus (*dotted white arrows*).

The third group (group 3) refers to individuals who are older than 65 to 70 years or physiologically older with a chronic full thickness rotator cuff tear or individuals of any age with a massive irreparable tear, with significant retraction, fatty degeneration, and humeral head superior migration and early articular arthritic change. These individuals have a limited capacity for rotator cuff healing after repair, and therefore, nonoperative treatment should be optimized, with little risk to the patient, because the irreversible changes are already present (see **Fig. 14**). MRI is not needed for this patient group initially, because the diagnosis is clearly delineated with the physical examination. If nonoperative treatment is not successful, it may be reasonable to consider surgical intervention and referral to a specialist but to also understand that the goals and outcomes may be limited. Taking medical cost accountability into mind, it is recommended that the specialist decide whether the patient needs MRI, because the decision to operate may be easily determined by the physical examination and plain films and may be an unnecessary cost if no surgical intervention is feasible.

MANAGEMENT OF AC JOINT ARTHRITIS

The treatment options for AC joint arthritis are similar to those for rotator cuff disorders. Activity modification, physical therapy, medication, and joint injection are the typical nonoperative options for treatment. The corticosteroid injection has 2 purposes: confirming the diagnosis and therapeutic treatment of the pain. AC joint injections are technically more difficult, because the space is narrow because it is a small joint (**Fig. 17**). The AC joint is identified by palpation and feeling the defect between the distal end of the clavicle and the acromion. Looking at the plain radiographs can also provide an idea of the orientation of the joint, because this can vary between individuals. Once the soft spot of the AC joint is identified, the local anesthetic is injected into the joint to confirm that the joint has been localized. The needle is then kept in place, and the syringe is exchanged with a syringe filled with no more than 1 mL of corticosteroid and exchanged again with local anesthetic to flush the corticosteroid into the joint. The AC joint is superficial and care should be taken to minimize the risk of skin depigmentation and subcutaneous fat atrophy.

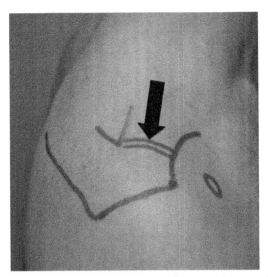

Fig. 17. AC joint injection. First localize the AC joint by palpation and feel the defect between the distal end of the clavicle and the acromion. Localize the soft spot and inject using a superior approach to the AC joint (*arrow*).

The nonoperative options are not so effective at permanently controlling the patient's pain, and these patients are more likely to require surgery. The surgical options for treatment include open and arthroscopic techniques for distal clavicle resection. The open technique requires a superior vertical or horizontal incision over the AC joint and division of the deep deltotrapezial fascia to elevate the muscle to expose the distal clavicle.[49] The distal 1 cm of the clavicle is excised, and meticulous closure of the deltotrapezial muscle and fascia is necessary. Careful postoperative follow-up is required to monitor for healing of the reattached deltoid and trapezius. Localized dehiscence of this soft tissue coverage can lead to ongoing persistent pain and weakness. Two arthroscopic techniques have been described: (1) direct and (2) indirect. The direct technique[50] uses 2 small incisions superiorly, anterior, and posterior to the joint to introduce instruments to resect the distal end of the clavicle. The indirect technique[51,52] uses a bursal approach in combination with an acromioplasty. The distal end of the clavicle is identified from the bursal surface and resected arthroscopically. The technique has the advantage of preserving the superficial AC ligaments and deltotrapezial musculature.

MANAGEMENT OF GLENOHUMERAL JOINT ARTHRITIS

The nonoperative treatment options include activity modification, physical therapy, medication, and intra-articular joint injection. Physical therapy may not be so effective for patients with advanced disease, because more activity and motion may aggravate their symptoms. Antiinflammatory medications are typically prescribed, whereas narcotic medications are usually avoided. Intra-articular injections can be effective in controlling arthritic symptoms. I prefer an anterior approach through the rotator interval, which is a natural space between the supraspinatus and the subscapularis (**Fig. 18**). The coracoid is marked out, and the injection is typically aimed just lateral to the coracoid, approximately 1 to 2 cm inferior to the clavicle. The local anesthetic is first injected to confirm the location. Leaving the needle in place, the syringe is exchanged and corticosteroid injected, followed by exchanging the syringe yet again

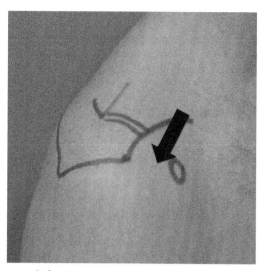

Fig. 18. Anterior approach for intra-articular joint injections. The coracoid is marked out and the injection is typically aimed just lateral to the coracoid, approximately 1 to 2 cm inferior to the clavicle. The injection is aimed to penetrate the joint through the rotator interval (*arrow*). First, local anesthetic is injected to confirm intra-articular location of the needle, and then leaving the needle in place, the syringe is exchanged and corticosteroid is injected. The syringe is exchanged yet again for local anesthetic to flush the steroid into the joint.

for local anesthetic to flush the steroid into the joint. When nonsurgical treatment fails and the pain is affecting the patient's quality of life, surgical intervention may be considered. For more advanced disease, the surgical treatment of choice is an anatomic total shoulder arthroplasty, with excellent results reported (**Fig. 19**).[53,54] In younger patients less than 40 years old, arthroscopic capsular release and extensive debridement may be considered, with guarded results.[55]

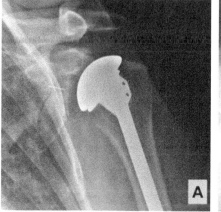
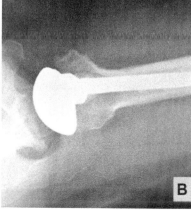

Fig. 19. Anatomic total shoulder arthroplasty for shoulder arthritis. (*A*) True AP view. (*B*) Axillary view.

SUMMARY

Rotator cuff disorders, AC joint arthritis, and glenohumeral joint arthritis each have their salient features during the history and physical examination. For instance, weakness during muscle strength testing is typical for rotator cuff disorders, localized pain over the AC joint for AC joint arthritis, and loss of passive external rotation with glenohumeral joint arthritis. Understanding these patterns can help to quickly guide the clinician to the appropriate treatment plan. In most instances, initial treatment may be focused on a nonoperative program, including physical therapy, medications such as NSAIDS, and joint injections. Surgical intervention is considered when nonsurgical treatment fails or in the second subgroup of rotator cuff disease, when nonsurgical treatment has a higher risk of causing further harm. This group of patients is typically the physiologically younger individuals who have an acute tear or who have a chronic rotator cuff tear with minimal irreversible changes on MRI. In this patient group, continued nonoperative treatment puts them at risk of rotator cuff tear progression, muscle fatty degeneration, tendon retraction increasing difficulty with tendon mobilization and repair, and potential for future arthritis.

REFERENCES

1. Greving K, Dorrestijn O, Winters JC, et al. Incidence, prevalence, and consultation rates of shoulder complaints in general practice. Scand J Rheumatol 2012; 41(2):150–5.
2. Armed Forces Health Surveillance Center (AFHSC). Arm and shoulder conditions, active component, US Armed Forces, 2003-2012. MSMR 2013;20(6):18–22.
3. Bruls VE, Bastiaenen CH, de Bie RA. Non-traumatic arm, neck and shoulder complaints: prevalence, course and prognosis in a Dutch university population. BMC Musculoskelet Disord 2013;14:8.
4. Buchberger DJ. Introduction of a new physical examination procedure for the differentiation of acromioclavicular joint lesions and subacromial impingement. J Manipulative Physiol Ther 1999;22(5):316–21.
5. Giphart JE, Brunkhorst JP, Horn NH, et al. Effect of plane of arm elevation on glenohumeral kinematics: a normative biplane fluoroscopy study. J Bone Joint Surg Am 2013;95(3):238–45.
6. Kibler WB, Sciascia A, Wilkes T. Scapular dyskinesis and its relation to shoulder injury. J Am Acad Orthop Surg 2012;20(6):364–72.
7. MacDonald PB, Clark P, Sutherland K. An analysis of the diagnostic accuracy of the Hawkins and Neer subacromial impingement signs. J Shoulder Elbow Surg 2000;9(4):299–301.
8. Hanchard NC, Lenza M, Handoll HH, et al. Physical tests for shoulder impingements and local lesions of bursa, tendon or labrum that may accompany impingement. Cochrane Database Syst Rev 2013;(4):CD007427.
9. Hegedus EJ, Goode AP, Cook CE, et al. Which physical examination tests provide clinicians with the most value when examining the shoulder? Update of a systematic review with meta-analysis of individual tests. Br J Sports Med 2012;46(14):964–78.
10. Myers JB, Laudner KG, Pasquale MR, et al. Glenohumeral range of motion deficits and posterior shoulder tightness in throwers with pathologic internal impingement. Am J Sports Med 2006;34(3):385–91.
11. Maenhout A, Van Eessel V, Van Dyck L, et al. Quantifying acromiohumeral distance in overhead athletes with glenohumeral internal rotation loss and the influence of a stretching program. Am J Sports Med 2012;40(9):2105–12.

12. Gillooly JJ, Chidambaram R, Mok D. The lateral Jobe test: a more reliable method of diagnosing rotator cuff tears. Int J Shoulder Surg 2010;4(2):41–3.
13. Hermans J, Luime JJ, Meuffels DE, et al. Does this patient with shoulder pain have rotator cuff disease?: The rational clinical examination systematic review. JAMA 2013;310(8):837–47.
14. Hurschler C, Wülker N, Windhagen H, et al. Evaluation of the lag sign tests for external rotator function of the shoulder. J Shoulder Elbow Surg 2004;13(3): 298–304.
15. Yoon JP, Chung SW, Kim SH, et al. Diagnostic value of four clinical tests for the evaluation of subscapularis integrity. J Shoulder Elbow Surg 2013;22(9):1186–92.
16. Scheibel M, Magosch P, Pritsch M, et al. The belly-off sign: a new clinical diagnostic sign for subscapularis lesions. Arthroscopy 2005;21(10):1229–35.
17. Walch G, Boulahia A, Calderone S, et al. The 'dropping' and 'hornblower's' signs in evaluation of rotator-cuff tears. J Bone Joint Surg Br 1998;80(4):624–8.
18. Chahal J, Mall N, MacDonald PB, et al. The role of subacromial decompression in patients undergoing arthroscopic repair of full-thickness tears of the rotator cuff: a systematic review and meta-analysis. Arthroscopy 2012;28(5):720–7.
19. Lashgari CJ, Yamaguchi K. Natural history and nonsurgical treatment of rotator cuff disorders. In: Norris TR, editor. Orthopaedic knowledge update: shoulder and elbow 2. Rosemont (IL): American Academy of Orthopaedic Surgeons; 2002. p. 155–62.
20. Maman E, Harris C, White L, et al. Outcome of nonoperative treatment of symptomatic rotator cuff tears monitored by magnetic resonance imaging. J Bone Joint Surg Am 2009;91(8):1898–906.
21. Safran O, Schroeder J, Bloom R, et al. Natural history of nonoperatively treated symptomatic rotator cuff tears in patients 60 years old or younger. Am J Sports Med 2011;39(4):710–4.
22. Fucentese SF, von Roll AL, Pfirrmann CW, et al. Evolution of nonoperatively treated symptomatic isolated full-thickness supraspinatus tears. J Bone Joint Surg Am 2012;94(9):801–8.
23. Yamaguchi K, Ditsios K, Middleton WD, et al. The demographic and morphological features of rotator cuff disease. A comparison of asymptomatic and symptomatic shoulders. J Bone Joint Surg Am 2006;88(8):1699–704.
24. Moosmayer S, Tariq R, Stiris M, et al. The natural history of asymptomatic rotator cuff tears: a three-year follow-up of fifty cases. J Bone Joint Surg Am 2013; 95(14):1249–55.
25. Mall NA, Kim HM, Keener JD, et al. Symptomatic progression of asymptomatic rotator cuff tears: a prospective study of clinical and sonographic variables. J Bone Joint Surg Am 2010;92(16):2623–33.
26. Tashjian RZ. Is there evidence in favor of surgical interventions for the subacromial impingement syndrome? Clin J Sport Med 2013;23(5):406–7.
27. Morrison DS, Frogameni AD, Woodworth P. Non-operative treatment of subacromial impingement syndrome. J Bone Joint Surg Am 1997;79(5):732–7.
28. Brox JI, Gjengedal E, Uppheim G, et al. Arthroscopic surgery versus supervised exercises in patients with rotator cuff disease (stage II impingement syndrome): a prospective, randomized, controlled study in 125 patients with a 2 1/2-year follow-up. J Shoulder Elbow Surg 1999;8(2):102–11.
29. Haahr JP, Østergaard S, Dalsgaard J, et al. Exercises versus arthroscopic decompression in patients with subacromial impingement: a randomised, controlled study in 90 cases with a one year follow up. Ann Rheum Dis 2005; 64(5):760–4.

30. Fukuda H, Hamada K, Nakajima T, et al. Partial-thickness tears of the rotator cuff. A clinicopathological review based on 66 surgically verified cases. Int Orthop 1996;20(4):257–65.
31. Cordasco FA, Backer M, Craig EV, et al. The partial-thickness rotator cuff tear: is acromioplasty without repair sufficient? Am J Sports Med 2002;30(2):257–60.
32. Harris JD, Pedroza A, Jones GL, et al. Predictors of pain and function in patients with symptomatic, atraumatic full-thickness rotator cuff tears: a time-zero analysis of a prospective patient cohort enrolled in a structured physical therapy program. Am J Sports Med 2012;40(2):359–66.
33. Koester MC, Dunn WR, Kuhn JE, et al. The efficacy of subacromial corticosteroid injection in the treatment of rotator cuff disease: a systematic review. J Am Acad Orthop Surg 2007;15(1):3–11.
34. Alvarez CM, Litchfield R, Jackowski D, et al. A prospective, double-blind, randomized clinical trial comparing subacromial injection of betamethasone and xylocaine to xylocaine alone in chronic rotator cuff tendinosis. Am J Sports Med 2005;33(2):255–62.
35. Adebajo AO, Nash P, Hazleman BL. A prospective double blind dummy placebo controlled study comparing triamcinolone hexacetonide injection with oral diclofenac 50 mg TDS in patients with rotator cuff tendinitis. J Rheumatol 1990;17(9):1207–10.
36. Petri M, Dobrow R, Neiman R, et al. Randomized, double-blind, placebo-controlled study of the treatment of the painful shoulder. Arthritis Rheum 1987; 30(9):1040–5.
37. Blair B, Rokito AS, Cuomo F, et al. Efficacy of injections of corticosteroids for subacromial impingement syndrome. J Bone Joint Surg Am 1996;78(11): 1685–9.
38. McWhorter JW, Francis RS, Heckmann RA. Influence of local steroid injections on traumatized tendon properties. A biomechanical and histological study. Am J Sports Med 1991;19(5):435–9.
39. Tillander B, Franzén LE, Karlsson MH, et al. Effect of steroid injections on the rotator cuff: an experimental study in rats. J Shoulder Elbow Surg 1999;8(3):271–4.
40. Mantone JK, Burkhead WZ Jr, Noonan J Jr. Nonoperative treatment of rotator cuff tears. Orthop Clin North Am 2000;31(2):295–311.
41. Wirth MA, Basamania C, Rockwood CA Jr. Nonoperative management of full-thickness tears of the rotator cuff. Orthop Clin North Am 1997;28(1):59–67.
42. Bassett RW, Cofield RH. Acute tears of the rotator cuff. The timing of surgical repair. Clin Orthop Relat Res 1983;(175):18–24.
43. Petersen SA, Murphy TP. The timing of rotator cuff repair for the restoration of function. J Shoulder Elbow Surg 2011;20(1):62–8.
44. Sugihara T, Nakagawa T, Tsuchiya M, et al. Prediction of primary reparability of massive tears of the rotator cuff on preoperative magnetic resonance imaging. J Shoulder Elbow Surg 2003;12(3):222–5.
45. Boileau P, Brassart N, Watkinson DJ, et al. Arthroscopic repair of full-thickness tears of the supraspinatus: does the tendon really heal? J Bone Joint Surg Am 2005;87(6):1229–40.
46. Goutallier D, Postel JM, Gleyze P, et al. Influence of cuff muscle fatty degeneration on anatomic and functional outcomes after simple suture of full-thickness tears. J Shoulder Elbow Surg 2003;12(6):550–4.
47. Gulotta LV, Nho SJ, Dodson CC, et al. Prospective evaluation of arthroscopic rotator cuff repairs at 5 years: part I–functional outcomes and radiographic healing rates. J Shoulder Elbow Surg 2011;20(6):934–40.

48. Cho NS, Lee BG, Rhee YG. Arthroscopic rotator cuff repair using a suture bridge technique: is the repair integrity actually maintained? Am J Sports Med 2011;39(10):2108–16.
49. Novak PJ, Bach BR Jr, Romeo AA, et al. Surgical resection of the distal clavicle. J Shoulder Elbow Surg 1995;4:35–40.
50. Flatow EL, Cordasco FA, Bigliani LU. Arthroscopic resection of the outer end of the clavicle from a superior approach: a critical, quantitative, radiographic assessment of bone removal. Arthroscopy 1992;8(1):55–64.
51. Gartsman GM. Arthroscopic resection of the acromioclavicular joint. Am J Sports Med 1993;21(1):71–7.
52. Kay SP, Ellman H, Harris E. Arthroscopic distal clavicle excision. Technique and early results. Clin Orthop Relat Res 1994;(301):181–4.
53. Denard PJ, Raiss P, Sowa B, et al. Mid- to long-term follow-up of total shoulder arthroplasty using a keeled glenoid in young adults with primary glenohumeral arthritis. J Shoulder Elbow Surg 2013;22(7):894–900.
54. Khan A, Bunker TD, Kitson JB. Clinical and radiological follow-up of the Aequalis third-generation cemented total shoulder replacement: a minimum ten-year study. J Bone Joint Surg Br 2009;91(12):1594–600.
55. Namdari S, Skelley N, Keener JD, et al. What is the role of arthroscopic debridement for glenohumeral arthritis? A critical examination of the literature. Arthroscopy 2013;29(8):1392–8.

Acute and Chronic Low Back Pain

Nathan Patrick, MD, Eric Emanski, MD, Mark A. Knaub, MD*

KEYWORDS

- Acute low back pain • Chronic low back pain • Patient education
- Treatment protocols

KEY POINTS

- Numerous factors put patients at risk for the development of chronic back pain, including age, educational status, psychosocial factors, occupational factors, and obesity.
- Evaluation of patients with back pain includes completing an appropriate history (including red-flag symptoms), performing a comprehensive physical examination, and, in some scenarios, obtaining imaging in the form of plain radiographs and magnetic resonance imaging.
- Treatment of an acute episode of back pain includes relative rest, activity modification, nonsteroidal anti-inflammatories, and physical therapy.
- Patient education is also imperative, as these patients are at risk for further episodes of back pain in the future.
- Chronic back pain (>6 months' duration) develops in a small percentage of patients. Clinicians' ability to diagnose the exact pathologic source of these symptoms is severely limited, making a cure unlikely. Treatment of these patients should be supportive, the goal being to improve pain and function rather than to "cure" the patient's condition.

MAGNITUDE OF THE PROBLEM

Low back pain is an extremely common problem that affects at least 80% of all individuals at some point in their lifetime, and is the fifth most common reason for all physician visits in the United States.[1–3] Approximately 1 in 4 adults in the United States reported having low back pain that lasted at least 24 hours within the previous 3 months, and 7.6% reported at least 1 episode of severe acute low back pain within a 1-year period.[4,5] In addition, low back pain is a leading cause of activity limitation and work absence (second only to upper respiratory conditions) throughout much of the world, resulting in a vast economic burden on individuals, families, communities, industry, and governments.[6–9] In 1998, total incremental direct health care costs attributable to low back pain in the United States were estimated at $26.3 billion.[10]

Department of Orthopaedic Surgery, Penn State–Milton S. Hershey Medical Center, 30 Hope Drive, Building A, Hershey, PA 17033, USA
* Corresponding author.
E-mail address: mknaub@hmc.psu.edu

Med Clin N Am 98 (2014) 777–789
http://dx.doi.org/10.1016/j.mcna.2014.03.005
0025-7125/14/$ – see front matter © 2014 Elsevier Inc. All rights reserved.

Furthermore, indirect costs related to days lost from work are substantial, with nearly 2% of the work force of the United States compensated for back injuries each year.[11]

RISK AND PROGNOSTIC FACTORS

Factors that play a role in the development of back pain include age, educational status, psychosocial factors, job satisfaction, occupational factors, and obesity. Age is one of the most common factors in the development of low back pain, with most studies finding the highest incidence in the third decade of life and overall prevalence increasing until age 60 to 65 years. However, there is recent evidence that prevalence continues to increase with age with more severe forms of back pain.[1,12] Other studies show that back pain in the adolescent population has become increasingly common.[13]

An increased prevalence of low back pain is associated with patients of low educational status.[1] Lower educational levels are a strong predictor of more prolonged episode duration and poorer outcomes.[14] Psychosocial factors such as stress, anxiety, depression, and certain types of pain behavior are associated with greater rates of low back pain. The presence of these conditions also increases the risk that a patient's episode of back pain will last long enough to be considered chronic.[1,15] Likewise, patients who are dissatisfied with their work situation are at risk of having an acute episode of back pain transition to a chronic situation.[16] Occupational factors, specifically the physical demands of work, are also associated with an increased prevalence of low back pain. Matsui and colleagues[17] found the point prevalence of low back pain to be 39% in manual workers, whereas it was found in only 18.3% of those with sedentary occupations. A more recent systematic review found manual handling, bending, twisting, and whole-body vibration to be risk factors for low back pain.[18] Lastly, obesity, or a body mass index of more than 30 kg/m^2, has been connected with an increased incidence of low back pain.[1,19]

PRESENTATION

For most patients, an episode of acute low back pain is a self-limited condition that does not require any active medical treatment.[5] Among those who do seek medical care, their symptoms and disability improve rapidly and most are able to return to work and normal activities within the first month.[20] Up to 1 in 3 of these patients, however, report persistent back pain of at least moderate intensity 1 year after an acute episode, and 1 in 5 reports substantial limitations in activity.[21]

Initial evaluation of patients with back pain should begin with a focused history. Key aspects of this should include: duration of symptoms; description of the pain (location, severity, timing, radiation, and so forth); presence of neurologic symptoms (weakness or alterations in sensation or pain) or changes in bowel and bladder function; evidence of any recent or current infection (fever, chills, sweats, and so forth); previous treatments; and pertinent medical history (cancer, infection, osteoporosis, fractures, endocrine disorders). Key facets of the history are listed in **Box 1**. Some historical facts, referred to by many as red-flag symptoms, may be a harbinger of a dangerous clinical situation (**Box 2**). When present, these symptoms should raise the level of suspicion of the provider that this patient is presenting with more than a simple, benign episode of acute low back pain. In patients presenting with 1 or more of these red flags, there is a 10% chance that they have a serious underlying source of their symptoms of low back pain. These patients should have plain radiographs taken of their lumbar spine to rule out serious structural abnormality. In a patient in whom an infectious cause is considered, plain radiographs may be normal early in the disease process. A white blood cell

---

Box 1
Historical factors that must be considered in the evaluation of a patient with low back pain

Duration

Acute low back pain: less than 4 weeks

Subacute low back pain: 4 weeks to 3 months

Chronic low back pain: more than 3 months

Pain Description

Location (cervical, thoracic, lumbar, sacral)

Severity (pain scale, type of pain, activities affected)

Timing (morning, evening, constant, intermittent)

Aggravating and relieving factors (ambulation/rest, sitting/standing/laying, inclines/declines, back flexion/extension)

Radiation (dermatomal or nondermatomal)

Deficits

Motor weakness

Sensory changes (numbness, tingling, paresthesias, dermatomal or nondermatomal)

Urinary or bowel incontinence, urgency, or frequency

Risk Factors

Age

Educational status

Psychosocial factors

Occupation

Body mass index

Medical History

Cancer

Recent or current infection

Osteoporosis and history of other fractures

Endocrine disorders

Previous spinal surgeries

---

count, erythrocyte sedimentation rate, and C-reactive protein should be obtained. Elevation of these inflammatory parameters should prompt evaluation with magnetic resonance imaging (MRI), with and without contrast, of the lumbar spine.

Patient-completed pain diagrams are useful adjuncts in evaluating patients with acute or chronic low back pain, and are especially useful for those with radicular complaints. Patient outcomes measures such as the Oswestry Disability Index can give insight into how patients' symptoms are affecting their life, and can be useful to track treatment progress.

PHYSICAL EXAMINATION

Physical examination of the patient with low back pain is a necessity during the office visit. The examination should focus on determining the presence and severity of

---

Box 2
Red-flag symptoms

The presence of any of these historical factors in a patient presenting with low back pain may indicate a serious underlying disorder and should prompt a more rapid and thorough evaluation of the patient.

Age >50 years

Systemic symptoms: fever, chills, night sweats, fatigue, decreased appetite, unintentional weight loss

History of malignancy

Nonmechanical pain (pain that gets worse with rest): night pain

Recent or current bacterial infection, especially skin infection or urinary tract infection

Immunosuppression

History of intravenous drug use

Failure of response to initial treatment/therapy

Prolonged corticosteroid use or diagnosis of osteoporosis

Trauma

---

neurologic involvement. At the conclusion of the visit, the clinician should also attempt to place the patient's back pain into 1 of 3 categories: nonspecific low back pain, back pain associated with radiculopathy or spinal stenosis, or back pain associated with a specific spinal cause.[22,23] **Table 1** lists common spinal causes of back pain with associated historical and physical examination findings, in addition to imaging recommendations. Although the physical examination is an essential part of the visit, it rarely provides the clinician with a specific diagnosis for the cause of the patient's symptoms. An examination begins with observation of the patient, typically starting when the clinician enters the examination room and involves noting how the patient acts during the history taking. Visual inspection of the patient's thoracic and lumbar spine, and the posterior pelvis, is accomplished by having the patient in a gown. Assessment for any skin abnormalities or asymmetry around the lumbar spine should be performed. Palpation of the bony elements of the spine and the posterior pelvis in addition to the paraspinal muscles can help localize the patient's complaints. Obvious deformities such as significant scoliosis or a high-grade spondylolisthesis may be discovered with observation and/or palpation in a nonobese patient. Assessment of spinal motion can be difficult in a patient with acute low back pain, but should be attempted. Limitations in specific directions should be noted, as should any worsening of symptoms with specific motions. Unfortunately, the assessment of motion has not proved to be reliable between observers and does not provide the clinician with a specific diagnosis.

A complete neurologic examination is performed, and should include both upper and lower extremity function. Subtle examination findings in the upper extremities, such as hyperreflexia or a positive Hofmann sign, could indicate a more proximal cause (cervical spinal cord compression/dysfunction) of a patient's lower extremity neurologic complaints or bowel/bladder dysfunction. Manual muscle strength testing should be performed of the major muscle groups of the lower extremity to include the myotomes of the lumbar nerve roots (**Table 2**). Muscle strength should be recorded using a scale of 0 to 5 (**Table 3**). Sensory examination should be performed with reference to the lumbar dermatomes (see **Table 2**). Side-to-side comparison of sensation to light touch and pinprick should be performed in all patients. Assessment of proprioception and vibration sense can be included in select patients in whom central processes or lesions are suspected. Patellar and Achilles deep tendon reflexes are helpful in differentiating central nervous system abnormalities (indicated by hyperactive reflexes) from lumbar nerve root or peripheral nerve problems (hypoactive reflexes expected). The presence of a Babinski sign (upward-moving great toe when the plantar-lateral surface of the foot is scraped) should alert the examiner to the probability of a more central issue. Functional muscle strength should be assessed by asking the patient to stand from a seated position without the assistance of the upper extremities (assessing functional strength of quadriceps). Asking the patient to squat from a standing position can also assess the functional strength of the quadriceps. Having the patient stand on the heels and toes can assess the strength of the ankle dorsiflexor and plantarflexor musculature. A single-leg toe raise can be used to diagnose subtle weakness of the gastrocnemius-soleus complex.

Straight-leg raise (SLR) and cross-SLR tests are not useful in patients with complaints of only low back pain. Nearly all patients with low back pain will have an increase in their symptoms with these maneuvers. These tests are helpful in patients with radiating leg pain in an attempt to differentiate true radiculopathy from other causes of leg pain. For an SLR test to be considered positive, the patient must have a reproduction of the radiating leg pain distal to the knee on the side that is being tested. A positive cross-SLR test occurs when the patient's radicular pain below the knee is reproduced while the contralateral leg is extended at the hip and knee. Positive results for the SLR test have high sensitivity (91%; 95% confidence interval [CI] 82%–94%) but is not specific (26%; 95% CI 16%–38%) for identifying a disc herniation. The cross-SLR test is more specific (88%; 95% CI 86%–90%) but not sensitive (29%; CI 24%–34%).[24] Both SLR and cross-SLR tests are designed to evaluate for compression of the lower (L4-S1) lumbar nerve roots. The femoral stretch test is a similar provocative maneuver that aims to create tension in the upper lumbar roots (L2 and L3) in an attempt to reproduce L2 or L3 radicular symptoms in the anterior thigh.

The physical examination must also evaluate for other potential sources of the patient's pain. Nonmusculoskeletal causes of back pain should be considered, as should nonspinal, musculoskeletal causes. A partial list of nonmusculoskeletal abnormalities that may cause back pain is shown in **Box 3**. The sacroiliac (SI) joints and the hips should be examined to assess whether these structures are contributing to a patient's symptoms. Simple internal and external rotation of the hip in either the supine or seated position places the hip joint through a range of motion that will likely reproduce the patient's pain if it is originating in the hip joint. The SI joint can be loaded or stressed with the Patrick test or the FABER test, whereby the patient's hip is placed into flexion, abduction, and external rotation. This test is typically performed with the patient in the supine position and the lower extremity placed into a "figure-4" position. The Patrick test is positive if it reproduces the patient's back pain on the side that is being examined. A positive test, though not diagnostic of an SI joint problem, should at least alert the examiner to the possibility that the SI joint may be contributing to the patient's symptoms.

Psychosocial issues play an important role in both acute and chronic low back pain. Patients with abnormal psychometric profiles are at greater risk for development of chronic back pain. In addition, they are more likely to be functionally affected (or disabled) by their symptoms of back pain. Screening for depression can be performed in an attempt to identify patients who are at risk. Psychological overlay is often found in these patients, which can cloud their physical examination. Assessing for Waddell signs can be useful in determining if there is a nonorganic cause of the patient's symptoms.[25,26] The presence of 1 or more of these findings on examination increases the

Table 1
Common spinal causes of back pain with associated historical factors, physical examination findings, recommended imaging modalities, and any additional diagnostic testing

Etiology	Key Features	Imaging	Additional Studies
Muscle strain	General ache or muscle spasms in the lower back, may radiate to buttock or posterior thighs; worse with increasing activity or bending	None	None
Disc herniation	Pain originating in the lower back with dermatomal radiation to the lower extremity; relieved by standing and worsened with sitting; may be accompanied by motor/sensory changes	Symptoms present <1 mo: none; Symptoms present >1 mo or severe/progressive: MRI	None
Lumbar spondylosis	Generalized back pain worse immediately after waking up; improvement throughout the day; pain fluctuates with activity and may worsen with extension of the spine	Symptoms present <1 mo: plain radiographs	None
Spinal stenosis with neurogenic claudication	Back pain with radiculopathy that is often worsened with extension/standing and improved with flexion/sitting; may be accompanied by motor/sensory changes	Symptoms present <1 mo: none; Symptoms present >1 mo or severe/progressive: MRI	None
Spondylolisthesis	Back pain that may radiate down one or both legs and is exacerbated by flexion and extension; may be accompanied by motor/sensory changes	Symptoms present <1 mo: none; Symptoms >1 mo or severe/progressive: plain radiographs	None
Spondylolysis: stress reaction or stress fracture of pars interarticularis	One of the most common causes of back pain in children and adolescents	Symptoms present <1 mo: none; Symptoms >1 mo or severe/progressive: plain radiographs	None

(continued on next page)

Table 1
(continued)

Etiology	Key Features	Imaging	Additional Studies
Ankylosing spondylitis	More common in young males; morning stiffness; low back pain that often radiates to the buttock and improves with exercise	Anterior-posterior pelvis radiographs	ESR, CRP, HLA-B27
Infection: epidural abscess ± osteomyelitis	Severe pain with an insidious onset that is unrelenting in nature; night pain; presence of constitutional symptoms; history of recent infection; may have radiculopathy or be accompanied by motor/sensory changes	Plain radiographs and MRI	CBC, ESR, CRP
Malignancy	History of cancer with new onset of low back pain; unexplained weight loss; age >50 y; may have radiculopathy or be accompanied by motor/sensory changes	Plain radiographs and MRI	CBC, ESR, CRP, PTH, TSH, SPEP, UA, UPEP
Cauda equina syndrome	Urinary retention or fecal incontinence; decreased rectal tone; saddle anesthesia; may be accompanied by weakness	MRI	None
Conus medullaris syndrome	Same as cauda equina, but often accompanied by upper motor neuron signs (hyperreflexia, clonus, etc)	MRI	None
Vertebral compression fracture	History of osteoporosis or corticosteroid use; older age	Plain radiographs	1,25-Dihydroxyvitamin D$_3$
Trauma	Variable examination pending the severity of the injury; may be accompanied by motor/sensory changes	Lumbosacral radiographs, CT, ± MRI	None

Abbreviations: CBC, complete blood count; CRP, C-reactive protein; CT, computed tomography; ESR, erythrocyte sedimentation rate; HLA-B27, human leukocyte antigen B27; MRI, magnetic resonance imaging; PTH, parathyroid hormone; SPEP, serum protein electrophoresis; TSH, thyroid-stimulating hormone; UA, urinalysis; UPEP, urine protein electrophoresis.

Table 2
Lower extremity myotomes, dermatomes, and reflexes by lumbar nerve root

Lumbar Nerve Root	Muscle Group	Sensory Distribution	Deep Tendon Reflex
L2	Hip flexor	Anterior medial thigh	None
L3	Quadriceps	Anterior thigh to knee	Patellar
L4	Anterior tibialis	Medial calf/ankle	Patellar
L5	Extensor hallicus longus	Lateral ankle/dorsum of foot	None
S1	Gastrocnemius/soleus/peroneals	Plantar-lateral foot	Achilles

possibility that the patient has a nonstructural source of the symptoms (**Box 4**). As a word of caution, the presence of Waddell signs does not exclude an organic cause of low back pain; rather, it points to the need for further psychological evaluation of the patient.

IMAGING

Evidenced-based treatment guidelines have long established that most patients presenting with an episode of acute low back pain do not need any imaging. Most of these patients will have improvement in their clinical symptoms within a few days to a week, even in the absence of any active treatment. In addition, imaging (including MRI) is not likely to reveal an exact pathologic diagnosis in the most patients. Overutilization of imaging in the evaluation of acute low back pain leads to increased health care expenditures in a patient population that will likely improve on its own. In addition, imaging in these patients frequently leads to the diagnosis of degenerative disc disease, which allows the patient to adopt the sick role. The thought that one has a "disease" leads the patient to change his or her behavior, and many begin to exhibit fear-avoidance behavior. This term refers to patients' fear that they are going to do something that will injury or worsen their "diseased" back; therefore they decrease their physical activity, which culminates in being detrimental to their recovery. The preferred approach is to reassure patients that they will likely get better without any active medical intervention and that imaging, including MRI, will not reveal an exact pathologic diagnosis in most patients.

Imaging is indicated in patients who present with red-flag symptoms or in those whose symptoms persist despite 4 to 6 weeks of conservative treatment. Standing plain radiographs of the lumbar spine are the initial imaging modality of choice. Though not likely to reveal the exact pathologic cause of a patient's symptoms, these

Table 3
Grading system for muscle power on manual muscle strength testing

Grade	Description
0	No contraction
1	Muscle flicker/twitch
2	Able to fire muscle with gravity removed
3	Able to fire muscle against force of gravity
4	Able to fire muscle against some resistance
5	Normal strength against resistance

Box 3
Nonmusculoskeletal causes of back pain

Nonmusculoskeletal causes of pain must be considered in patients being evaluated for back pain.

Genitourinary
  Nephrolithiasis
  Pyelonephritis
  Prostatitis
  Endometriosis
  Ovarian cysts

Gastrointestinal
  Esophagitis
  Gastritis and peptic ulcer disease
  Cholelithiasis and cholecystitis
  Pancreatitis
  Diverticulitis
  Other intra-abdominal infections

Cardiovascular
  Abdominal or thoracic aortic aneurysm
  Cardiac ischemia or myocardial infarction

Neurologic
  Intramedullary spinal cord tumors

---

images will rule out troubling disorder such as fracture, tumor, or infection. With these diagnoses largely excluded with plain radiographs, most patients with low back pain do not require further imaging. MRI should be used in patients with neurologic complaints or in those for whom the clinician has a high level of suspicion for an occult

---

Box 4
Signs of nonorganic abnormality

Waddell's signs, when present, can indicate a psychological component of chronic low back pain.

Tenderness tests: superficial and/or diffuse tenderness and/or nonanatomic tenderness

Simulation tests: based on movements, which produce pain, without actually causing that movement, such as axial loading on the top of the head causing low back pain and pain on simulated lumbar spine rotation

Distraction tests: positive tests are rechecked when the patient's attention is distracted, such as a straight leg raise test with the patient in a seated position

Regional disturbances: regional strength or sensory changes that do not follow accepted neuroanatomy

Overreaction: subjective signs regarding the patient's demeanor and overreaction to testing

From Waddell G, McCulloch J, Kummel E, et al. Nonorganic physical signs in low-back pain. Spine 1980;5:117–25.

fracture, tumor, or early infection. MRI is a highly sensitive imaging modality, but lacks specificity when a patient's complaint is axial pain. Degenerative changes are found in many asymptomatic subjects, and these changes increase in frequency with increasing age. Therefore, it is impossible to attribute a patient's back pain to a degenerative disc or an arthritic facet joint, given that they are present in most asymptomatic subjects.

Other imaging modalities that are used in patients with back pain include computed tomography, myelography, and bone scans. The indications for these tests are limited and fall outside the scope of this article. Provocative lumbar discography is a highly debated topic within the community of spine care providers. The senior author believes that discography has poor positive predictive value for successful surgical outcomes when it is used to determine whether a patient is a candidate for surgical intervention for axial low back pain. As a result, discography is not used during the evaluation of patients with chronic low back pain. Other spine surgeons routinely use discography to determine if a patient is a candidate for spinal fusion for "discogenic" low back pain, and many patients agree to have this diagnostic test performed and subsequently undergo spinal fusion in an attempt to improve their axial low back pain. Successful outcomes occur in only 40% to 60% of patients undergoing this type of procedure. Because of these poor results, the senior author does not perform spinal fusion procedures on patients with isolated low back pain and only degenerative changes on imaging.

TREATMENT

An exhaustive discussion of the treatment options available for acute and chronic low back pain is beyond the scope of this article. Most acute episodes of low back pain will resolve within 6 to 8 weeks even in the absence of active treatment. Relative rest, activity modification, nonsteroidal anti-inflammatory drugs (NSAIDs), chiropractic manipulation, and physical therapy are all treatment options in the acute and subacute phase of this clinical syndrome. These treatment modalities probably do not result in a significant change in the natural history of the condition, but do provide the patient with some active treatment modalities while the episode runs its natural course. Initial management of an episode of low back pain should include relative rest, cessation of pain-provoking activities, and a limited course of medications. NSAIDs, acetaminophen, tramadol, muscle relaxants, antidepressants, and opioids are frequently used in the treatment of both acute and chronic back pain. In patients with chronic axial pain, the use of simple analgesics, such as acetaminophen or tramadol, in combination with an antidepressant, appears to have the greatest efficacy.[27] Long-term opioid use for the treatment of chronic low back pain appears to be safe but only modestly effective in this patient group. These patients have only small functional improvements from the use of the medication, and are at risk for the adverse effects of opioid use including central nervous system depression, constipation, development of tolerance, and aberrant behavior. NSAIDs are perhaps the most commonly used single class of medications for back pain symptoms. NSAIDs are as effective as other medication classes but harbor the potential for gastrointestinal side effects. Their safety for long-term use in the setting of hypertension and/or cardiovascular disease has been questioned.

Adjunctive treatment options include physical therapy, a period of immobilization, and local treatment modalities that may include heat, ice, ultrasound, massage, and transcutaneous electrical nerve stimulation. Alternative treatment options may include spinal manipulation, acupuncture, yoga, and other exercise-based therapy programs.

These alternative therapies lack conclusive scientific evidence supporting their efficacy in the treatment of acute or chronic back pain. Despite this, there are patients who pursue these options, and many benefit to at least some extent. Physical therapy or exercise-based programs tend to focus on core muscle strengthening and aerobic conditioning. No differences have been found when comparing the effectiveness of supervised with home-based exercise programs.

Spinal injections have a limited role in the treatment of chronic, mechanical low back pain. There is some evidence that intralaminar epidural steroid injections may play a small role in the short-term treatment of this patient population. Some patients may also benefit from facet injections or facet blocks when other conservative treatment modalities have been exhausted.

For those unfortunate few who fail to improve and fall into the category of chronic back pain, modern medicine has failed to provide any effective treatments. Despite many advances in medicine, clinicians' ability to diagnose the exact source of a patient's axial back pain is extremely limited. Therefore, our ability to treat this clinical entity is poor. Many surgeons believe that there are some patients who suffer from chronic back pain who would improve with surgical treatment of their symptoms. The problem lies in our inability to determine which individual patient will benefit from surgery and which will be left with ongoing pain and disability. The goals of treatment for these patients should move away from a "cure" and focus on lessening symptoms and the effects they have on the patient, in addition to improving function.

SUMMARY

Back pain is an extremely common presenting complaint that occurs in upward of 80% of persons. The natural history of acute episodes of back pain is favorable in most patients. Numerous factors put patients at risk for the development of chronic back pain, including age, educational status, psychosocial factors, occupational factors, and obesity. Evaluation of these patients includes completing an appropriate history (including red-flag symptoms), performing a comprehensive physical examination, and, in some scenarios, obtaining imaging in the form of plain radiographs and MRI. Treatment of an acute episode of back pain includes relative rest, activity modification, NSAIDs, and physical therapy. Patient education is also imperative, as these patients are at risk for further episodes of back pain in the future. Chronic back pain (>6 months' duration) develops in a small percentage of patients. Clinicians' ability to diagnose the exact pathologic source of these symptoms is severely limited, making a cure unlikely. Treatment of these patients should be supportive, the goal being to improve pain and function rather than to "cure" the patient's condition.

REFERENCES

1. Hoy D, Brooks P, Blyth F, et al. The epidemiology of low back pain. Best Pract Res Clin Rheumatol 2010;24:769–81.
2. Chou R, Qaseem A, Snow V, et al, Clinical efficacy assessment Subcommittee of the American College of Physicians, American College of Physicians, American Pain Society Low Back Pain Guidelines Panel. Diagnosis and treatment of low back pain: a joint clinical practice guideline from the American College of Physicians and the American Pain Society. Ann Intern Med 2007;147(7):478–91.
3. Hart LG, Deyo RA, Cherkin DC. Physician office visits for low back pain. Frequency, clinical evaluation, and treatment patterns from a U.S. National Survey. Spine 1995;20:11–9.

4. Deyo RA, Mirza SK, Martin BI. Back pain prevalence and visit rates: estimates from U.S. national surveys, 2002. Spine 2006;31:2724–7.

5. Carey TS, Evans AT, Hadler NM, et al. Acute severe low back pain. A population-based study of prevalence and care-seeking. Spine 1996;21:339–44.

6. Lidgren L. The bone and joint decade 2000-2010. Bull World Health Organ 2003; 81(9):629.

7. Steenstra IA, Verbeek JH, Heymans MW, et al. Prognostic factors for duration of sick leave in patients sick listed with acute low back pain: a systematic review of the literature. Occup Environ Med 2005;62(12):851–60.

8. Kent PM, Keating JL. The epidemiology of low back pain in primary care. Chiropr Osteopat 2005;13:13.

9. Thelin A, Holmberg S, Thelin N. Functioning in neck and low back pain from a 12-year perspective: a prospective population-based study. J Rehabil Med 2008; 40(7):555–61.

10. Luo X, Pietrobon R, Sun SX, et al. Estimates and patterns of direct health care expenditures among individuals with back pain in the United States. Spine 2004;29: 79–86.

11. Andersson GB. Epidemiological features of chronic low-back pain. Lancet 1999; 354:581–5.

12. Dionne CE, Dunn KM, Croft PR. Does back pain prevalence really decrease with increasing age? A systematic review. Age Ageing 2006;35(3):229–34.

13. Jeffries LJ, Milanese SF, Grimmer-Somers KA. Epidemiology of adolescent spinal pain: a systematic overview of the research literature. Spine 2007;32(23): 2630–7.

14. Dionne CE, Von Korff M, Koepsell TD, et al. Formal education and back pain: a review. J Epidemiol Community Health 2001;55(7):455–68.

15. Linton SJ. A review of psychological risk factors in back and neck pain. Spine 2000;25(9):1148–56.

16. van Tulder M, Koes B, Bombardier C. Low back pain. Best practice & research. Clin Rheumatol 2002;16(5):761–75.

17. Matsui H, Maeda A, Tsuji H, et al. Risk indicators of low back pain among workers in Japan: association of familial and physical factors with low back pain. Spine 1997;22(11):1242–8.

18. Hoogendoorn WE, van Poppel MN, Bongers PM, et al. Systematic review of psychosocial factors at work and private life as risk factors for back pain. Spine 2000; 25(16):2114–25.

19. Webb R, Brammah T, Lunt M, et al. Prevalence and predictors of intense, chronic, and disabling neck and back pain in the UK general population. Spine 2003; 28(11):1195–202.

20. Pengel LH, Herbert RD, Maher CG, et al. Acute low back pain: systematic review of its prognosis. BMJ 2003;327:323.

21. Von Korff M, Saunders K. The course of back pain in primary care. Spine 1996; 21:2833–7 [discussion: 2838–9].

22. Deyo RA, Rainville J, Kent DL. What can the history and physical examination tell us about low back pain? JAMA 1992;268:760–5.

23. Bigos S, Bowyer O, Braen G, et al. Acute low back problems in adults. Clinical practice guideline No. 14. AHCPR Publication No. 95–0642. Rockville (MD): Agency for Health Care Policy and Research, Public Health Service, U.S. Department of Health and Human Services; 1994.

24. Devillé WL, van der Windt DA, Dzaferagić A, et al. The test of Lasègue: systematic review of the accuracy in diagnosing herniated discs. Spine 2000;25:1140–7.

25. Waddell G, McCullock JA, Kummel E, et al. Nonorganic physical signs in low-back pain. Spine 1980;5(2):117–25.
26. Hoppenfeld S. Physical examination of the spine and extremities. Norwalk (CT): Appleton-Century-Crofts; 1976. p. 164–229.
27. Malanga G, Wolff E. Evidence-informed management of chronic low back pain with nonsteroidal anti-inflammatory drugs, muscle relaxants, and simple analgesics. Spine J 2008;8(1):173–84.

Cervical Radiculopathy

Deanna Lynn Corey, MD[a],*, Douglas Comeau, DO, CAQSM[b,c,d]

KEYWORDS

- Cervical radiculopathy • Neck pain • Shoulder pain • Spurling test

KEY POINTS

- Evaluation of shoulder pain should prompt examination of the cervical spine.
- Patient history and physical examination are often sufficient to make a diagnosis of cervical radiculopathy.
- Always correlate radiologic findings with clinical findings.
- A multimodal treatment approach may help to alleviate symptoms.

INTRODUCTION

Neck and shoulder pain are common presenting complaints for primary care providers, sports medicine physicians, and orthopedists. Shoulder pain may be a referred symptom of cervical pathology. The age-adjusted incidence of cervical radiculopathy is 83 per 100,000 persons, making it less common than lumbar radiculopathy.[1] In a recent study of United States military personnel, female gender and white race were implicated as potential risk factors.[2] Cigarette smoking, axial load bearing, and prior lumbar radiculopathy may also predispose patients to cervical radiculopathy.[3]

Nerve roots C6 and C7 are most commonly affected. Radicular pain develops as inflammatory mediators, changes in vascular response, and intraneural edema combine in response to nerve compression. Spondylosis resulting in foraminal encroachment causes 70% of cases. Decreased disk height or degenerative changes of the uncovertebral joints anteriorly or zygopophyseal joints posteriorly are common contributors. Disk herniation is not seen as frequently in cervical radiculopathy compared with lumbar radiculopathy.[1] Compression alone does not necessarily lead to radicular pain unless the dorsal root ganglion is affected.[4]

Disclosures: None.
[a] Department of Family Medicine, Boston Medical Center, Boston University, 1 BMC Place, Boston, MA 02118, USA; [b] Sports Medicine, Ryan Center for Sports Medicine, Boston Medical Center, Boston University, 915 Commonwealth Avenue Rear, Boston, MA 02215, USA; [c] Family Medicine, Boston University School of Medicine, Boston University, 1 BMC Place, Boston, MA 02118, USA; [d] Department of Sports Medicine, Boston College, 140 Commonwealth Avenue, Chestnut Hill, MA 02467, USA
* Corresponding author.
E-mail address: deanna.corey@bmc.org

PATIENT PRESENTATION

Symptoms related to radiculopathy tend to be unilateral. This is particularly true of neck pain relating to cervical radiculopathy. Bilateral symptoms are more consistent with arthritis of the cervical spine. Radiation of pain depends on the involved nerve root. The absence of radiating symptoms does not eliminate cervical radiculopathy as a potential diagnosis. Presenting pain may be isolated to the shoulder. Pain is not always the presenting complaint, because sensory or motor deficits may present without pain.

Certain modifying factors are consistent in cervical radiculopathy. Activities that decrease the size of the neural foramen, such as extension and rotation to the affected side, exacerbate symptoms. Abducting the shoulder tends to alleviate symptoms.

Distribution of sensory and motor deficits may overlap with other neuropathic conditions, including carpal tunnel syndrome or ulnar nerve entrapment. Although these conditions may coexist in some patients, an appropriate physical examination can help differentiate the level at which the nerve is affected.

History should include questions to determine if there are signs or symptoms of myelopathy. Problems with manual dexterity (dropping objects and difficulty writing) are symptoms of myelopathy. Examination findings consistent with myelopathy include upper motor neuron signs, such as Hoffmann sign, Babinski sign, hyperreflexia, and clonus. Differentiation between radicular and myelopathic symptoms is critical, because the latter is caused by spinal cord compression, which is best relieved with surgical decompression. Therefore, this is an important distinction to make.

Red flags should also be evaluated in the history, because they may suggest other diagnoses. Symptoms, such as fevers, chills, unexplained weight loss, night pain, previous cancer, immunosuppression, and intravenous drug abuse, are not associated with radiculopathy. The presence of these symptoms is more suggestive of malignancy or infection. Other factors of the history that make a diagnosis of cervical radiculopathy less likely include age younger than 20 or older than 50 years, constant and progressive signs and symptoms, neck rigidity without trauma, dysphasia, altered consciousness, and central nervous signs and symptoms.[5]

Systemic disorders should also be considered potential causes. Down syndrome is associated with atlantoaxial instability. Heritable connective tissue disorders carry an increased risk of ligament laxity.

PHYSICAL EXAMINATION

Findings vary depending on the level of nerve root involved. Evaluation should include neck range of motion, with careful observation of movements that result in worsening symptoms. Neurologic examination of the upper extremities should include motor testing at the shoulders, elbows, wrists, and hands to assess for any weakness and sensory testing of all dermatomes to assess for variations. Reflex testing should be considered abnormal when there is asymmetry between the affected and unaffected side. Any deficits noted can help to determine the compressed nerve root (**Table 1**).

Provocative testing must also be included. Spurling test is designed to exacerbate encroachment of exiting nerve roots by decreasing the dimensions of the foramen. The patient is asked to extend and laterally rotate the neck to the suspected side while the provider applies an axial load. A positive test recreates radiating pain. Equivocal tests are notable for discomfort only. Recent studies have shown this test to be highly sensitive (95%) and specific (94%).[6] Shoulder abduction sign, where the arm is raised above the head, should alleviate or relieve symptoms of cervical radiculopathy. Cervical traction should produce similar effects.

Table 1
Patterns of cervical radiculopathy

Root	Pain Distribution	Motor Abnormalities	Sensory Deficits	Reflexes
C4	Lower neck and trapezius	N/A	Cape distribution	N/A
C5	Neck, shoulder, lateral arm	Deltoid, elbow flexion	Lateral arm	Biceps
C6	Neck, radial arm, thumb	Biceps, wrist extension	Radial forearm, thumb	Brachioradialis
C7	Neck, dorsal forearm, long finger	Triceps, wrist flexion	Dorsal forearm, long finger	Triceps
C8	Neck, medial forearm, ulnar digits	Finger flexors	Medial forearm, ulnar digits	N/A

DIAGNOSTIC TESTS/IMAGING STUDY

History and physical examination are often enough to diagnose cervical radiculopathy. Laboratory studies are expected to be normal in cervical radiculopathy. These studies should be ordered if other etiologies are more clinically suspicious.

Radiography, to include anterioposterior lower cervical and neutral lateral views, may be indicated for patients with suspected cervical radiculopathy. Loss of the normal cervical lordosis, osteophyte formation, and neuroforaminal narrowing responsible for symptoms can be observed (**Fig. 1**).

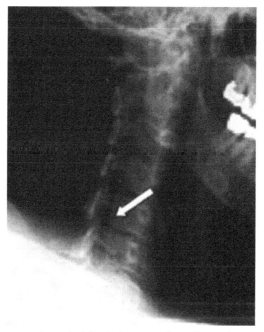

Fig. 1. Loss of the normal cervical lordosis, osteophyte formation, and neuroforaminal narrowing responsible for symptoms can be observed in the radiography.

For patients with normal radiography who fail a nonoperative course of treatment, additional diagnostic studies should be considered. MRI is the preferred modality to evaluate for disk herniations with or without nerve root compression (**Fig. 2**). MRI findings should be correlated with clinical findings, because both false-positive and false-negative rates are high.[7] CT may be used in patients with contraindications to MRI, such as pacemakers or stainless steel hardware. If nerve entrapment at the carpal or cubital tunnel is suspected, electromyelography should be pursued.

DIFFERENTIAL DIAGNOSIS

The differential for neck and shoulder pain is broad, including diagnoses related to neurologic, cardiac, infectious, and musculoskeletal causes. A summary of the differential diagnosis is provided in **Table 2**.

Malignancy that may result in presenting symptoms similar to cervical radiculopathy include, but are not limited to, schwannoma, osteochondromas, Pancoast tumors, thyroid tumors, esophageal tumors, lymphomas, and carcinomatous meningitis.[8,9]

TREATMENT

Pain relief, improvement of neurologic function, and prevention of recurrence are the treatment objectives. Nonoperative treatment modalities for cervical radiculopathy have not been compared in large-scale, randomized control trials. Recommendations are based on current available evidence, including case series and anecdotal experience. Patient preference and potential compliance should be considered when making treatment decisions.[4]

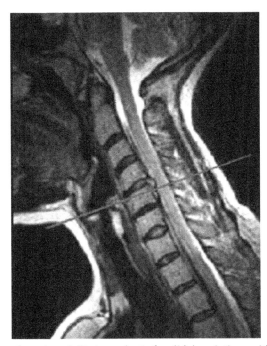

Fig. 2. MRI is the preferred modality to evaluate for disk herniations with or without nerve root compression.

Table 2
Differential diagnosis of cervical radiculopathy

Condition	Characteristics
Cardiac pain	Radiating upper extremity pain, typically to left shoulder and arm
Cervical spondylotic myelopathy	Difficulties with manual dexterity, gait changes, bowel or bladder dysfunction, upper motor neuron findings
Complex regional pain syndrome/reflex sympathetic dystrophy	Pain and tenderness of the extremity out of proportion with examination, skin changes, vasomotor fluctuations, dysthermia
Entrapment syndromes	Weakness and sensory deficits consistent with median or ulnar nerve distributions, direct stimulation of nerve recreates symptoms
Herpes zoster (shingles)	Dermatomal radicular pain associated with reactivation of viral infection
Malignancy	Consider with presence of red flag symptoms, intra- and extraspinal tumors, presentations vary depending on primary tumor
Parsonage-Turner syndrome	Acute onset of upper extremity pain, usually followed by weakness and sensory disturbances
Rotator cuff impingement	Pain and weakness in the shoulder and lateral arm
Thoracic outlet syndrome	Lower brachial plexus nerve root dysfunction due to compression by vascular or neurogenic causes

PHARMACOLOGIC TREATMENT OPTIONS

Pharmacotherapy may be helpful in the management and relief of symptoms. The effectiveness of medications is extrapolated from their effectiveness in the treatment of lumbar radiculopathy and low back pain. As discussed previously, however, the etiology behind radiculopathy is not typically the same in both locations.

Nonsteroidal anti-inflammatory drugs (NSAIDs) may help alleviate symptoms in the acute setting. A 2-week trial at a therapeutic dose can be effective in relieving symptoms or reducing pain to a degree that other treatment modalities can be better tolerated. These medications make a good choice for first-line therapy, because they are readily available and affordable. Appropriate considerations should be made when suggesting NSAID treatment, including patient age, medication interactions, and other comorbidities.[10]

Muscle relaxants, including cyclobenzaprine (Flexeril) and tizanidine (Zanaflex), may help alleviate neck pain caused by increased muscle tension at insertion sites.[8] These medications are most effective in the acute setting. Their long-term use in treatment of cervical radiculopathy is unclear.

Tramadol may provide significant relief of neuropathic pain based on systematic review findings.[11] This makes it useful in managing acute exacerbations of cervical radiculopathy.

Oral steroids, in particular dose packs, are often used to manage acute episodes. High-quality evidence to support this practice is, however, lacking.[12] In addition, recurrent use of oral steroids can lead to avascular necrosis, hyperglycemia, weight gain, and mood swings. The degree to which oral steroids improve symptoms may be an indicator for further treatment with corticosteroid injection. Another systematic review suggests that tricyclic antidepressants and venlafaxine (Effexor) may provide moderate relief of radicular pain in patients who have declined surgery or continue to have pain after surgical intervention.[13]

Studies on neuropathic pain suggest opioids may be an effective treatment course for up to 8 weeks. These findings are not specific to cervical radiculopathy, and there is insufficient evidence to support their use beyond a 2-month period.[13,14]

NONPHARMACOLOGIC TREATMENT OPTIONS

Many modalities beyond pharmacotherapy exist for the treatment of cervical radiculopathy. A short course of immobilization has been suggested to reduce symptoms in the inflammatory phase, although this has not been proved beneficial.[8,12,15,16]

Traction may be performed at home or in conjunction with physical therapy and manipulation. Distracting the neural foramen leads to decompression of the nerve root and improvement in symptoms. This modality works best when acute muscular pain has subsided. It should be avoided in patients with signs of myelopathy. Insufficient evidence exists to support the use of traction, especially in the home setting.[17]

Physical therapy helps restore range of motion and strengthen neck musculature. Doing this alleviates pain and prevents recurrence. Early on in the treatment of cervical radiculopathy, gentle range-of-motion and stretching exercises may be combined with additional modalities, including heat, ice, and electrical stimulation. As pain improves, isometric strengthening, active range-of-motion, and resistance exercises may be added as tolerated.[12,15]

Manipulative therapy lacks high-quality evidence to support its use in the long-term management of cervical radiculopathy. There is evidence, however, to suggest short-term benefit.[15,18] Manipulative therapy is not without risk. Rare complications include worsening radiculopathy, myelopathy, and spinal cord injury.[12]

Cervical steroid injections may also be considered in the management of cervical radiculopathy. These procedures should be performed under radiographic guidance. Patients who are good candidates for this modality include those with confirmed pathology by advanced imaging (MRI or CT) who had improvement while taking and after completing an oral steroid dose pack. Injections may consist of translaminar or transforaminal epidurals or selective nerve blocks. Evidence suggests that corticosteroid injection may lead to short-term, symptomatic improvement of radicular symptoms.[12,19–23] Retrospective and prospective studies show up to 60% of patients with relief of radicular symptoms and neck pain and return to usual activity.[4,19]

SURGICAL TREATMENT OPTIONS

Surgery may relieve intractable symptoms of cervical radiculopathy in appropriate patients. Evidence is lacking to guide optimal timing of surgical intervention.[4] The presence of myelopathy, as discussed previously, is a sign of spinal cord compression and an indication for surgery.

Emotional and cognitive factors should be considered when addressing treatment decisions for cervical radiculopathy. Patient expectations, postoperative limitations, and job satisfaction are areas that should be discussed prior to choosing an intervention course.[24–36]

Surgical intervention should be reserved for patients with radiographic evidence of nerve compression on MRI or CT with corresponding signs and symptoms, persistence of symptoms despite 12 weeks of nonoperative management, or progressive or functionally important motor deficit.[4] Various techniques exist, including anterior and posterior approaches, but evidence comparing them is lacking. A majority of patients have substantial relief of their symptoms. Complications are uncommon but may include iatrogenic injury of the spinal cord, nerve root injury, recurrent nerve palsy, esophageal perforation, and failure of instrumentation.[4]

There is a lack of high-quality evidence comparing nonoperative and surgical intervention in the treatment of cervical radiculopathy.

SUMMARY

Cervical radiculopathy is a commonly seen condition across many patient populations. It results from the compression of a cervical nerve root as it exits the neural foramen. Presentation may include pain, weakness, and sensory deficits. This diagnosis should be considered for all patients presenting with neck and shoulder pain. A thorough history and physical examination are often sufficient for diagnosis. Radiologic studies are often helpful to confirm cervical radiculopathy.

There is no high-quality evidence comparing medical and surgical interventions. Nonoperative treatment is the first course, unless there are signs of myelopathy. If patients fail to improve with nonoperative treatment or exhibit progressively worsening symptoms, surgical intervention should be considered.

REFERENCES

1. Radhakrishnan K, Litchy WJ, O'Fallon WM, et al. Epidemiology of cervical radiculopathy. A population-based study from Rochester, Minnesota, 1976 through 1990. Brain 1994;117(Pt 2):325–35.
2. Schoenfeld AJ, George AA, Bader JO, et al. Incidence and epidemiology of cervical radiculopathy in the United States military: 2000 to 2009. J Spinal Disord Tech 2012;25(1):17–22.
3. Roth D, Mukai A, Thomas P, et al. Cervical radiculopathy. Dis Mon 2009;55: 737–56.
4. Carrette S, Fehlings M. Cervical radiculopathy. N Engl J Med 2005;353(4):392–9.
5. Bussieres AE, Taylor JA, Peterson C. Diagnostic imaging practice guidelines for musculoskeletal complaints in adults – an evidence-based approach – part 3: spinal disorders. J Manipulative Physiol Ther 2008;31(1):33–88.
6. Shabat S, Leitner Y, Rami D. The correlation between Spurling test and imaging studies in detecting cervical radiculopathy. J Neuroimaging 2012;22:375–8.
7. Kuijper B, Tan J, van der Kallen B, et al. Root compression on MRI compared with clinical findings in patients with recent onset cervical radiculopathy. J Neurol Neurosurg Psychiatry 2011;82:561–3.
8. Levine MJ, Albert TJ, Smith MD. Cervical radiculopathy: diagnosis and nonoperative management. J Am Acad Orthop Surg 1996;4(6):305–16.
9. Polston DW. Cervical radiculopathy. Neurol Clin 2007;25(2):373–85.
10. Liantonio J, Simmons B. NSAIDs and the geriatric patient: a cautionary tale. Clin Geriatr 2013;21(5).
11. Hollingshead J, Duhmke RM, Cornbiath DR. Tramadol for neuropathic pain. Cochrane Database Syst Rev 2006;(3):CD003726.
12. Eubanks J. Cervical radiculopathy: nonoperative management of neck pain and radicular symptoms. Am Fam Physician 2010;81(1):33–40.
13. Saarto T, Wiffen PH. Antidepressants for neuropathic pain. Cochrane Database Syst Rev 2007;(4):CD005454.
14. Eisenberg E, McNicol ED, Carr DB. Efficacy and safety of opioid agonists in the treatment of neuropathic pain of nonmalignant origin: systematic review and mata-analysis of randomized controlled trials. JAMA 2005;293(24):3043–52.

15. Rhee JM, Yoon T, Riew KD. Cervical radiculopathy. J Am Acad Orthop Surg 2007; 15(8):486–94.
16. Naylor JR, Mull GP. Surgical collars: a survey of their prescription and cuse. Br J Rheumatol 1991;30(4):282–4.
17. Graham N, Gross A, Goldsmith CH, et al. Mechanical traction for neck pain with or without radiculopathy. Cochrane Database Syst Rev 2008;(3):CD006408.
18. Haneline M. Chiropractic manipulation in the presence of acute cervical intervertebral disc herniation. Dyn Chiropract 1999;17(25).
19. Vallee JN, Feydy A, Carlier RY, et al. Chronic cervical radiculopathy: lateral approach periradicular corticosteroid injection. Radiology 2001;218(3):886–92.
20. Kolstad F, Leivseth G, Nygaard OP. Transforaminal steroid injections in the the treatment of cervical radiculopathy: a prospective outcome study. Acta Neurochir (Wien) 2005;147(10):1065–70.
21. Anderberg L, Annertz M, Persson L, et al. Transforaminal steroid injections for the treatment of cervical radiculopathy: a prospective and randomized study. Eur Spine J 2007;16(3):321–8.
22. Cicala RD, Thoni K, Angel JJ. Long-term results of cervical epidural steroid injections. Clin J Pain 1989;5:143–5.
23. Slipman CW, Lipetz JS, Jackson HB, et al. Therapeutic selective nerve root in the nonsurgical treatment of atraumatic cercival spondylotic radicular pain: a retrospective analysis with independent clinical review. Arch Phys Med Rehabil 2000;81:741–6.
24. Bono CM, Ghiselli G, Gilbert TJ, et al. An evidence-based clinical guideline for the diagnosis and treatment of cervical radiculopathy from degenerative disorders. Spine J 2011;11:64–72.
25. Apelby-Albrecht M, Anderson L, Kleiva I, et al. Concordance of upper limb neurodynamic test with medical examination and magnetic resonance imaging in patients with cervical radiculopathy: a diagnostic cohort study. J Manipulative Physiol Ther 2013;36(9):626–31.
26. Abbed KM, Coumans JV. Cervical radiculopathy: pathophysiology, presentation, and clinical evaluation. Neurosurgery 2007;60(1 Suppl 1):28–34.
27. Rubenstein SM, Pool JJ, van Tulder MW, et al. A systematic review of the diagnostic accuracy of provocative tests of the neck for diagnosing cervical radiculopathy. Eur Spine J 2007;16:307–19.
28. Tampin B, Briffa NK, Hall T, et al. Inter-therapist agreement in classifying patients with cervical radiculopathy and patients with non-specific neck-arm pain. Man Ther 2012;17:445–50.
29. Tampin B, Slater H, Hall T, et al. Quantitative sensory testing somatosensory profriles in patients with cervical radiculopathy are distinct from those in patients with non-specific neck-arm pain. Pain 2012;153:2403–14.
30. Anekstein Y, Blecher R, Smorgick Y, et al. What is the best way to apply the Spurling test for cervical radiculopathy? Clin Orthop Relat Res 2012;(470):2566–72.
31. Shah KC, Rajshekhar V. Reliability of diagnosis of soft cervical disc prolapse using Spurling's test. Br J Neurosurg 2004;18:480–3.
32. Spurling RS, Scoville WB. Lateral rupture of the cervical intervertebral discs: a common cause of shoulder and arm pain. Surg Gynecol Obstet 1944;78:350–8.
33. Tong HC, Haig AJ, Yamakawa K. The Spurling test and cervical radiculopathy. Spine (Phila Pa 1976) 2002;27:156–9.
34. Kuijper B, Beelen A, van der Kallen BF, et al. Interobserver agreement on MRI evaluation of patients with cervical radiculopathy. Clin Radiol 2011;66:25–9.

35. Waldrop MA. Diagnosis and treatment of cervical radiculopathy using a clinical prediction rule and a multimodal intervention approach: a case series. J Orthop Sports Phys Ther 2006;36(3):152–9.
36. Mamula CJ, Erhard RE, Piva SR. Cervical radiculopathy or Parsonage-Tuerner syndrome: differential diagnosis of a patient with neck and upper extremity symptoms. J Orthop Sports Phys Ther 2005;35(10):659–64.

Evaluation and Treatment of Chronic Hand Conditions

Michael Darowish, MD*, Jyoti Sharma, MD

KEYWORDS

- Carpal tunnel • Cubital tunnel • Trigger finger • de Quervain tenosynovitis
- Ganglion cyst • Hand arthritis

KEY POINTS

- Carpal tunnel syndrome and cubital tunnel syndrome are common causes of hand numbness, and can be diagnosed by history taking and physical examination. Ergonomic adjustments and nocturnal splinting can be very helpful.
- Many tendinopathies of the hand and wrist are caused by friction between the tendon and their overlying sheaths. Diagnosis is made by history taking and physical examination; many patients can be successfully treated with bracing or injection.
- Arthritis of the carpometacarpal joint of the thumb is a common source of pain and dysfunction, particularly in middle-aged women. Nonoperative measures including splinting and injection can provide significant relief.
- Ganglion cysts can form on the volar or dorsal wrist, or can arise from the flexor sheath of the finger. Many patients can be treated with simple reassurance. Aspiration or injection can be considered, as can surgical excision, for symptomatic cysts.

GENERAL PRINCIPLES

Patient Evaluation

The evaluation begins with a complete history, including hand dominance, onset of symptoms (antecedent injury/trauma), duration and specific localization of symptoms, exacerbating or relieving factors, and discussion of comorbid conditions that may contribute to or confound the diagnosis (eg, neck pain, diabetic neuropathy, cane/walker use). Getting patients to localize their symptoms can be difficult. To help with this, the authors often ask patients to place one finger on one spot that most bothers them; this can be immensely helpful in beginning to narrow the diagnosis. Previous treatments that have been successful or unhelpful should be reviewed. The nature of patients' employment can significantly affect their condition, and should be documented.

Neither Dr J. Sharma nor Dr M. Darowish has any financial conflicts to disclose.
Penn State Bone and Joint Institute, Penn State Milton S. Hershey Medical Center, 30 Hope Drive, PO Box 859, Hershey, PA 17033, USA
* Corresponding author.
E-mail address: mdarowish@hmc.psu.edu

Med Clin N Am 98 (2014) 801–815
http://dx.doi.org/10.1016/j.mcna.2014.03.006
0025-7125/14/$ – see front matter © 2014 Elsevier Inc. All rights reserved.

Physical examination of the hand and wrist can be daunting, as the anatomy is complex and many structures are in close proximity to one another, making differentiation of one condition from another challenging. Examination begins with inspection: looking for masses, obvious deformities, skin coloration, hair loss, or swelling. The bulk of the hand muscles should be evaluated, looking for atrophy, particularly at the thenar eminence and first web space.

Range of motion should be evaluated by asking the patient to make a fist and fully extend the fingers, looking for lack of full flexion or extension. Passive motion should be compared with active motion; lack of passive motion shows a mechanical block to motion, whereas full passive but deficient active motion can be a result of pain, weakness, or loss of tendon or nerve function. Range of motion of the wrist includes flexion, extension, and rotation. Pronation and supination should be evaluated with the patient's elbow against the side to avoid substitution of shoulder motion for forearm rotation.

Testing the motor function of the hand can be accomplished quickly. Start by having the patient make a fist and extend the fingers. Then have the patient make an "OK" sign, looking specifically for flexion of the distal interphalangeal (DIP) joint of the index finger and flexion of the interphalangeal joint of the thumb. The muscles responsible for these motions, the flexor digitorum profundus (FDP) and the flexor pollicis longus (FPL), respectively, are innervated by the anterior interosseous nerve, the motor portion of the median nerve in the forearm. Care must be taken to confirm that the patient is truly making an "OK" sign and not a key pinch, which uses the ulnar-innervated intrinsic muscles of the hand (**Fig. 1**). Ask the patient to give a thumbs-up sign (a function of the extensor pollicis longus and abductor pollicis longus), which demonstrates posterior interosseous nerve function, the terminal motor branch of the radial nerve. Although finger extension can be used to assess the radial nerve, it is important to remember that extension of the metacarpophalangeal (MCP) joints relies on innervated muscles of the radial nerve. The intrinsic muscles of the hands serve to extend the proximal interphalangeal and DIP joints, and are innervated by the ulnar nerve.

Ulnar nerve function is assessed by asking the patient to cross the index and long fingers; this can be difficult for patients with ulnar neuropathy. It is more sensitive and specific, and more difficult to "fake out" the examiner than finger abduction and adduction; the patient may appear to abduct and adduct the fingers with finger flexion.[1]

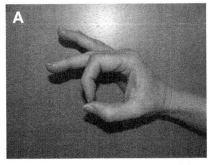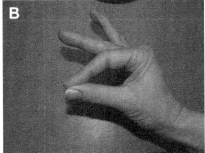

Fig. 1. When evaluating the function of the anterior interosseous nerve, the patient is asked to make an "OK" sign. Careful note must be made for flexion of the interphalangeal joint of the thumb and distal interphalangeal joint of the index finger (A). Patients without anterior interosseus nerve function will replace this with a key pinch, which is accomplished with the use of ulnar nerve innervated muscles (B).

Finally, ask the patient to palmarly abduct the thumb, assessing the function of the recurrent motor branch of the median nerve, which can be affected in carpal tunnel syndrome (**Fig. 2**). The entire process can be completed in a few seconds and can provide a substantial amount of information to the examiner.

Sensory testing needs to evaluate the radial, ulnar, and median nerves. There is significant overlap of the nerve distributions; however, the pulp of the thumb is predictably innervated by the median nerve and the small-finger pulp is reliably ulnarly innervated. The radial nerve provides sensation to the dorsal skin of the first web space. Various sensibilities can be evaluated, including light touch, pressure, pinprick, and 2-point discrimination. Pressure sensibility, as evaluated with Semmes-Weinstein monofilaments, is affected much earlier than loss of 2-point discrimination, which is a very late finding.

Following this, specific provocative testing is performed based on the specific complaints and differential diagnoses; these are discussed in each subsection.

HAND NUMBNESS
History and Physical Examination

Patients will often present with complaints of hand numbness. Over time this can progress to pain, loss of coordination, or difficulty holding objects. Patients may also describe hand weakness. Dropping objects can occur from either loss of strength or loss of feeling (ie, the patient cannot feel the object in the hand and it falls out).

During documentation of the history, it is important to ask about the distribution of the numbness. Many patients do not closely pay attention to which part of their hand is numb. Clearly delineating the fingers involved will help to narrow the diagnosis. In particular, the inclusion of the ulnar side of the hand (and specifically the small finger) will suggest the ulnar nerve, whereas the radial side of the hand is more consistent with median nerve involvement.

Inquiring about comorbid conditions that can contribute to numbness is important. Such conditions include neck pain or pain/numbness radiating from the neck down the arm, which can point to a possible cervical radiculopathy, leg numbness or weakness indicating an abnormality more related to the central nervous system, history of stroke or transient ischemic attack with residual symptoms, or other causes of

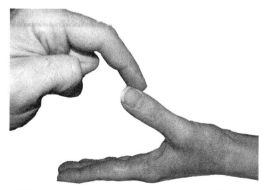

Fig. 2. Evaluation of the recurrent motor branch of the median nerve is performed by asking the patient to palmarly abduct the thumb, most easily accomplished by having the patient touch the examiner's finger above the palm.

peripheral neuropathy including diabetes, vitamin deficiency, alcoholism (which can lead to vitamin B_{12} deficiency), human immunodeficiency virus, chemotherapeutics, or hypothyroidism. Other diseases that can contribute to carpal or cubital tunnel syndrome include rheumatoid arthritis, amyloidosis, or other space-occupying lesions, such as ganglia or elbow arthritis with osteophyte formation in the area of the cubital tunnel.

Exacerbating factors should be questioned. Carpal tunnel syndrome is exacerbated by wrist flexion, which occurs while driving, reading a newspaper, or sleeping. Cubital tunnel syndrome causes hand numbness when pressure is placed on the ulnar nerve, such as when leaning on the arms of a chair or when the elbow is held in a flexed posture for a prolonged time. Activities when this occurs include sleeping, reading, talking on the telephone, texting/using a tablet computer, using a keyboard, or styling/blow drying one's hair.

Physical Examination

Physical examination should start with cervical spine range of motion, and testing for a Spurling sign. The Spurling sign is elicited by having the patient rotate the head and extend the neck, and applying axial force to the head. A positive test reproduces shock-like symptoms down the arm toward which the patient is facing. Generation of neck pain without arm symptoms is not a positive test. Provocative tests for carpal tunnel syndrome include the Tinel sign, the Phalen test, the Durkan compression test, and a wrist compression-flexion test. A Tinel test is performed by striking directly over the carpal tunnel; a positive test produces electric-shock–like sensations into the median innervated fingers. A Phalen test is performed by allowing the wrist to passively flex with gravity (**Fig. 3**). It is critical to perform this with the elbow extended to avoid concomitant traction on the ulnar nerve, which can also cause hand numbness. The Durkan test is performed by directly compressing the median nerve at the carpal tunnel with reproduction of paresthesias. The authors prefer to use the wrist compression-flexion test, which combines Phalen and Durkan tests. With the elbow extended, the wrist is passively flexed and pressure is held over the carpal tunnel (**Fig. 4**). Again, a positive test reproduces paresthesias in the median nerve distribution, and has the greatest specificity and sensitivity (92% and 80%, respectively) (**Table 1**).

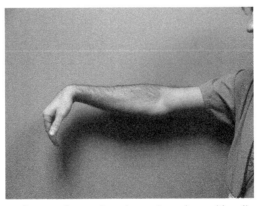

Fig. 3. The Phalen test for carpal tunnel syndrome is performed by allowing gravity to flex the wrist with the elbow extended. A positive test causes reproduction of paresthesias in the median nerve distribution. It is essential to perform this with the elbow extended so as to avoid producing hand paresthesias because of traction on the ulnar nerve at the elbow.

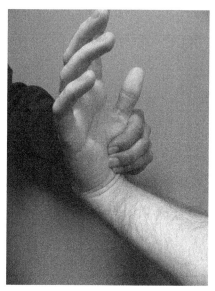

Fig. 4. Wrist compression-flexion test for carpal tunnel syndrome. With the patient's elbow extended, the examiner flexes the patient's wrist while simultaneously compressing the median nerve at the carpal tunnel. A positive test reproduces paresthesias in the median nerve distribution.

Provocative maneuvers for cubital tunnel syndrome include the Tinel test (**Fig. 5**), which again is performed by percussing directly over the ulnar nerve at the postero-medial elbow. The equivalent of the Phalen test can be performed by having the patient hold the elbow flexed with the wrist in neutral position for up to 30 seconds. One must bear in mind that this test is positive in at least 10% of the normal population.[2] Combining this with direct pressure over the nerve at the cubital tunnel (elbow compression-flexion test) increases sensitivity and specificity of the diagnosis

Table 1
Diagnosing carpal tunnel syndrome using physical maneuvers

Test	Technique	Positive Test	Sensitivity (%)	Specificity (%)
Phalen	Patient holds wrist flexed 90° with elbow in full extension	Pain or paresthesia ≤60 s	68	73
Tinel	Clinician repetitively taps wrist directly over median nerve	Pain or paresthesia	50	77
Durkan	Clinician applies direct pressure over the transverse carpal ligament	Pain or paresthesia ≤30 s	64	83
Wrist compression-flexion test	As median nerve compression, with wrist held in flexion	Pain or paresthesia ≤30 s	80	92

Adapted from Wipperman J, Potter L. Carpal tunnel syndrome—try these diagnostic maneuvers. J Fam Pract 2012;61(12):726–32.

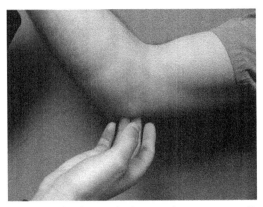

Fig. 5. The Tinel sign at the cubital tunnel. The examiner percusses directly over the ulnar nerve at the posteromedial elbow. A positive test causes electrical shock in the ulnar nerve distribution. This test is positive in at least 10% of normal individuals.

(**Fig. 6**).[3] Early in the course of the disease, these may be the only positive findings on examination, as sensation and motor function may be normal in the absence of pressure or tension on the nerve (**Table 2**).

Other signs that may be present on examination include the Froment sign (**Fig. 7**) whereby the patient replaces key pinch (ulnar innervated) with tip pinch (median innervated).

Testing

The diagnoses of carpal tunnel and cubital tunnel syndromes are clinical, based on history and physical examination. However, electrodiagnostic testing can be helpful in confirming diagnoses or evaluating for concomitant causes of hand numbness such as neuropathy or radiculopathy. In addition, electromyography (EMG) and nerve conduction studies (NCS) can help to localize the site of abnormality based on the site of slowed conduction or the pattern of muscles affected on EMG. This localization can

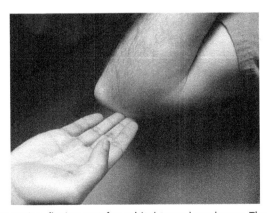

Fig. 6. Elbow compression-flexion test for cubital tunnel syndrome. The patient's elbow is passively flexed with the wrist held in neutral alignment (to avoid any confounding median neuropathy). The examiner then places pressure directly over the ulnar nerve at the posteromedial elbow. Reproduction of paresthesias in the ulnar nerve distribution is a positive test.

Table 2
Physical examination for cubital tunnel syndrome

Test	Sensitivity (%)	Specificity (%)	Positive Predictive Value (%)	Negative Predictive Value (%)
Tinel	98	70	94	87
Elbow flexion 30 s	99	32	93	74
Elbow flexion 60 s	99	75	97	89
Elbow compression 30 s	98	55	92	81
Elbow compression 60 s	98	89	95	95
Elbow compression-flexion 30 s	97	91	96	93
Elbow compression-flexion 60 s	95	98	91	99

Adapted from Novak CB, Lee GW, Mackinnon SE, et al. Provocative testing for cubital tunnel syndrome. J Hand Surg Am 1994;19(5):817–20.

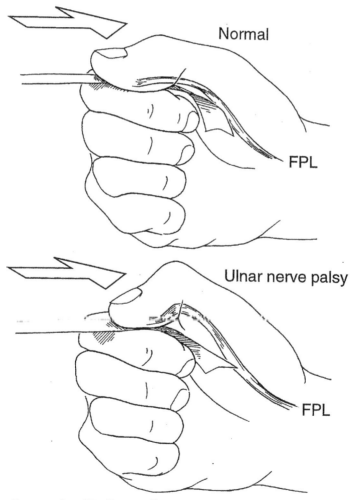

Fig. 7. The Froment sign. FPL, flexor pollicis longus. (*From* Trumble TE. Principles of hand surgery and therapy. Philadelphia: Saunders; 2000. p. 15; with permission.)

be useful in trying to differentiate proximal from distal sites of nerve compression (eg, cubital tunnel vs Guyon canal).

Similarly, the results of electrodiagnostic testing must be interpreted with care, as the clinical picture may not correlate with the test results, with either clinically irrelevant positive findings or negative electrodiagnostic test results in a classic clinical presentation. This scenario particularly occurs in cubital tunnel syndrome, for which electrodiagnostic testing is often negative because cubital tunnel syndrome is a dynamic problem, highly influenced by arm position. As such, cubital tunnel syndrome may be clinically present but not advanced enough to be detected by EMG/NCS. EMG/NCS can be obtained as a preoperative baseline for comparison should symptoms persist or worsen following surgical intervention.

Treatment

Carpal tunnel syndrome

Splinting of the wrist is beneficial, particularly for improving nocturnal symptoms. By avoiding wrist flexion or extension, pressure on the median nerve is decreased. Weiss and colleagues[4] showed that the lowest pressure was measured in the carpal tunnel with the wrist in $2° \pm 9°$ of extension. This finding has been confirmed by multiple other investigators. Wrist flexion and extension have been associated with increases in pressure within the carpal tunnel from 3 to 9 mm Hg to 20 to 60 mm Hg; in patients with carpal tunnel syndrome, resting pressures were 15 to 30 mm Hg, increasing to 150 to 200 mm Hg with wrist and finger extension.[5]

However, there is discrepancy regarding the optimal position and duration of splinting. One study attempted to compare cock-up and neutral splinting. Depending on the interpretation of the data, equivalent results or slightly better results were seen with neutral splints; depending on how success is defined, significant differences can be created or eliminated.[6] A second study compared outcomes between full-time and nighttime-only use; in this small study (24 patients), there was more improvement in distal nerve conduction velocities in the full-time wear group.[7] However, one must be cautious in recommending full-time wear so as to avoid development of weakness, stiffness, or dependence on the braces.

Cortisone injections for carpal tunnel syndrome have been shown to improve symptoms in the short term. By decreasing inflammation within the carpal tunnel, compression of the median nerve is lessened. A recent randomized, placebo-controlled trial showed improvement with methylprednisolone injection in comparison with placebo at 10 weeks. However, relief was temporary and incomplete; three-fourths of patients had surgery within 1 year.[8] Patients who had 80 mg methylprednisolone were less likely to have surgery than those on placebo, and had a longer time to surgery than both patients on placebo and recipients of 40 mg. Patients with more advanced carpal tunnel syndrome (thenar atrophy, 2-point discrimination >8 mm) were excluded; surgery should be recommended to these patients to prevent progressive sensory or motor loss. Injections can also be used diagnostically when the clinical presentation is atypical or when confounding factors such as concomitant cervical abnormality are present.

Cubital tunnel syndrome

Nonoperative treatment of cubital tunnel syndrome focuses on avoidance of pressure over the elbow and avoidance of prolonged elbow flexion. Patient education is key, and explaining the course of the ulnar nerve and the goals of treatment are essential in achieving patient compliance with recommendations.

Ergonomic adjustments include removing armrests from desk chairs to prevent leaning on the ulnar nerve while typing, and assuring that the keyboard is further from the patient to avoid holding the elbows flexed while typing. Use of hands-free telephone headsets or shoulder cradles can be helpful.

In patients for whom pressure on the elbow is unavoidable, such as those confined to wheelchairs, the use of elbow pads can be beneficial.

To avoid nocturnal symptoms, instructing patients to either wrap a towel around their elbow or turn an elbow pad backward so the padding is in the antecubital fossa is an effective way to prevent prolonged elbow flexion while sleeping, and is better tolerated than rigid splints.

Patients with severe symptoms (wasting, increased 2-point discrimination) or who fail to achieve relief with nonoperative measures should be referred for surgical consultation.

HAND MASSES

Masses of the hand can be the cause of pain, numbness, or concern for malignancy. The most common enlargements are ganglion cysts, volar retinacular cysts, mucous cysts, or changes associated with arthritis such as Heberden or Bouchard nodes. Other masses encountered include knuckle pads, tumors, or dermatologic conditions such as verruca. Cysts of the hand and wrist are the focus of this review.

Presentation

Ganglion cysts are fluid-filled masses stemming from the joints of the hand or wrist, which can arise from many articulations; however, the most common locations are the volar radial wrist immediately adjacent to the radial artery and the dorsal radial wrist. Ganglia can occur through either degeneration or tearing of the joint capsule, resulting in an outpouching of fluid from the joint, through a 1-way valve. Their size can increase or decrease, often in conjunction with activity level. These lesions may be asymptomatic but can cause pain, particularly during activity or with pressure over the area. As ganglia enlarge they can exert pressure on surrounding structures, resulting in symptoms.

Cysts can also arise from the sheaths surrounding tendons. Most commonly this is encountered in the flexor retinaculum of the fingers. A small mass is palpable in the flexion crease at the base of the finger. Patients complain of pain when grasping objects, often noting pain when driving, as the steering wheel strikes the hand at the mass.

Cysts at the dorsal DIP are given the name mucous cysts, which develop from arthritic changes and osteophytes in the underlying joint. Complaints may be simply cosmetic, or pain related. The cyst can exert pressure on the germinal matrix, resulting in fingernail ridging distal to the mass. The skin overlying mucous cysts can be markedly thin, and spontaneous drainage can occur. Increasing redness or pain may represent an infected mucous cyst. This may be managed with antibiotics, although these cases should be referred urgently because progressive infection can result in septic arthritis of the underlying DIP.

Physical Examination

On examination ganglia are smooth, mildly tender masses, which may be single or multilobular. Dorsal wrist ganglia are typically located over the scapholunate interval, and are more prominent with wrist flexion. Volar masses arise between the flexor carpi radialis and radial artery, and are more noticeable with wrist extension. Transillumination can help to differentiate solid and cystic masses. Occasionally a patient's history will be consistent with a ganglion, but with no visible mass; a small or occult ganglion may be present. Swelling in the area is typically present; however, diagnosis may depend on advanced imaging such as magnetic resonance imaging or ultrasonography.

Volar retinacular cysts are firm, small masses in the flexion crease at the base of the finger. These cysts do not move with flexion and extension of the finger, thus differentiating enlargement of the tendon itself from these cysts. Tapping over the mass should not elicit electric shocks, as would be seen with digital nerve abnormality.

Mucous cysts appear over the dorsum of the DIP joint, and can be difficult to differentiate from Heberden nodes. Mucous cysts can be more distal than Heberden nodes, resulting in fingernail ridging. The differentiation can be aided by history of enlargement, drainage, or transillumination.

Treatment

Most ganglia are asymptomatic, and reassurance that these are not malignancies is sufficient for many patients. Spontaneous resolution can occur; a recent study showed 42% of untreated dorsal ganglia resolved over 6 years.[9] However, if persistently symptomatic, treatment may be indicated.

Volar wrist ganglia should be approached with care, as the radial artery is located immediately adjacent, and sometimes directly over, the mass. For this reason, it is the authors' practice to not offer aspiration of volar wrist ganglia.

Dorsal ganglia or volar retinacular cysts can be treated with attempts at either aspiration or injection. After cleaning the overlying skin, the subcutaneous tissue is anesthetized with a small volume of local anesthetic. In the case of volar retinacular cysts, local anesthetic should be injected proximally; if injected at the site, the physician may not be able to palpate the mass within the swelling caused by the local anesthetic, and puncture is less likely to be successful. Care should be taken to remain central so as to avoid the nearby digital neurovascular bundles that run adjacent and parallel to the flexor sheath. A large-bore needle (18 or 20 gauge) is then inserted into the mass. Fluid can be withdrawn, or multiple perforations made and a large volume of lidocaine injected into the cyst to "pop" it. Following aspiration or injection, the area is massaged and palpated for residual masses. Dorsal ganglia have a 30% to 40% chance of resolution with aspiration; volar retinacular ganglia are more likely to be successfully treated with injection.

Dorsal injection of mucous cysts is not recommended because of the risk of introducing infection into the underlying joint. In addition, clipping, freezing, or topical treatments are not effective, and can result in skin breakdown or infection.

Surgery is indicated for symptomatic volar ganglia and symptomatic or recurrent dorsal wrist or volar retinacular ganglia, or for patients who prefer a more definitive intervention or who wish to defer attempts at aspiration/injection. Recurrence rates following surgical intervention vary widely, with rates from 0% to 40% reported in the literature. Surgery may be considered for symptomatic mucous cysts or unacceptable cosmesis; typically reassurance is adequate. An infected mucous cyst should be referred for urgent evaluation by a hand surgeon, owing to the possibility of septic arthritis of the underlying DIP.

TENDINOPATHIES
Trigger Finger

Presentation
Stenosing tenosynovitis is hypertrophy and narrowing of the flexor sheath, typically the A1 pulley, which results in rubbing against the flexor tendon. In its earliest stages, stenosing tenosynovitis presents with pain and difficulty in fully flexing the digit. Pain

can be volar, or can also be dorsal because of overexertion of the extensors to overcome the increased friction of the flexor tendons. As the tendon becomes inflamed a nodule may form, which can impinge or frankly lock at the proximal edge of the A1 pulley, resulting in painful catching or "triggering." As the trigger worsens, manual manipulation may be required to straighten the digit.

Middle-aged women are up to 6 times more likely than men to suffer from trigger digits.[10] The thumb is the most frequently involved when multiple digits are affected. Patients with diabetes, rheumatoid arthritis, gout, and renal disease may suffer from secondary trigger finger, and carry a worse prognosis. The incidence of trigger digits, the mechanism of which remains unclear, is 4 times more common in diabetic patients than in nondiabetics.[11]

Physical examination

Visual inspection of the affected hand may demonstrate some swelling at the distal palm. Tenderness is often elicited over the A1 pulley. A palpable nodule may be present within the flexor tendon; this can be differentiated from cysts by the fact that it moves with excursion of the tendon. Triggering or locking of the digit may be seen with active flexion; triggering can be provoked by bringing the hand into a full fist (this may be painful in and of itself for the patient) and having the patient clench the fist repeatedly, then extend the fingers. Advanced-stage disease can cause the finger to remain in a fixed, flexed position. It is critical to evaluate for other causes of inability to extend the finger, including subluxation of the extensor tendon, which can be seen on the dorsum of the hand; Dupuytren contracture, which is a painless condition associated with a visible and palpable cord on the palm; and arthritic contractures. Neither Dupuytren nor arthritic contractures are passively correctable.

Imaging

Radiographs of the hand are not required for diagnosis, which is largely based on history and physical examination, although they may be obtained to rule out any other bony abnormality.

Nonoperative treatment

Several studies have demonstrated successful treatment of primary trigger finger with corticosteroid injections, upwards of 95% at 3 months' follow-up.[12,13] Injections have been found to be highly effective in nondiabetic patients with single-digit involvement presenting with a palpable nodule. Injections are also effective in diabetic patients, although success rates are lower.[14] To perform the injection the digit is extended, the metacarpal head is palpated, and a 25-gauge needle is introduced directly into the flexor sheath and through the tendon, down to the metacarpal. The needle is withdrawn until loss of resistance is felt. A lidocaine-steroid mixture (1–2 mL) is then injected into the flexor sheath.

Splinting can be used for patients who decline injections. A consensus does not exist regarding the best method of splinting, but recent studies have demonstrated success with custom-made thermoplastic splints designed to limit MCP joint flexion for 6 weeks.[15]

Referral

Patients with fixed flexion deformity of the digit(s) or continued symptoms despite appropriate nonoperative treatment should be referred to a hand surgeon. Repeat steroid injections can be performed, and surgical treatment options may be discussed.

De Quervain Tenosynovitis

Presentation

Six extensor compartments, which contain specific tendons, exist in the forearm and hand. The first dorsal compartment contains the abductor pollicis longus (APL) and extensor pollicis brevis (EPB) tendons, making the volar aspect of the anatomic snuffbox. At the radial styloid, the tendons run through a fibro-osseous tunnel that holds them against the bone. Tendon entrapment in this first extensor compartment can be a source of pain and disability. Studies have shown that most patients with this disease have multiple septa, or tunnels, within the extensor compartment, which can predispose them to this disease.[16]

Patients present with complaints of radial-sided wrist pain associated with thumb movement or lifting, often of duration of several weeks to months. Middle-aged women are most commonly afflicted. This condition is also common in new parents, brought about by repeated lifting of their growing infants.

Physical examination

Disease of the first extensor compartment can be detected with specific physical examination maneuvers. Tenderness to palpation directly over the compartment is present. Swelling 1 to 2 cm proximal to the radial styloid along the course of the tendons may be seen. The Finkelstein test, reproduction of pain with ulnar deviation of the wrist with the thumb clasped in the palm of the hand, is pathognomonic for de Quervain tenosynovitis. Other sources of radial wrist pain, including arthritis of the carpometacarpal (CMC) or scaphoid-trapezoid-trapezium (STT) joint of the thumb (see the section on arthritis for specific examination), trigger thumb, or radial sensory neuritis, should be evaluated. Radial sensory neuritis typically presents with burning or electric pain in the radial wrist and first web space, and is provoked with a Tinel sign over the radial wrist just dorsal to the first compartment.

Imaging

de Quervain tenosynovitis is a clinical diagnosis; however, when the diagnosis is unclear, radiographs of the hand or wrist may be necessary to evaluate for arthritic changes at the CMC or STT joint, or, in cases of trauma, to rule out fractures of the scaphoid or distal radius.

Nonoperative treatment

Use of a forearm-based thumb spica splint during aggravating activities can provide relative rest to the involved tendons. Oral anti-inflammatory medications should be used consistently for several weeks. Corticosteroid injections have reported success of 62% to 93%.[17] A combination of local anesthetic and steroid can be injected into the first dorsal extensor compartment. The thumb is extended and abducted, and the tendons are localized approximately 1 cm proximal to the radial styloid. A 25-gauge needle is inserted directly into and through the tendons, down to the radial styloid. The needle is pulled back until a change in resistance is felt, and the medication is injected. If relief is short lived, a second injection may be considered 6 to 8 weeks after the first; care should be taken with further injections. It must be noted that this injection is in a very subcutaneous location; patients should be warned of the risk of local depigmentation or subcutaneous fat atrophy. The authors prefer to use dexamethasone for this injection, which in their experience has a lower incidence of depigmentation than other depot steroids.

Referral

For patients who fail to receive sustained relief from splinting or injections, referral to a hand surgeon is recommended. In many of these patients, the APL and EPB tendons are contained within separate subsheaths within the first compartment, resulting in failure of corticosteroid injections. This disorder is seen in 20% to 60% of patients, with a higher incidence seen at the time of surgery for de Quervain tenosynovitis than in the general population.[18]

Arthritis

The discussion of hand arthritis is too vast for this review; however, a few words are offered regarding osteoarthritis of the CMC joint of the thumb, a common source of pain and disability.

Thumb basal joint arthritis (carpometacarpal joint arthritis)

Presentation As with any osteoarthritic joint, patients with osteoarthritis of the basal joint of the thumb present with varying degrees of symptoms and can present with a spectrum of disease. This form of arthritis is one of the most common in the hand after DIP joint arthritis, and is the most common form of osteoarthritis in the hand that requires surgery. Patients, who tend to be middle-aged or elderly women, often complain of pain at the base of the thumb with vigorous activity or with continuous grasping and pinching activities. Opening jars or turning doorknobs becomes difficult. Fine motor activities also become more difficult and painful. Often symptoms occur in the nondominant hand, which is used to stabilize objects during activities. Patients will also complain of and/or present for evaluation for deformity at the base of the thumb. Over time the base of the thumb enlarges owing to dorsoradial subluxation of the metacarpal, and compensatory metacarpal adduction and hyperextension of the MCP joint ensue. This visible deformity worsens with time.[19]

Physical examination In early-stage disease, visual inspection of the thumb appears relatively benign. Range of motion is usually normal. Tenderness at the CMC joint and occasional swelling are present. Translational movement of the CMC joint can reveal increased laxity and crepitus. Observation of pinch can relay subtle hyperextension of the MCP joint with collapse of the joint. These changes become more evident with advancing disease, as fixed deformity can result. As the stage of the disease progresses, the patient can start to lose motion secondary to osteophyte formation. With increasing pain and deformity, loss of strength can also be noted on examination when compared with the contralateral hand. The grind test of the CMC joint, which involves axial loading with circular motions of the thumb metacarpal, indicates CMC joint abnormality **(Fig. 8)**.[20]

Patients can also have concomitant STT joint arthritis, which can also be a source of pain. Physical examination should also include volar palpation of this joint, which is located 1 cm proximal to the thumb CMC joint.

Imaging Standard radiographs of the hand including posteroanterior, lateral, and oblique views are often satisfactory for identifying and diagnosing osteoarthritic changes to the CMC joint. Changes noted on radiographs include narrowing or obliteration of the CMC joint space, osteophyte or loose body formation, or hyperextension of the MCP joint. Stress views of the thumb basilar joint can aid in surgical planning for patients who pursue that route. Radiographs are used to stage disease and also to identify STT joint involvement. A stress view is obtained by a 30° posteroanterior view centered on the thumbs with the patient pressing the thumb tips together.

Nonoperative treatment Success of various treatments is patient dependent and multifactorial. Activity level, stage of disease, radiographic findings, and severity of presenting symptoms all play a role in treatment outcomes. Treatment options include

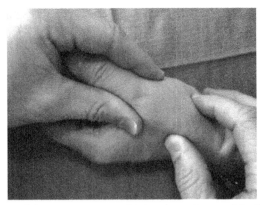

Fig. 8. The grind test of the carpometacarpal joint. (*From* Barron OA, Catalano LW. Thumb basal joint arthritis. In: Wolfe SW, Hotchkiss RN, Pederson WC, editors. Green's operative hand surgery. 6th edition. Philadelphia: Elsevier; 2011. p. 408; with permission.)

activity modifications, thumb splinting, oral anti-inflammatory medications, and intra-articular steroid injections.[20]

Patient education is a key factor in successful nonoperative treatment in the early stage of disease. Once patients understand the origin of the thumb pain, they can modify activities accordingly. For example, using a proper pinch technique to prevent MCP joint collapse and using larger writing tools can help reduce daily symptoms. For patients with more advanced or worse pain, more aggressive treatment with splints and oral anti-inflammatory medication may be warranted. Although specifics of regarding duration of use and type of splinting are not completely agreed upon, starting with full-time thumb spica-type splinting, which immobilizes the wrist, CMC joint, and MCP joint, is a reasonable route. Initially splints should be worn at all times and then can gradually be weaned. A 3- to 6-week full-time trial is reasonable. Oral anti-inflammatory use for 2 to 3 weeks is also an option for adjunctive treatment of symptoms. Patients should be warned of the side effects of these medications before use.[21]

If these treatment modalities do not provide the patient with sustained relief, an intra-articular steroid injection is an option. Because of the degenerate condition of the joint, performing these injections in the clinic setting is difficult and requires expertise. Referring these patients to either a hand surgeon or orthopedic surgeon trained in these techniques is appropriate. Otherwise, referral for fluoroscopic-guided injection into the CMC joint is advised if such services are available.

Referral For patients who continue to have symptoms secondary to their CMC joint arthritis despite a trial of nonoperative treatment modalities, referral to a hand specialist or orthopedic surgeon is appropriate. Often these patients are surgical candidates. A variety of surgical treatment options exist, which can be further discussed between the surgeon and patient as necessary.

REFERENCES

1. Earle AS, Vlastou C. Crossed fingers and other tests of ulnar nerve motor function. J Hand Surg Am 1980;5(6):560–5.
2. Brumback RA, Bobele GB, Rayan GM. Electrodiagnosis of compressive nerve lesions. Hand Clin 1992;8(2):241–54.

3. Novak CB, Lee GW, Mackinnon SE, et al. Provocative testing for cubital tunnel syndrome. J Hand Surg Am 1994;19(5):817–20.
4. Weiss ND, Gordon L, Bloom T, et al. Position of the wrist associated with the lowest carpal-tunnel pressure: implications for splint design. J Bone Joint Surg Am 1995;77(11):1695–9.
5. Werner R, Armstrong TJ, Bir C, et al. Intracarpal canal pressures: the role of finger, hand, wrist and forearm position. Clin Biomech (Bristol, Avon) 1997; 12(1):44–51.
6. Burke DT, Burke MM, Stewart GW, et al. Splinting for carpal tunnel syndrome: in search of the optimal angle. Arch Phys Med Rehabil 1994;75(11):1241–4.
7. Walker WC, Metzler M, Cifu DX, et al. Neutral wrist splinting in carpal tunnel syndrome: a comparison of night-only versus full-time wear instructions. Arch Phys Med Rehabil 2000;81(4):424–9.
8. Atroshi I, Flondell M, Hofer M, et al. Methylprednisolone injections for the carpal tunnel syndrome: a randomized, placebo-controlled trial. Ann Intern Med 2013; 159(5):309–17.
9. Dias JJ, Dhukaram V, Kumar P. The natural history of untreated dorsal wrist ganglia and patient reported outcome 6 years after intervention. J Hand Surg Eur Vol 2007;32(5):502–8.
10. Fahey JJ, Bollinger JA. Trigger-finger in adults and children. J Bone Joint Surg Am 1954;36-A(6):1200–18.
11. Koh S, Nakamura S, Hattori T, et al. Trigger digits in diabetes: their incidence and characteristics. J Hand Surg Eur Vol 2010;35(4):302–5.
12. Salim N, Abdullah S, Sapuan J, et al. Outcome of corticosteroid injection versus physiotherapy in the treatment of mild trigger fingers. J Hand Surg Eur Vol 2012; 37(1):27–34.
13. Peters-Veluthamaningal C, van der Windt DA, Winters JC, et al. Corticosteroid injection for trigger finger in adults. Cochrane Database Syst Rev 2009;(1):CD005617.
14. Stahl S, Kanter Y, Karnielli E. Outcome of trigger finger treatment in diabetes. J Diabetes Complications 1997;11(5):287–90.
15. Tarbhai K, Hannah S, von Schroeder HP. Trigger finger treatment: a comparison of 2 splint designs. J Hand Surg Am 2012;37(2):243–9, 249.e1.
16. Gousheh J, Yavari M, Arasteh E. Division of the first dorsal compartment of the hand into two separated canals: rule or exception? Arch Iran Med 2009;12(1): 52–4.
17. Ilyas AM. Nonsurgical treatment for de Quervain's tenosynovitis. J Hand Surg Am 2009;34(5):928–9.
18. Kulthanan I, Chareonwat B. Variations in abductor pollicis longus and extensor pollicis brevis tendons in the Quervain syndrome: a surgical and anatomical study. Scand J Plast Reconstr Surg Hand Surg 2007;41(1):36–8.
19. Armstrong AL, Hunter JB, Davis TR. The prevalence of degenerative arthritis of the base of the thumb in post-menopausal women. J Hand Surg Br 1994;19(3): 340–1.
20. Matullo KS, Ilyas A, Thoder JJ. CMC arthroplasty of the thumb: a review. Hand (N Y) 2007;2(4):232–9.
21. Barron OA, Glickel SZ, Eaton RG. Basal joint arthritis of the thumb. J Am Acad Orthop Surg 2000;8(5):314–23.

Osteoporosis and Its Complications

Matthew A. Varacallo, MD*, Ed J. Fox, MD

KEYWORDS

- Osteoporosis • Fragility fractures • Vertebral compression fractures • Hip fractures
- Bisphosphonates

KEY POINTS

- At least 10 million individuals in the United States are diagnosed with osteoporosis, and more than half of the United States population older than 50 years has low bone density.
- The 2 most devastating orthopedic complications of osteoporosis are the hip fracture and the vertebral compression fracture.
- Osteoporosis is underdiagnosed in the outpatient setting, resulting in an increased rate of fragility fractures.
- There is a demonstrated overall benefit and decreased fracture risk for patients with osteoporosis who are placed on 3 to 5 years of bisphosphonate therapy.

OSTEOPOROSIS: THE BIG PICTURE

Osteoporosis is a condition in which there is compromised bone strength caused by deterioration in bone mass and quality.[1–4] Consequently, it is predominantly a condition found in the elderly, with 10 million individuals currently diagnosed in the United States.[5] It is estimated that more than 3 times as many individuals have low bone mass and are at risk for the disease.[5] This figure equates to more than half of the United States population older than 50 years.[6] The common manifestation of osteoporosis is the fragility fracture. Roughly 2 million osteoporotic fractures occur each year in the United States.[2] This number is of great concern, considering that those who sustain such fractures increase their chance of having a future fracture by 3- to 4-fold.[5,7] In fact, future fracture risk in the elderly may increase by up to 9.5-fold.[8] For the average 50-year-old Caucasian woman sustaining a fragility fracture, a 40% lifetime risk for a repeat fragility fracture is inherited.[1]

Osteoporosis and fragility fractures significantly compromise patients' quality of life and financially devastate the health care system. In 2005, the direct cost of fragility fractures was $19 billion; a compilation of 2.5 million medical office visits, 430,000

Penn State Hershey Department of Orthopaedics and Rehabilitation, College of Medicine, 30 Hope Drive, Building A, Hershey, PA 17033, USA
* Corresponding author.
E-mail address: Matt.varacallo@tenethealth.com

Med Clin N Am 98 (2014) 817–831
http://dx.doi.org/10.1016/j.mcna.2014.03.007
0025-7125/14/$ – see front matter © 2014 Elsevier Inc. All rights reserved.

medical.theclinics.com

hospital admissions, and 180,000 nursing home admissions.[5,9] Studies suggest that about 22% of patients move to nursing home care within 1 year of their fragility fracture.[10] By 2025, the osteoporosis burden in the United States is expected to grow by nearly 50%, culminating in excess of 3 million fractures and $25.3 billion each year in direct and indirect costs.[9] Despite this obvious burden, current literature demonstrates that there is a significant care gap with respect to diagnosis, treatment, and management of osteoporosis. In fact, rates of follow-up care received by patients experiencing fragility fractures are reported to be anywhere in the range of 1% to 25%.[1,3,5,8,11–20]

FRAGILITY FRACTURES

A fragility fracture is defined as a fracture that occurs as a result of a low-energy force that is insufficient to break normal bone.[2,21] The most common locations for these fractures are the spine, hip, pelvis, proximal humerus, forearm, and wrist.[21] Current estimates state that for the average Caucasian woman older than 50, the lifetime risk of a fragility fracture ranges from 33% to 45%.[1,2,21] The incidence of these fractures increases dramatically in persons older than 65.[2] This fact is particularly concerning given that in the year 2040, the worldwide population of individuals in this age bracket is predicted to increase from 37.1 million to 77.2 million.[22] Thus, a diagnostic protocol that identifies these high-risk patients before they fracture is invaluable. Depending on fracture location and patient characteristics, fragility fractures can present as either acute, debilitating events or as part of a chronic, subtle course eventually leading to a patient's inability to carry out activities of daily living.

Hip Fractures

Hip fractures remain the most serious fragility fractures in terms of morbidity and mortality; about half of these individuals never regain their previous functional capacity.[23] One-year mortality rates are estimated to be in the range of 14% to 36%.[22,23]

Hip fractures in patients with osteoporosis often result from a fall (**Fig. 1**).[2] The nature of the fall must be determined, as these patients often have multiple medical comorbidities; possible causes of the fall, such as stroke, myocardial infarction, or dehydration, must be delineated because circumstances have an impact on medical optimization for surgery. One must also question a history of metastases. Patients often present with groin pain and/or pain with hip motion.[2] Depending on fracture pattern and degree of displacement, the leg will be shortened and rotated.[2]

In general, hip fractures devastate patients' quality of life and place a huge financial burden on the health care system. Most these fractures occur in women 65 years of age or older[22] with or without a current diagnosis of osteoporosis. The total cost of a hip fracture is estimated to be about $40,000 for both acute and chronic care.[23] At present, 330,000 hip fractures occur yearly in the United States.[2] Projected future estimates on the impact of hip fractures on the health care system are staggering. In the United States alone there are expected to be at least 550,000 hip fractures by 2040, culminating in $62 billion in costs.[2] By 2050, when 1 in every 5 individuals will be older than 60, the World Health Organization (WHO) estimates that 6 million hips will be fractured each year worldwide,[24] a striking increase considering that in 1992 there were 1.7 million hip fractures.[25]

Vertebral Compression Fractures

Vertebral compression fractures (VCFs) are very common in patients with osteoporosis (**Fig. 2**). Most cases occur in asymptomatic patients.[26] Reports estimate that

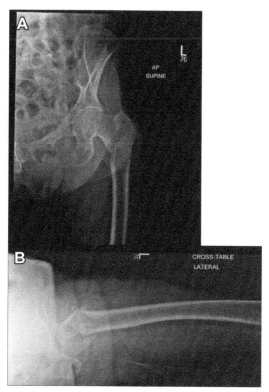

Fig. 1. Anteroposterior (AP) (*A*) and lateral (*B*) radiographs of the left hip, showing a hip fracture in a 94-year-old woman with a history of osteoporosis.

anywhere from 750,000 to 1.5 million VCFs occur yearly in the United States,[2,27] approximately 85% of which are linked to osteoporosis.[28] In severe osteoporosis, the cortical and trabecular bone of the vertebral body weakens to the point where simple activities such as changing postural positions, lifting light objects, or even sneezing can cause a break in the bone.[2,26] It has been suggested that about 30% of VCFs in patients with severe osteoporosis occur while the patient is in bed.[27] Regardless of the mechanism, the theory behind the increased load across the vertebral bodies is due to contraction of the paraspinal muscles.[27] When patients younger than 55 years present with a VCF in the absence of severe trauma, underlying malignancy must be considered.[27]

When symptomatic, a patient with a VCF experiences acute onset of back pain with or without radiculopathy. A list of common symptoms related to VCFs is provided in **Table 1**. However, most patients will either be asymptomatic or will initially overlook the acute symptoms; this is especially true when there is minimal or no pain in the absence of neurologic complications.[26] The chronic and subtle course often turns out to be a debilitating condition that severely limits function.[2,26] VCFs can lead to segmental instability when the vertebral body collapse is greater than 50% of the initial height.[27] Some compression fractures propagate from the initial microfracture in the anterior column of the vertebra, and result in wedging. Others may be due to a larger force of impact and result in failure of the trabeculae, which causes initial collapse of the entire vertebral body.[2] Subsequently the segmental instability increases the load

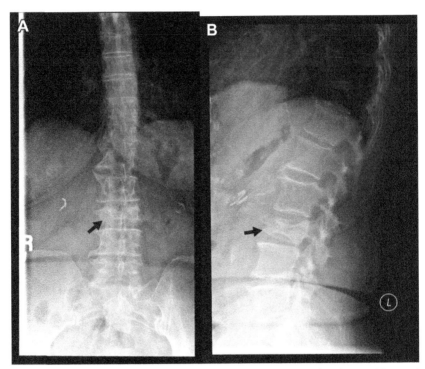

Fig. 2. AP (*A*) and lateral (*B*) radiographs of the lumbar spine, showing an L3 vertebral compression fracture in an 86-year-old woman with a history of osteoporosis.

on adjacent levels. One study suggested that regardless of an individual's bone mineral density (BMD), having 1 VCF increases the risk of a subsequent VCF by 5-fold.[27] Over time, as the kyphotic deformity worsens, contraction of the paraspinal muscles to maintain posture continuously increases the load across the vertebral bodies, and subsequent VCFs occur even after the initial one has healed.[27] This process perpetuates an unfortunate cycle as kyphotic deformity worsens and progressively limits

Table 1
Common presenting symptoms and complications of vertebral compression fracture

Symptoms	Complications
Acute-onset back pain	Low-grade back pain
Back pain increases on postural changes	Thoracic kyphosis and lumbar lordosis
Back pain decreases when lying on back	Decreased pulmonary function, respiratory
Tenderness to palpation over affected level	capacity, and increased prevalence of
Decreased spinal mobility secondary to pain	atelectasis pneumonia
	Gastrointestinal problems, decreased appetite, weight loss
	Disuse osteoporosis
	Deep venous thrombosis due to inactivity
	Low self-esteem and emotional, social problems

Modified from Alexandru D, So W. Evaluation and management of vertebral compression fractures. Perm J 2012;16:46–51.

function, decreases quality of life, increases future fracture risk, reduces lung function, impairs balance, and increases the incidence of falls.[28]

DIAGNOSING OSTEOPOROSIS

Given that osteoporosis is a disease that affects the microarchitecture of bone and that routine bone biopsy is not used in clinical practice, BMD testing is the gold standard for diagnosis. One of the biggest problems that fuels this osteoporosis burden is the lack of a universally adopted BMD screening protocol. There still remains some controversy in regard of how cost-effective such a protocol can be made. The National Osteoporosis Foundation (NOF), in agreement with the US Preventive Services Task Force, recommends BMD testing for all women aged 65 years and older. In addition, the NOF recommends the following individuals for BMD testing: men aged 70 years or older, men or women 50 years or older who have had a fragility fracture, men between 50 and 70 years old with 1 or more risk factors for osteoporosis, and postmenopausal women younger than 65 years with 1 or more risk factors for osteoporosis.[29] Although this remains a legitimate set of recommendations, physicians must also rely on each individual's fracture-risk assessment. The WHO developed a fracture-risk algorithm (FRAX), which is an estimate of a patient's 10-year absolute hip/fragility fracture score. Some of the documented parameters include age, gender, race, body mass index, history of prior fractures, family history of fractures, medication use, and current smoking and drinking history.[23] The diagnosis of osteoporosis is often established clinically once a patient sustains a fragility fracture, and is subsequently confirmed via BMD measurements by dual-energy x-ray absorptiometry (DEXA) of the spine, hip, and/or wrist. A DEXA scan measures the central bone mass, and a patient's T score represents the standard deviation from the mean peak value in the age-matched population. The WHO set a T score less than −2.5 as diagnostic for osteoporosis, with scores between −1 and −2.5 indicating osteopenia and a score greater than −1 being normal.[27]

ADDRESSING THE OSTEOPOROSIS CARE GAP
Barriers to Identification of Patients at Risk

In an era of chronic illnesses, the unfortunate reality is that osteoporosis is commonly overlooked in the outpatient setting. Many patients at the highest risk for osteoporosis often will have some combination of chronic conditions such as congestive heart failure, chronic obstructive pulmonary disease, diabetes, and/or dementia[30,31]; these issues ultimately consume the entire office visit. Thus, not all patients meeting the NOF criteria for BMD testing actually receive a DEXA scan. Furthermore, even fewer are treated for their low bone density.[8,17,23]

There is clear evidence that treatment with calcium, vitamin D, and a bisphosphonate helps prevent future fractures.[8] Despite this common knowledge, the follow-up rates for treatment after a fragility fracture are extremely low. Some of the major barriers to diagnosis and treatment include lack of knowledge and awareness from both the physician and the patient,[8,23] the perception by the orthopedic surgeon that the diagnosis and treatment is not his or her responsibility,[8] low rates of referral to the appropriate osteoporosis service,[17] the cost of therapy, side effects of medications, and multiple medical comorbidities.[8] In fact, one study reported that only 27% of eligible women between 66 and 70 years of age received DEXA testing. The same study reported that only 16% of women between the ages of 81 and 85 received testing, and only 9.7% of women between 86 and 90 years of age had DEXA testing.[23] As a result, not only does the quality of life of these patients suffer but there also is a high cost associated with long-term complications.

Providing Solutions

Given the morbid nature of this condition combined with the overall financial impact on the health care system, more efficient approaches and protocols have been studied and are starting to be implemented worldwide.[1,3,5,8,11–20] Some reports have even detailed the financial savings from fracture prevention versus the cost of implementing such programs.[23] These protocols are geared toward efficiently identifying patients at high risk for osteoporosis and improving follow-up rates in the clinic. By and large, there is a wide range of systems in place geared toward recognizing these patients both in the inpatient setting and in the outpatient arena. Although the programs differ in many ways, the underlying goals are undisputed: (1) improve the efficiency for identifying patients at risk for osteoporosis and enhance the rate of postfracture diagnosis and treatment initiation; and (2) improve patients' quality of life and relieve the financial burden of osteoporosis on the health care system.

Unfortunately, owing to the lack of a universal standardized protocol for BMD screening and the failure to address osteoporosis in the clinic, one of the more common ways to identify these high-risk patients is postfragility fracture. In many ways, these fractures serve as the initial screening protocol to identify those currently not on treatment.

Once these patients are identified, it is crucial that they are managed as efficiently as possible while in the hospital. Quick diagnosis, early medical management, surgical intervention (when necessary), and limiting the patient's stay in hospital all require a cohesive management plan that spans multiple specialties and hospital departments. Bugata and colleagues[2] reported excellent outcomes after implementing a "Geriatric Fracture Program" based on a comanaged care model that has become standard protocol at multiple institutions. The fracture patient is rapidly assessed in the emergency department (ED) and is admitted to the orthopedic surgery service once medically stable. The orthopedic team works in conjunction with the geriatric medicine hospitalist service to assess the candidate's current medical stability, and optimizes the patient for early surgery. Most patients are operated on within 24 hours, and postoperative care follows a standard protocol with the medicine and surgical services. The stable patient is discharged by the third day.[2]

Transitioning to the outpatient setting, the next step is to encourage a follow-up appointment in the clinic for BMD testing. There are reports that less than 30% of postmenopausal women and less than 10% of men with prior fragility fractures are treated for osteoporosis.[19] In general, current literature cites the rate of follow-up care for all patients experiencing fragility fractures as anywhere from 1% to 25%.[3] In a study by Varacallo and colleagues,[3] patients at high risk for osteoporosis were identified on arrival to the ED based on ICD-9 diagnostic fracture codes. An automated protocol was developed that captured patients older than 50 years who visited the ED for a fragility fracture. These patients were sent a follow-up letter after the initial visit to the ED that advised them to follow up with a medical provider to obtain a DEXA scan and directly address his or her risk for osteoporosis. These types of programs are fiscally responsible, easy to implement, and have documented significant improvements in the follow-up rate in the outpatient setting on discharge from the hospital. Another example reported by Sugi and colleagues[19] demonstrated a nearly identical protocol with similar success.

As mentioned previously, osteoporosis diagnosis and BMD testing is often overlooked in the outpatient setting. In today's age of increasing patient medical comorbidities, osteoporosis tends to fall by the wayside. Bogoch and colleagues[8] reported the successful implementation of an Osteoporosis Exemplary Care Program for the education, investigation, and treatment of high-risk patients. A central coordinator was hired to integrate the outpatient fracture clinic, the inpatient orthopedic unit, the metabolic bone disease clinic, and the nuclear medicine unit for the evaluation and management of patients sustaining a fragility fracture. Three hundred fifty-nine patients were identified as at high risk after the fragility fracture and more than 95% were appropriately diagnosed, treated, and referred for care. Vaile and colleagues[20] created a First Fracture Project with a dedicated Osteoporosis Nurse (ON). The ON attended the fracture clinic daily, and ensured that high-risk patients were educated and up-to-date on blood work and BMD testing. The ON also coordinated follow-up with the family physician. Before the intervention, less than 12% of patients were taking calcium, vitamin D, or other antiosteoporosis medications, and new treatment had been commenced in a very small percentage. Only 9% were taking calcium, 11% vitamin D, and 11% bisphosphonate. After 6 months of intervention, one-third of patients were taking calcium and/or a bisphosphonate and one-quarter were taking vitamin D.

In reality, the care for a patient at high risk of osteoporosis can be managed by many types of physicians across a wide range of specialties. If a primary care provider (PCP) is comfortable prescribing osteoporosis medications and monitoring appropriate laboratory tests and DEXA scans, the patient does not need to be seen at a specialty facility. If at any time there is doubt regarding the treatment and follow-up regimen, the patient should be referred to a specialist with an osteoporosis clinic (ie, endocrinology, rheumatology, orthopedics, obstetrics/gynecology). The patient may then be referred back to the PCP for continued follow-up.

Once the gaps that exist between recognition and treatment are bridged, patients' quality of life will improve and the health care system will experience less financial burden; in fact this has already been demonstrated on an institution-by-institution level. For example, Kaiser Permanente's Healthy Bones Program uses a closed-panel Health Maintenance Organization component that has demonstrated efficiency in each of these areas.[2] Furthermore, automated programs are promising, given their potential to be universally adopted at any hospital.[3]

TREATMENT

Treatment protocols have been well established to date. On the most basic level, most adults older than 50 years should be receiving 1200 to 1500 mg of calcium per day. Most are only getting about half of this recommendation.[2] Although there is a modest benefit in fracture prevention associated with supplementation,[32] it is important to be aware of the risk of routine calcium supplementation in certain patient subgroups. For example, calcium supplements accelerate vascular calcification and mortality in patients with renal failure, including both dialysis and predialysis individuals.[33–35]

Vitamin D is recommended at 800 to 2000 IU per day or enough to maintain a serum 25-OH vitamin D level of at least 32 ng/mL.[2] The amount of vitamin D required is based on diet, sunlight exposure, age, obesity, skin pigmentation, concurrent medication use, and time of year. Older adults require 2000 IU.[2] Several trials have shown that inadequate intake of calcium and vitamin D is an important risk factor for developing osteoporosis and experiencing fragility fractures.[21] Patients experiencing low-energy hip fractures have demonstrated a 70% to 90% vitamin D insufficiency rate.[2] Vitamin D can also improve parameters beyond bone strength. One study noted its effect on balance, lower extremity muscle strength, gait speed, and performance in individuals older than 65 years.[36]

Beyond basic supplements, there are many different categories of medications approved for the treatment of osteoporosis (**Tables 2** and **3**). Each category fulfills some component of maintaining bone mass, limiting bone loss, and reducing fracture risk.[2]

Bisphosphonates are the most commonly prescribed medication.[37] These agents are hydroxyapatite analogues that directly deposit into bone and interfere with osteoclast bone resorptive function, and ultimately induce their apoptosis.[4] In 1995, alendronate became the first bisphosphonate to be approved by the Food and Drug Administration (FDA) for the treatment of osteoporosis.[4] The Fracture Intervention Trial (FIT) reported a relative risk reduction for all fractures across all age groups,[38] and another found BMD measurements to improve at both the spine and hip in elderly women residing in long-term care facilities.[39] There is a plethora of evidence reporting that the use of bisphosphonates results in reduction of fracture risk. However, there is some variation when comparing different types of bisphosphonates, the fragility fractures they help prevent, and the patient populations for which they have demonstrated efficacy (see **Table 3**). For example, alendronate, risedronate, and ibandronate all reduce the incidence of vertebral fractures (see **Table 3**).[29] However, alendronate and risedronate are approved for both prevention and treatment of osteoporosis in men and postmenopausal women, and in osteoporosis secondary to excessive glucocorticoids; ibandronate is only approved for treatment in postmenopausal women (see **Table 2**).[29]

Beyond bisphosphonates, selective estrogen receptor modulators are also approved for the treatment of osteoporosis; raloxifene was the first on the market. The Multiple Outcomes of Raloxifene Evaluation (MORE) trial demonstrated a decrease in the risk of vertebral fractures.[40]

Teriparatide is the lone anabolic agent. A recombinant form of parathyroid hormone (PTH), this agent primarily stimulates osteoblasts to produce bone.[2,4] Because persistently high levels of PTH or a continuous infusion of PTH favors bone resorption,[41] teriparatide is FDA-approved as a once-weekly injection for use in patients at high risk for osteoporotic fracture. Unlike bisphosphonates, the protective effects of PTH begin to

Table 2
Indications for bone-active agents approved by the Food and Drug Administration (FDA)

Drug	Postmenopausal Osteoporosis		Glucocorticoid-Induced Osteoporosis		Men
	Prevention	Treatment	Prevention	Treatment	
Estrogen	X				
Calcitonin (Miacalcin, Fortical)		X			
Raloxifene (Evista)	X	X			
Ibandronate (Boniva)	X	X			
Alendronate (Fosamax)	X	X		X	X
Risedronate (Actonel)	X	X	X	X	X
Zoledronate (Reclast)	X	X	X	X	X
Denosumab		X			X
Teriparatide (Forteo)		X		X	X
Risedronate (Atelvia)		X			

Modified from Diab DL, Watts NB. Diagnosis and treatment of osteoporosis in older adults. Endocrinol Metab Clin North Am 2013;42:305–17.

Table 3
FDA-Approved agents and evidence of fracture-risk reduction

Drug	Vertebral Fracture	Nonvertebral Fracture	Hip Fracture
Calcitonin (Miacalcin, Fortical)	X	No effect demonstrated	No effect demonstrated
Raloxifene (Evista)	X	No effect demonstrated	No effect demonstrated
Ibandronate (Boniva)	X	No effect demonstrated	No effect demonstrated
Alendronate (Fosamax)	X	a	X
Risedronate (Actonel, Atelvia)	X	X	a
Zoledronate (Reclast)	X	X	X
Denosumab	X	X	X
Teriparatide (Forteo)	X	X	No effect demonstrated

a Evidence for effect, but not currently an FDA-approved indication.

Modified from Diab DL, Watts NB. Diagnosis and treatment of osteoporosis in older adults. Endocrinol Metab Clin North Am 2013;42:305–17.

decline shortly after discontinuation of therapy, and use of the former before use of the latter has been demonstrated to delay the anabolic response of teriparatide. However, currently it remains difficult to obtain insurance coverage for teriparatide until a treatment course of bisphosphonates is attempted.[42]

BISPHOSPHONATE COMPLICATIONS AND THE ATYPICAL FEMUR FRACTURE

Bisphosphonates directly inhibit osteoclast function and halt bone turnover.[43] As with any medication, there is an inherent risk of side effects. Two major clinical side effects related to bisphosphonate therapy are osteonecrosis of the jaw and the atypical femur fracture. Although a detailed review of the former is beyond the scope of this discussion, bisphosphonate-related osteonecrosis of the jaw (BRONJ) is a rare yet devastating complication first reported in the literature in 2003.[44] According to a systematic review of the literature by Woo and colleagues,[44] the most important predisposing risk factors for developing BRONJ are the type, dose, and route of administration of the bisphosphonate, and a history of trauma, dental surgery, or dental infection. Ninety-four percent of cases involved intravenous administration of primarily pamidronate and zoledronic acid. Furthermore, 85% of patients were receiving high-dose therapy for multiple myeloma or metastatic breast cancer. The dosing for oncologic indications is up to 12 times higher than doses used for osteoporosis. The oral lesions associated with BRONJ were documented as early as 4 months and up to 39 months after treatment induction.

Bisphosphonates have long been praised for their ability to improve BMD scores and reduce the risk for fragility fracture.[45] However, safety and efficacy have only been rigorously evaluated in short-term studies over a 3- to 5-year time period.[43] Beyond 5 years, the evidence for benefit against nonvertebral fractures is limited; recent literature has highlighted reports of atypical femur fractures with prolonged bisphosphonate therapy. This finding is thought to be related to severely suppressed bone turnover rates and decreased mineralization.[37] In normal bone physiology, cyclic loading leads to the accumulation of microdamage in bone. Such microdamage normally would stimulate bone remodeling. Prolonged suppression of bone turnover via bisphosphonate therapy is believed to play a part in the susceptibility of these bones to fracture.[46]

The femur is the only bone reported in the literature to fracture from prolonged bisphosphonate use. The classic atypical fracture affects the subtrochanteric or diaphyseal region following a low-energy trauma, and displays a distinct morphology characterized radiographically (**Fig. 3**C).[45–47] This fracture differs from typical hip fractures found in the femoral neck, trochanteric, and intertrochanteric regions of the femur.[6] Atypical fractures demonstrate simple transverse or oblique, noncomminuted patterns with a medial spike and lateral cortical thickening.[46] Furthermore, they often occur bilaterally, may clinically present as anterior thigh pain in the prodrome, and often lack inciting trauma (see **Fig. 3**B, C).[48] In 2009, the American Society of Bone and Mineral Research rendered a task force that reviewed all available data correlating bisphosphonate use with these fractures, and the committee decided on major and minor criteria and radiographic features that would improve the identification and characterization of these atypical femur fractures (**Box 1**).[49]

Much attention should be given to the patient presenting with mild thigh discomfort while on bisphosphonates. Anterior thigh pain can be associated with a periosteal stress reaction before the fracture (see **Fig. 3**B).[46] These patients can present in the clinic weeks to months before sustaining the complete fracture (see **Fig. 3**C).[45] However, not all patients will present in this fashion, and currently there are no clinical criteria to aid the physician in early detection of fractures in asymptomatic patients.[45]

Studies have shown that the incidence of atypical femur fractures while on bisphosphonate therapy is relatively low. For example, one study demonstrated an

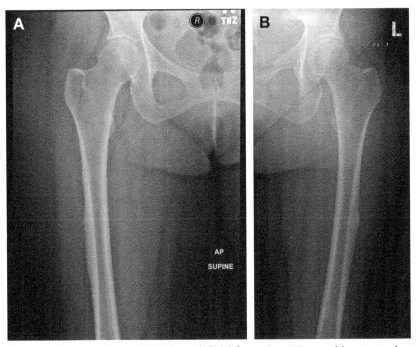

Fig. 3. AP radiographs of the right (A) and left (B) femur in a 55-year-old woman who was referred to the clinic 2 years after sustaining a fall, with continuing pain in her left leg and on bisphosphonate therapy for 10 years. The patient suffered from a bisphosphonate-induced atypical stress fracture (B), and subsequently developed an atraumatic, atypical fracture of the left femur 3 weeks later (C). She was treated with a cephalomedullary nail (D) for fracture fixation. (E) Follow-up radiograph at 1 year shows fracture healing.

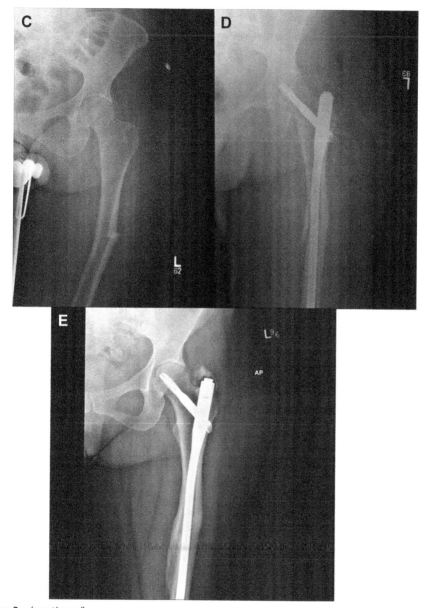

Fig. 3. (*continued*)

incidence of 1 per 1000 patients,[50] and another reported 0.61 fractures per 1000 patients per year. Tamminen and colleagues[47] found the combined rate of subtrochanteric or diaphyseal femur fractures in patients taking bisphosphonates to be 2.3 per 10,000 patient-years. These statistics should be analyzed alongside the expected rate of hip fractures in elderly osteoporotic patients who are not taking bisphosphonates. For example, Dell and colleagues[48] found that the age-adjusted incidence rate for atypical femur fractures was 1.78 per 100,000 per year with treatment duration

---

Box 1
American Society of Bone and Mineral Research major and minor criteria for atypical femoral fractures

Major features of atypical fractures

Location: subtrochanteric and shaft

Orientation: transverse or oblique

Trauma: minimal to none

Other: medial spike when fracture is complete, absence of comminution

Minor features of atypical fractures

Cortical thickening

Periosteal reaction of lateral cortex

Prodromal pain

Bilateral, delayed healing

Concomitant drugs: bisphosphonates, steroids, proton-pump inhibitors

---

of up to 2 years. The incidence rate increased to 113.1 per 100,000 per year when treatment duration exceeded 8 years. Incidence of hip fracture in all women 45 years of age or older in this same study population was 224 per 100,000 per year. This study agrees with previous work analyzing the placebo arms of bisphosphonate trials with treatment durations of 3 to 4 years. Hip-fracture incidence in placebo groups was 750,[38] 833[51] (vertebral fractures), 1390[52] (age 70–79 years with osteoporosis), and 4200[52] (age >80 years with osteoporosis) per 100,000 per year. Thus, hip-fracture rates are reduced by 20% to 50% with bisphosphonate therapy.

Several articles have investigated the appropriate duration of bisphosphonate treatment. As mentioned earlier, the safety and efficacy in the initial 3- to 5-year time period has been thoroughly evaluated, and there is a clear benefit in fracture reduction experienced by patients on treatment. Although no clear consensus has been reached outside of this time frame, individual risk factors such as age, race, BMD, family history, and fracture history will always play a part in the risk-to-benefit ratio. For example, individuals of Asian descent have demonstrated an increase in prevalence for atypical femur fractures.[37] Patients at a lower risk of fracture may not benefit beyond the initial 5 years of therapy.[43,48]

There are situations whereby the decision to stop treatment is more straightforward. For example, a few studies have reported that there is a significant correlation between continued bisphosphonate use after an initial atypical femur fracture and a subsequent contralateral atypical femur fracture. Specifically, one study in California noted that the incidence of a contralateral atypical femur fracture was 41% in patients who continued with treatment for 3 years after the first fracture. The rate in the group that discontinued treatment after the initial fracture was 19%.[53] Another study demonstrated a 70% reduction in the relative risk of developing atypical femur fractures per year after bisphosphonate withdrawal.[36]

Although the incidence of both BRONJ and atypical femur fractures is low, it should be a component of the physician's discussion with the patient in regard of initiating bisphosphonate therapy. The decision to treat should always be based on an educated and informed decision between the physician and the patient. It is imperative to remain cognizant but nonjudgmental regarding the potential for a patient's media-driven bias toward bisphosphonate complications. Education and transparency are essential.

Patients may fail to realize the true benefits of fracture-risk reduction while on treatment, compared with the rare chance of having a devastating complication while on a bisphosphonate. Each patient needs to be educated about the importance of secondary prevention of fragility fractures. Rates of patient compliance and adherence to treatment are already low,[54] and failure to address this aspect of bisphosphonate therapy may further exacerbate the communication barrier between the physician and patient that is a large component of noncompliance.

REFERENCES

1. Bessette L, Ste-Marie LG, Jean S, et al. Recognizing osteoporosis and its consequences in Quebec (ROCQ): background, rationale, and methods of an antifracture patient health-management programme. Contemp Clin Trials 2008;29: 194–211.
2. Bukata SV, Sieber FE, Tyler KW, et al. A guide to improving the care of patients with fragility fractures. Geriatr Orthop Surg Rehabil 2011;2:5–39.
3. Varacallo MA, Fox EJ, Hassenbein SE, et al. Patients' response toward an automated osteoporosis intervention program. Geriatr Orthop Surg Rehabil 2013; 4(3):89–98.
4. Diab DL, Watts NB. Diagnosis and treatment of osteoporosis in older adults. Endocrinol Metab Clin North Am 2013;42:305–17.
5. Ekman E. The role of the orthopaedic surgeon in minimizing mortality and morbidity associated with fragility fractures. J Am Acad Orthop Surg 2010;18:278–85.
6. Gedmintas L, Solomon DH, Kim SC. Bisphosphonates and risk of subtrochanteric, femoral shaft, and atypical femur fracture: a systematic review and meta-analysis. J Bone Miner Res 2013;28:1729–37.
7. Johnell O, Kanis JA, Oden A, et al. Fracture risk following an osteoporotic fracture. Osteoporos Int 2004;15:175–9.
8. Bogoch ER, Elliot-Gibson V, Beaton DE, et al. Effective initiation of osteoporosis diagnosis and treatment for patients with a fragility fracture in an orthopaedic environment. J Bone Joint Surg Am 2006;88:25–34.
9. Burge R, Dawson-Hughes B, Solomon DH, et al. Incidence and economic burden of osteoporosis-related fractures in the united states, 2005-2025. J Bone Miner Res 2006;22:465–75.
10. Salkeld G, Cameron ID, Cumming RG, et al. Quality of life related to fear of falling and hip fracture in older women: a time trade off study. BMJ 2000;320:341–6.
11. Bogoch ER, Elliot-Gibson V, Wang RY, et al. Secondary causes of osteoporosis in fracture patients. J Orthop Trauma 2012;26:e145–52.
12. Byszewski A, Lemay G, Molnar F, et al. Closing the osteoporosis care gap in hip fracture patients: an opportunity to decrease recurrent fractures and hospital admissions. J Osteoporos 2011;2011:404969.
13. Edwards BJ, Bunta AD, Anderson J, et al. Development of an electronic medical record based intervention to improve medical care of osteoporosis. Osteoporos Int 2012;23:2489–98.
14. Harrington T, Lease J. Osteoporosis disease management for fragility fracture patients: new understanding base on three years' experience with an osteoporosis care service. Arthritis Rheum 2007;57:1502–6.
15. Khan SA, de Geus C, Holroyd B, et al. Osteoporosis follow-up after wrist fractures following minor trauma. Arch Intern Med 2001;161:1309–12.
16. Leslie WD, LaBine L, Klassen P, et al. Closing the gap in postfracture care at the population level: a randomized controlled trial. CMAJ 2012;184:290–6.

17. Marsh D, Akesson K, Beaton DE, et al, IOF CSA Fracture Working Group. Coordinator-based systems for secondary prevention in fragility fracture patients. Osteoporos Int 2011;22:2051–65.
18. Rozental TD, Makhni EC, Day CS, et al. Improving evaluation and treatment for osteoporosis following distal radial fractures. A prospective randomized intervention. J Bone Joint Surg Am 2008;90:953–61.
19. Sugi MT, Sheridan K, Lewis L, et al. Active referral intervention following fragility fractures leads to enhanced osteoporosis follow-up care. J Osteoporos 2012; 2012:234381.
20. Vaile J, Sullivan L, Bennett C, et al. First fracture project: addressing the osteoporosis care gap. Intern Med J 2007;37:717–20.
21. Gosch M, Kammerlander C, Roth T, et al. Surgeons save bones: an algorithm for orthopedic surgeons managing secondary fracture prevention. Arch Orthop Trauma Surg 2013;133:1101–8.
22. Miyamoto RG, Kaplan KM, Levine BR, et al. Surgical management of hip fractures: an evidence-based review of the literature. I: femoral neck fractures. J Am Acad Orthop Surg 2008;16:596–607.
23. Dell R, Green D. Is osteoporosis disease management cost effective? Curr Osteoporos Rep 2010;8:49–55.
24. Anonymous. Chronic diseases and health promotion. Geneva, Switzerland: World Health Organization; 2012. Available at: http://www.who.int/chp/topics/rheumatic/en/. Accessed September 1, 2012.
25. Cumming RG, Nevitt MC, Cummings SR. Epidemiology of hip fractures. Epidemiol Rev 1997;19:244–57.
26. Picazo DR, Villaescusa JR, Martinez EP, et al. Late collapse osteoporotic vertebral fracture in an elderly patient with neurological compromise. Eur Spine J 2013. http://dx.doi.org/10.1007/s00586-013-2751-3.
27. Alexandru D, So W. Evaluation and management of vertebral compression fractures. Perm J 2012;16:46–51.
28. Bayliss M, Miltenburger C, White M, et al. A conceptual and disease model framework for osteoporotic kyphosis. Osteoporos Int 2013;24:2423–32. http://dx.doi.org/10.1007/s00198-013-2317-6.
29. National Osteoporosis Foundation. Clinician's guide to prevention and treatment of osteoporosis. Washington, DC: National Osteoporosis Foundation; 2013.
30. Menzies IB, Mendelson DA, Kates SL, et al. Prevention and clinical management of hip fractures in patients with dementia. Geriatr Orthop Surg Rehabil 2010;2:63–72.
31. Brauner DJ, Muir JC, Sachs GA. Treating nondementia illnesses in patients with dementia. JAMA 2000;283:3230–5.
32. Recker RR, Hinders S, Davies KM, et al. Correcting calcium nutritional deficiency prevents spine fractures in elderly women. J Bone Miner Res 1998;13: 168–74.
33. Goodman WG, Goldin J, Kuizon BD, et al. Coronary-artery calcification in young adults with end-stage renal disease who are undergoing dialysis. N Engl J Med 2000;342:1478–83.
34. Block GA, Raggi P, Bellasi A, et al. Mortality effect of coronary calcification and phosphate binder choice in incident hemodialysis patients. Kidney Int 2007;71: 438–41.
35. Russo D, Miranda I, Ruocco C, et al. The progression of coronary artery calcification in predialysis patients on calcium carbonate or sevelamer. Kidney Int 2007;72:1255–61.

36. Wicherts IS, van Schoor NM, Boeke AJP, et al. Vitamin D status predicts physical performance and its decline in older persons. J Clin Endocrinol Metab 2007;92: 2058–65.
37. Unnanuntana A, Saleh A, Mensah KA, et al. Atypical femoral fractures: what do we know about them? J Bone Joint Surg Am 2013;95:e8.1–8.13.
38. Black DM, Cummings SR, Karpf DB, et al. Randomised trial of effect of alendronate on risk of fracture in women with existing vertebral fractures: Fracture Intervention Trial Research Group. Lancet 1996;348:1535.
39. Greenspan SL, Schneider DL, McClung MR, et al. Alendronate improves bone mineral density in elderly women with osteoporosis residing in long-term care facilities: a randomized, double-blind, placebo-controlled trial. Ann Intern Med 2002;136:742.
40. Ettinger B, Black DM, Mitlak BH, et al. Reduction of vertebral fracture risk in post-menopausal women with osteoporosis treated with raloxifene: results from a 3-year randomized clinical trial. Multiple Outcomes of Raloxifene Evaluation (MORE) Investigators. JAMA 1999;282:637.
41. Bukata SV, Puzas E. Orthopedic uses of teriparatide. Curr Osteoporos Rep 2010;8:28–33.
42. Augustine M, Horwitz MJ. Parathyroid hormone and parathyroid hormone-related protein analogs as therapies for osteoporosis. Curr Osteoporos Rep 2013;11:400–6.
43. Hermann AP, Abrahamsen B. The bisphosphonates: risks and benefits of long term use. Curr Opin Pharmacol 2013;13:435–9.
44. Woo SB, Hellstein JW, Kalmar JR. Systematic review: bisphosphonates and osteonecrosis of the jaws. Ann Intern Med 2006;144:753–61.
45. Allison MB, Markman L, Rosenberg Z, et al. Atypical incomplete femoral fractures in asymptomatic patients on long term bisphosphonate therapy. Bone 2013;55:113–8.
46. Saleh A, Hegde VV, Potty AG, et al. Bisphosphonate therapy and atypical fractures. Orthop Clin North Am 2013;44:137–51.
47. Tamminen IS, Yli-Kyyny T, Isaksson H, et al. Incidence and bone biopsy findings of atypical femoral fractures. J Bone Miner Metab 2013. http://dx.doi.org/10.1007/s007744-013-0448-7.
48. Dell RM, Adams AL, Greene DF, et al. Incidence of atypical nontraumatic diaphyseal fractures of the femur. J Bone Miner Res 2012;27:2544–50.
49. Honig S, Chang G. Osteoporosis: an update. Bull NYU Hosp Jt Dis 2012;70:140–4.
50. Schilcher J, Aspenberg P. Incidence of stress fractures of the femoral shaft in women treated with bisphosphonate. Acta Orthop 2009;80:413–5.
51. Black DM, Delmas PD, Eastell R, et al. Once-yearly zoledronic acid for treatment of postmenopausal osteoporosis. N Engl J Med 2007;356:1809–22.
52. McClung MR, Geusens P, Miller PD, et al. Effect of risedronate on the risk of hip fracture in elderly women. Hip Intervention Program Study Group. N Engl J Med 2001;344:333–40.
53. Dell R, Greene D, Tran D. Stopping bisphosphonate treatment decreases the risk of having a second atypical femur fracture. Read at the annual meeting of the American Academy of Orthopaedic Surgeons. San Francisco, February 7–11, 2012. Paper 190.
54. Sale JE, Gignac Monique AM, Hawker G, et al. Decision to take osteoporosis medication in patients who have had a fracture and are 'high' risk for future fracture: a qualitative study. BMC Musculoskelet Disord 2011;12:92.

Elbow Tendinopathy

Michael E. Pitzer, MD, Peter H. Seidenberg, MD*,
Dov A. Bader, MD

KEYWORDS

- Elbow tendinopathy • Tennis elbow • Golfer's elbow • Lateral epicondylitis
- Medial epicondylitis • Elbow overuse injuries

KEY POINTS

- Epicondylitis is thought to be an angiofibroblastic tendinosis and not an inflammatory condition. As such, epicondylosis and tendinosis are more appropriate terms.
- Epicondylosis is a clinical diagnosis and further investigations (radiographs, magnetic resonance images, and nerve conduction tests) are used after a failure of conservative therapy to rule out other clinical entities.
- Most patients improve with time and conservative therapy.
- Corticosteroid injection may reduce pain in the early stages of epicondylosis but has not been shown to be better than placebo for long-term treatment.
- Patients may benefit from a trial of platelet-rich plasma or autologous blood injection prior to consideration of surgical intervention in recalcitrant epicondylosis.

INTRODUCTION

The elbow is a three-joint complex formed by the humerus, radius, and ulna.[1] It allows for flexion and extension of the elbow and flexion, extension, pronation, and supination of the wrist (**Fig. 1**, **Table 1**). The wrist extensors originate from the lateral epicondyle of the humerus, whereas the flexors originate from the medial epicondyle (**Figs. 2–4**, **Tables 2** and **3**). Epicondylar pain is a frequent patient complaint. Commonly referred to as tennis elbow and golfer's elbow, respectively, these overuse injuries are related to sport, recreational, and/or occupational activities.

PREVALENCE

The prevalence of medial and lateral epicondylitis is variable depending on the population. In a Finnish study of 4783 persons, the prevalence of lateral epicondylitis was determined to be 1.3% and the prevalence of medial epicondylitis was determined to

Disclosures: None.
Penn State Sports Medicine, Penn State University, State College, 1850 East Park Avenue, Suite 112, State College, PA 16803, USA
* Corresponding author.
E-mail address: pseidenberg@hmc.psu.edu

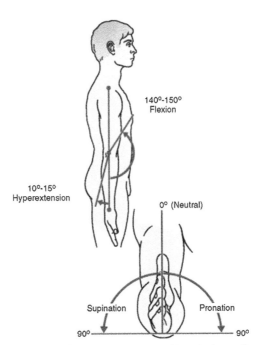

140°-150°
Flexion

10°-15°
Hyperextension

0° (Neutral)

Supination   Pronation

90°   90°

Fig. 1. Elbow range of motion. (*From* Magee DJ, Sueki D. Orthopedic physical assessment. Philadelphia: Elsevier; 2011; with permission.)

be 0.4%.[5] In a recent study of the US military, incident rates for lateral and medial epicondylitis were 2.98 and 0.81 per 1000 person-years.[6] In an occupational health study of 1757 subjects performing repetitive upper extremity movements as part of their occupation, the prevalence of medial epicondylitis was 3.8% (68 of 1757) at the beginning of the study.[7] Three years later this same study found prevalence in the same population to be 5.2% (31 of 598) and calculated the annual incidence of medial epicondylitis in this occupational population to be 1.5%.[7] Lateral epicondylitis has long been associated with racquet sports, and an estimated 10% to 50% of tennis players develop lateral epicondylitis over their careers.[15] Although the incidence of lateral epicondylitis is equal in men and women in the general population, male tennis players are more often affected than female players.[16] Medial epicondylitis predominantly occurs in the fourth and fifth decades with rates in males and females nearly equal, affecting the dominant arm in 75% of patients.[17] Overall, lateral epicondylitis is 7 to 10 times more common than medial epicondylitis.[4]

Table 1 Active movements of elbow complex	
Motion	**Degrees of Motion**
Flexion of elbow	140–150
Extension of elbow	0–10 (hyperextension)
Supination of forearm	90
Pronation of forearm	80–90

From Magee DJ. Elbow. Orthopedic physical assessment. 5th edition. Philadelphia: WB Saunders; 2002. p. 368.

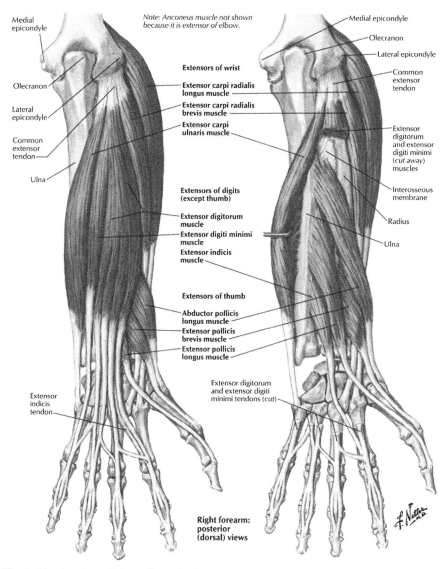

Note: Anconeus muscle not shown because it is extensor of elbow.

Right forearm: posterior (dorsal) views

Fig. 2. Muscles that originate from the lateral epicondyle. (*Courtesy of* www.netterimages. com. © Elsevier Inc. All rights reserved.)

MECHANISM OF INJURY

Overuse and repetitive microtrauma of the wrist flexor and extensor tendons is thought to be the mechanism for injury of medial and lateral epicondylitis (**Table 4**). Repetitive movements with eccentric contraction (muscle-tendon unit lengthening while contracting) increase susceptibility to epicondylitis.[10,14,18] This theory was supported by Van Hofwegen who discovered via computer analysis and magnetic resonance imaging that novice tennis players with improper backhand technique underwent eccentric contraction of very lengthened extensor muscles and suggested the microtrauma caused by this technique to be the cause for lateral epicondylitis.[14]

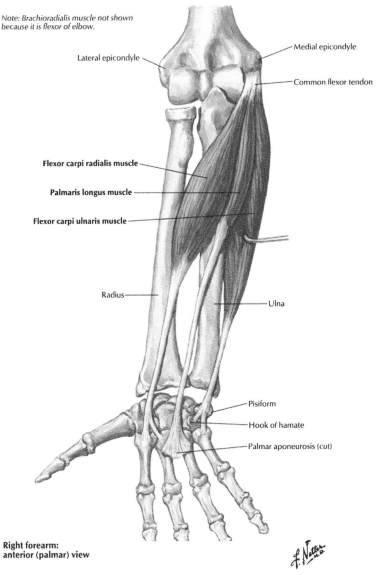

Note: Brachioradialis muscle not shown because it is flexor of elbow.

Lateral epicondyle

Medial epicondyle

Common flexor tendon

Flexor carpi radialis muscle

Palmaris longus muscle

Flexor carpi ulnaris muscle

Radius

Ulna

Pisiform

Hook of hamate

Palmar aponeurosis (cut)

**Right forearm:
anterior (palmar) view**

Fig. 3. Muscles that originate from the medial epicondyle (superficial). (*Courtesy of* www. netterimages.com. © Elsevier Inc. All rights reserved.)

Although lateral epicondylitis is associated with sports involving repetitive movements of the upper extremity, it is also recognized as an occupational disorder involving overuse of the hand, wrist, and forearm.[8–10] In a prospective cohort study of 45 auto assembly workers with known lateral epicondylitis, Werner and colleagues[18] found that older workers with jobs requiring more repetition and awkward wrist postures were less likely to have resolution of their elbow tendonitis.

Medial epicondylitis is less common and, as such, fewer investigations into the mechanism of injury have been performed. However, repetitive wrist flexion during

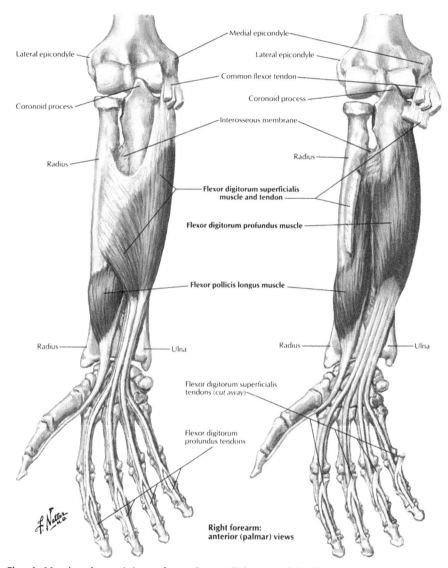

Fig. 4. Muscles that originate from the medial epicondyle (deep). (*Courtesy of* www. netterimages.com. © Elsevier Inc. All rights reserved.)

eccentric contraction is theorized to cause similar tendon injury as has been demonstrated in the common extensor tendon of the lateral elbow.

PATHOPHYSIOLOGY

Despite the suggestive name, epicondylitis is an inflammatory process only in the earliest stage of the disease.[16] Rather, the hallmark of this disease is microvascular damage, degenerative cellular processes, and disorganized healing. For this reason "tendinosis" is considered a more appropriate name for this clinical entity.[19] A microvascular dysregulation and degenerative cause for lateral epicondylitis was first

Table 2
Muscles that originate on the lateral epicondyle of the humerus

Name	Function
Extensor digitorum communis[a]	Wrist and digit extension
Extensor digiti minimi	Wrist and fifth digit extension
Extensor carpi ulnaris	Wrist extension and ulnar deviation of the wrist
Extensor carpi radialis longus	Wrist extension and radial deviation of the wrist
Extensor carpi radialis brevis[a]	Wrist extension and radial deviation of the wrist
Brachioradialis	Elbow flexion
Anconeus	Elbow extension

[a] Injury to the extensor carpi radialis brevis muscle[2] and, less often, the extensor digitorum communis muscle are involved in lateral epicondylitis.[3]

Table 3
Muscles that originate on the medial epicondyle of the humerus

Name	Function
Pronator teres[a]	Elbow flexion and forearm pronation
Flexor carpi radialis[a]	Wrist flexion and radial deviation of the wrist
Palmaris longus	Wrist flexion
Flexor carpi ulnaris	Wrist flexion and ulnar deviation of the wrist
Flexor digitorum superficialis	Digit flexion at the proximal interphalangeal joint (PIP) joint and wrist flexion

[a] Injury to the pronator teres and flexor carpi radialis muscles are commonly involved in medial epicondylitis.[4]

Table 4
Risk factors for lateral and medial epicondylitis

Lateral Epicondylitis	Medial Epicondylitis
Overuse in athletics	Overuse in athletics
Tobacco smoking	Repetitive movement
Obesity	Forceful activity off the upper extremity
Age 45–54 y	White race
Repetitive movement (at least 2 h daily)	Other tendinopathies/tenosynovitis
Oral steroid use	Eccentric contraction
Other tendinopathies/tenosynovitis	
Diabetes	
White race	
Female	
Eccentric contraction	

Data from Refs.[5–14]

supported by reports of pathologic changes in tissue removed at operation in recalcitrant epicondylitis.[20] Very few inflammatory cells were noted in these early tissue samples. Further evidence against an inflammatory cause for epicondylitis came by using microdialysis to study the concentration of substances in the extensor carpi radialis brevis (ECRB) tendon in patients with lateral epicondylitis. Using this technique, Alfredson and colleagues[21] found there were no inflammatory biomarkers in the ECRB of patients with lateral epicondylitis. Moreover, histologic examination of the ECRB in lateral epicondylitis has demonstrated chronic degeneration with few inflammatory cells, many immature fibroblasts, disorganized vascular elements, and disorganized collagen.[19,22] This chronic degeneration and failed healing after microtrauma is thought to be secondary to poor blood supply to the tendons. A 2007 study by Bales and colleagues[23] demonstrated areas of hypovascularity in the lateral elbow and suggested that these areas may lack a blood supply sufficient to generate a normal inflammatory cycle and a robust healing response. Furthermore, in studying lateral epicondylitis from a cellular and molecular perspective, Chen and colleagues[24] found a markedly elevated rate of apoptosis and autophagic cell death in the ECRB tendon in 10 patients with chronic recalcitrant lateral epicondylitis. Overall, based on these vascular, histologic, and cellular findings, epicondylitis is most appropriately termed an angiofibroblastic tendinosis[15] or epicondylosis.

PATIENT HISTORY

Elbow pain is the presenting complaint in patients with epicondylitis. This pain can be acute in onset related to a specific event, injury, or trauma. However, epicondylitis pain is more likely to be gradual and insidious in onset.[16] Initially, the pain is worse with activity and relieved by rest. The pain may or may not radiate down the forearm in the distribution of the wrist flexors or extensors. Patients may experience weakness in the hand or difficulty carrying items.[16] Pain severity can vary with some patients experiencing very mild symptoms and other patients experiencing disabling symptoms. In 1992, Nirschl[15] suggested seven phases of tendinosis pain with the earliest phase being mild pain after activity that resolves within 24 hours and the latest phase having constant rest pain and pain that disturbs sleep.

PHYSICAL EXAMINATION

After a thorough history is taken and the differential diagnosis is narrowed, then a careful physical examination aids in making the correct diagnosis. In considering the differential diagnosis of epicondylitis, a full evaluation of the upper extremity is necessary including cervical spine, shoulder, elbow and wrist. Physical examination of the elbow includes inspection, palpation, range of motion, elbow and wrist strength testing, and ligamentous stability assessment.

Palpation of the lateral aspect of the elbow aids in distinguishing lateral epicondylitis from other pathologies affecting the lateral elbow. Tenderness with palpation of the lateral epicondyle and the origin of the wrist extensor muscles is suggestive of lateral epicondylitis. Care should be taken to determine the distribution of any tenderness because posterior interosseous nerve syndrome may also have tenderness to palpation over the lateral epicondyle that extends into the volar forearm.[25] The radial collateral ligament can be palpated from its origin in the lateral epicondyle to its insertion on the annular ligament and the lateral ulna.

Palpation of the medial aspect of the elbow aids diagnosing medial epicondylitis, an ulnar nerve entrapment or neuritis, an ulnar collateral ligament (UCL) sprain, or a combination of the three entities. Palpation of the medial epicondyle and muscle bellies of the wrist flexor tendons elicits tenderness in a case of medial epicondylitis. The UCL may be palpated from its origin on the medial epicondyle to its insertions on the coronoid process and the olecranon process. Palpation of the cubital tunnel, just posterior to the medial epicondyle, may cause pain or altered sensorium stemming from ulnar nerve pathology.

In examining flexion and extension of the wrist, pain with resisted wrist extension is suggestive of lateral epicondylitis and pain with resisted wrist flexion is suggestive of medial epicondylitis. These findings on physical examination along with the following specialized tests aids in the diagnosis of epicondylitis.

> Lateral epicondylitis test, type 1[26]: The patient should be seated with the elbow at approximately 110 degrees, the forearm supinated, and the hand forming a fist. The examiner should stabilize the patient's elbow with the thumb resting against the patient's lateral epicondyle and should place his or her other hand over the patient's fist to resist motion. The patient is then directed to pronate the forearm. While the examiner resists pronation, the patient should radially deviate the fist and extend at the wrist. The test is positive if the patient experiences pain at the location of the lateral epicondyle (**Fig. 5**).
>
> Lateral epicondylitis test, type 2[25]: With the patient seated and the elbow at approximately 90 degrees, the examiner should position a hand over the patient's elbow

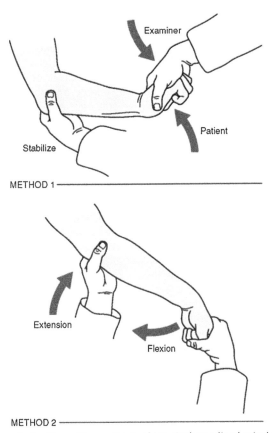

Fig. 5. Tennis elbow tests. (*From* Magee DJ, Sueki D. Orthopedic physical assessment. Philadelphia: Elsevier; 2011; with permission.)

with the thumb resting on the lateral epicondyle. The examiner passively pronates the patient's forearm while the wrist is simultaneously flexed and the elbow is extended. The test is positive if the patient experiences pain at the location of the lateral epicondyle (see **Fig. 5**).

Lateral epicondylitis test, type 3[25]: The patient should be seated with the elbow flexed and the wrist and fingers extended. In this test, the examiner resists extension of the third digit distal to the proximal interphalangeal joint of the patient. The test is positive if the patient experiences pain at the location of the lateral epicondyle (see **Fig. 5**).

Thomsen maneuver[16]: With the patient seated, the elbow in full extension, and the forearm pronated, the examiner actively resists extension of the patient's wrist. The test is positive if the patient experiences pain at the location of the lateral epicondyle.

Medial epicondylitis test[25]: With the patient seated and the elbow flexed, the examiner applies one hand to the elbow with thumb over the medial epicondyle and then passively supinates the forearm of the patient while extending both the wrist and the elbow. The test is positive if the patient experiences pain at the location of the medial epicondyle (**Fig. 6**).

Milking maneuver[25]: With the patient seated and their shoulder extended, their elbow flexed at 90 degrees, and their forearm supinated, the physician pulls on the patients thumb. The test is positive for damage to the UCL with pain in the medial elbow and a sensation of apprehension and instability with this valgus tension. Further information can be gained about possible damage to the UCL if the milking maneuver is performed dynamically. While grasping the patient's thumb, the examiner provides valgus stress to the forearm while moving the elbow through its full range of motion. With this dynamic examination the examiner is able to identify at what point in the range of motion the stress and pain occurs in the UCL (**Fig. 7**).[27]

Tinel sign at elbow: With the elbow flexed, the examiner taps the ulnar nerve as it lies within the cubital tunnel. It is considered positive if the patient experiences tingling in the distribution of the ulnar nerve with this maneuver. Because medial epicondylitis has been found in 60% of patients with ulnar neuritis, it is

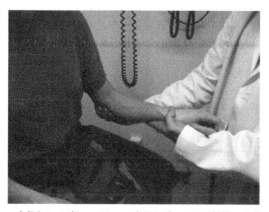

Fig. 6. Medial epicondylitis test. (*From* Howard TM, Shaw JL, Phillips J. Physical examination of the elbow. In: Seidenberg PH, Beutler AI, editors. The sports medicine resource manual. Philadelphia: Saunders-Elsevier; 2008; with permission.)

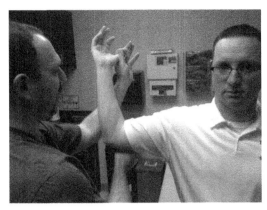

Fig. 7. Milking maneuver.

important to include evaluation of the ulnar nerve as part of the examination (**Fig. 8**).[13]

Elbow flexion test for ulnar neuritis[17]: With the patient seated, the affected elbow is placed in maximum flexion with pronation of the forearm and wrist extension. This position is held for 30 to 60 seconds. The test is positive if elbow pain is experienced with numbness or tingling in the fourth and fifth digits.

IMAGING AND FURTHER DIAGNOSTIC TESTING

Epicondylitis is a clinical diagnosis and further investigations are used after a failure of conservative therapy to rule out other clinical entities (**Table 5**). Radiographs are recommended if the patient presents with epicondylar pain with a traumatic mechanism of injury instead of the overuse pattern that is typical with epicondylosis. Radiographs with contralateral comparison views should be obtained in the skeletally immature patient even with a history of repetitive motion. In this population, growth plates are more likely to be injured than tendons.

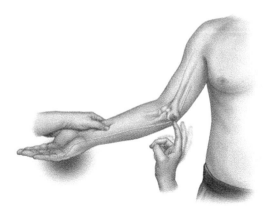

Fig. 8. Tinel sign at elbow. (*From* Waldman SD. Atlas of pain management injection techniques. Philadelphia: Elsevier; 2013.)

Table 5
Differential diagnosis for elbow pain

Lateral Pain	Medial Pain
Epicondylitis	Epicondylitis
Loose bodies	Ulnar nerve entrapment
Posterior interosseous nerve syndrome	Ulnar neuritis
Radiocapitellar osteochondral defect or arthritis	Ulnar collateral ligament sprain
Valgus extension overload	Osteochondritis dissecans
Lateral synovial plica	Little Leaguer's elbow
Cervical radiculopathy	Arthritis
	Cervical radiculopathy

Magnetic resonance imaging is not indicated in the evaluation of epicondylosis. However, in recalcitrant cases, it can be used to rule out loose bodies, osteochondral lesions, and ligamentous injury.

Musculoskeletal ultrasound is gaining popularity in the evaluation of medial and lateral elbow pain. Tendinosis is seen as a loss of the tendon's normal fibrillar pattern with neovascularization visualized with the use of power Doppler. Dynamic examination can be used to evaluate muscle or tendon tears, subluxation of the ulnar nerve, and tears of the UCL.[28] Diagnostic musculoskeletal ultrasound should be reserved for patients with atypical presentations or inadequate response to conservative measures.

Radial nerve entrapment presents as lateral elbow pain that is often confused for lateral epicondylosis. Nerve conduction and electromyography studies are used to help clarify the diagnosis.[29]

TREATMENT

The cornerstone of treatment of epicondylosis is summarized in the pneumonic PRICEMM (*P*rotection, *R*est, *I*ce, *C*ompression, *E*levation, *M*edication, *M*odalities). Protection signifies that the patient should avoid the offending overuse activity that resulted in tendon injury so as to prevent further damage. Rest is better termed relative rest, because therapeutic exercise can help heal the damaged tendon. Ice, especially ice massage, can assist in pain control. A counterforce elbow strap can be used for compression. Placed approximately 2 cm below the painful epicondyle, this can help offload the proximal tendon during wrist extension or flexion.[30,31] In addition, a nighttime volar wrist splint can prevent excessive epicondylar stress caused by sleep position.[32]

Medications are used for pain control. Tylenol is first line. Nonsteroidal anti-inflammatory drugs are often preferred by patients but there is debate as to whether anti-inflammatories actually inhibit tendon healing. A short-term course may be indicated to increase comfort so that patients can tolerate therapy exercise. Topical anti-inflammatory drugs are also used but there is scant research on their efficacy in elbow tendinopathy. Topical nitroglycerin therapy has shown some promise but studies have shown mixed results.[33–35] Oral corticosteroids are not indicated in the treatment of medial or lateral epicondylosis.

Physical therapy modalities, such as electrical stimulation, phonophoresis, and iontophoresis, are effective in assisting in pain control but are unable to correct the underlying tendinosis. To accomplish this, exercises are performed on the flexor-pronator group or the extensor-supinator group in medial and lateral epicondylosis, respectively. This includes tendon stretching and strengthening exercises. Progression to eccentric exercises is the goal, because this is thought to reestablish normal tendon architecture.[36]

Use of corticosteroid injections is considered by many practitioners to be safe for trial in refractory cases of epicondylitis. Although epicondylosis is not considered to be an inflammatory disease, increased levels of neurogenic pain markers have been documented in lateral epicondylosis and corticosteroids have been shown to relieve pain of neurogenic origin.[37] A 2009 meta-analysis by Gaujoux-Viala colleagues[38] found evidence supporting short-term pain benefits from injection of glucocorticoids for epicondylitis (up to 8 weeks). Later, a 2013 meta-analysis agreed that corticosteroid injections are successful in providing short-term pain relief that is better than naproxen, placebo, physical therapy, or a wait-and-see approach.[39–41] However, the same meta-analysis found that long-term benefits of glucocorticoid injection were not better than placebo in the treatment of lateral epicondylitis.[41] Moreover, there is concern that the temporary pain relief by corticosteroid injections might weaken the wrist flexor or extensor tendons or allow patients to further aggravate their tendinosis. This was supported by Smidt's study, which discovered worse outcomes at 1 year of follow-up with corticosteroid injections for epicondylitis compared with no intervention or physiotherapy.[40] Overall, glucocorticoid injections are reasonable for use in severe epicondylitis pain, but the natural course of epicondylar disease may be unaltered or potentially worsened by this intervention.

Autologous blood injections and platelet-rich plasma (PRP) injections have been used to treat epicondylitis, and the results are promising but inconsistent.[42–46] These injections may be performed with or without ultrasound guidance. The success of these treatments couples well with a hypovascular and noninflammatory cause to epicondylitis. Both autologous blood injections and PRP injections are thought to use platelet-derived growth factors and angiogenic mediators to aid in the healing response by recruiting vascularity to the damage tissue.[23] Historically, forcefully releasing the tendinous insertion at the lateral epicondyle[47] and percutaneous release of the ECRB tendon[48] improved outcomes in cases of refractory epicondylitis, and now these practices are thought to have been successful because of the degree of bleeding in the affected areas and the mitomorphogenic properties of blood.[43] In a study of 28 patients who failed prolonged conservative treatment, 79% had complete relief of lateral epicondylitis pain after autologous blood injection therapy. The average time to maximal benefit was 3 weeks, which is consistent with a healing process, but some patients required up to 8 weeks to achieve maximal benefit from a single injection.[43] In a 2006 study by Suresh and colleagues,[44] 20 patients with refractory medial epicondylitis with symptom duration of 12 months underwent rigorous dry needling to fenestrate the tendon causing local bleeding and fibril disruption before autologous blood injection. Overall, this study showed a significant improvement in pain scores and reported only treatment failure in three patients.[44] In another small study that compared PRP injections with bupivacaine injections, after 8 weeks 60% of patients treated with PRP injection had improvements in pain scores compared with only 16% of the patients treated with bupivacaine. More impressively, at 6 months there was an 81% improvement in pain scores in the PRP-treated group and a 93% improvement in pain scores at final follow-up.[45] The results of this study and other autologous blood and PRP studies show promise in the treatment of epicondylosis. However, a recent meta-analysis found the studies on PRP and autologous blood injections to likely be highly biased toward favoring the procedure.[41] For this reason and because of the inconsistent response to autologous blood injections and PRP in prior studies, more work is needed to determine the true benefit of this intervention in epicondylosis.

Botulinum toxin has been studied as a treatment of epicondylosis. The rationale for its use comes from the reversible inhibition of muscle contraction by blocking the neuromuscular end plates and prevention of repetitive microtrauma.[49] Botulinum toxin A may also have direct analgesic properties.[50] Injection of botulinum toxin A into the origin of the forearm extensor muscles in the treatment of lateral epicondylosis was first reported in a trial of 14 patients in 1997.[51] In this study, there was a significant reduction in pain from lateral epicondylosis; however, side effects of weakness in the extensors of the third and fourth digits were also noted. Several studies have shown pain reduction with this treatment method.[49,52,53] The evidence of using botulinum toxin A in the treatment of epicondylosis remains controversial because other studies have not shown long-term improvement in pain, grip strength, or quality of life.[54] Kalichman and colleagues[55] reviewed 10 studies on the use of botulinum toxin A injections for treatment of chronic lateral epicondylosis through November 2009 and found a moderate benefit to this treatment. A later meta-analysis suggested that the noted benefits from botulinum toxin A should be viewed cautiously. The analysis determined the results to be unreliable and reported lacking data on maximum grip strength, pain during maximum grip, and on function and quality of life.[41]

Extracorporeal shock wave therapy (ECSWT) has been used in the treatment of lateral epicondylosis that is refractory to conservative treatment. The procedure uses acoustic waves to treat tendinosis. The exact mechanism of action for ECSWT is unknown but is thought to be caused by the activation of the inflammatory cycle, release of local growth factors, and the recruitment of appropriate stem cells to the affected area.[56] A 2005 randomized, double-blind, placebo-controlled study of 114 patients found a 50% pain reduction in most patients in the active treatment group at 12 weeks of follow-up.[57] The authors of this study concluded that ECSWT can significantly improve pain scores, functional scores, and a patient's subjective impression of epicondylosis.[57] Similarly, a study in 2005 concluded that ECSWT reduced pain and functional impairment, and increased pain-free grip strength in lateral epicondylitis.[58] However, other studies have not found benefit of ECSWT over placebo.[59,60] A recent systematic review of ECSWT concluded that there was little to no benefit from this procedure in the treatment of lateral elbow pain.[61]

Prolotherapy is a complementary therapy that involves the injection of a local irritant into ligamentous or tendinous attachments in peppering fashion to elicit an inflammatory response and lead to induction of tissue growth factors.[62] It has been used in common chronic musculoskeletal conditions including tendinopathy, knee osteoarthritis, and low back pain.[63] The most common injectant is dextrose 15%.[63] There are few trials of prolotherapy as an intervention in epicondylosis, but in a study of 24 adults with at least 6 months of refractory lateral epicondylosis, prolotherapy with 50% dextrose and 5% sodium morrhuate had a significant improvement in pain scores compared with baseline and compared with a control group at 16 weeks postinjection. In addition, clinical improvement in the prolotherapy subjects was maintained at 52 weeks follow-up.[64,65] Further work is needed to determine the value of prolotherapy in epicondylosis.

ECSWT, autologous blood injections, prolotherapy, and PRP treatments are less invasive interventions than surgery and are extensions of more conservative therapies. Surgical interventions can be considered if these therapies fail. Open, arthroscopic, and percutaneous release are all surgical options in recalcitrant cases of lateral epicondylosis.

Patients with epicondylosis who have failed the above mentioned conservative therapies warrant further evaluation with the previously mentioned diagnostic studies. If the diagnosis is confirmed as tendinosis, the patient may benefit from surgical debridement of the diseased tendons.

REFERENCES

1. Sarwark JF. Essentials of musculoskeletal care. 4th edition. Rosemont (IL): American Academy of Orthopaedic Surgeons; 2010. p. 345–6.
2. Nirschl RP. Prevention and treatment of elbow and shoulder injuries in the tennis player. Clin Sports Med 1998;7:289–308.
3. LaBelle H, Guidbert R, Joncas J, et al. Lack of scientific evidence for the treatment of lateral epicondylitis of the elbow. An attempted meta-analysis. J Bone Joint Surg Br 1992;74:646–51.
4. Leach RE, Miller JK. Lateral and medial epicondylitis of the elbow. Clin Sports Med 1987;6:59–72.
5. Shiri R, Viikari-Juntura E, Varonen H, et al. Prevalence and determinants of lateral and medial epicondylitis: a population study. Am J Epidemiol 2006; 164:1065–74.
6. Wolf JM, Mountcastle S, Burks R, et al. Epidemiology of lateral and medial epicondylitis in a military population. Mil Med 2010;175(5):336–9.
7. Descatha A, Leclerc A, Chastang JF, et al. Medial epicondylitis in occupational settings: prevalence, incidence, and associated risk factors. J Occup Environ Med 2003;45:993–1001.
8. Gruchow HW, Pelletier D. An epidemiologic study of tennis elbow. Incidence, recurrence, and effectiveness of prevention strategies. Am J Sports Med 1979;7:234–8.
9. Szabo SJ, Savoie FH, Field LD, et al. Tendinosis of the extensor carpi radialis brevis: an evaluation of three methods of operative treatment. J Shoulder Elbow Surg 2006;15:721–7.
10. Croisier JL, Foidart-Dessalle M, Tinant F, et al. An isokinetic eccentric programme for the management of chronic lateral epicondylar tendinopathy. Br J Sports Med 2007;41:269–75.
11. Titchener AG, Fakis A, Tambe AA, et al. Risk factors in lateral epicondylitis (tennis elbow): a case-control study. J Hand Surg Eur Vol 2013;38(2):159–64.
12. Gabel GT, Morrey BF. Operative treatment of medial epicondylitis. Influence of concomitant ulnar neuropathy at the elbow. J Bone Joint Surg Am 1995;77:1065–9.
13. Field LD, Savoie FH. Common elbow injuries in sport. Sports Med 1998;26: 193–205.
14. Riek S, Chapman AE, Milner T. A simulation of muscle force and internal kinematics of extensor carpi radialis brevis during backhand tennis stroke: implications for injury. Clin Biomech 1999;14:477–83.
15. Nirschl RP. Elbow tendinosis/tennis elbow. Clin Sports Med 1992;11:851–70.
16. Van Hofwegen C, Baker CL III, Baker CL Jr. Epicondylitis in the athlete's elbow. Clin Sports Med 2010;29:577–97.
17. Ciccotti MG. Diagnosis and treatment of medial epicondylitis of the elbow. Clin Sports Med 2004;23:693–705.
18. Werner RA, Franzblau A, Gell N, et al. Predictors of persistent elbow tendonitis among auto assembly workers. J Occup Rehabil 2005;15:393–400.
19. Kraushaar BS, Nirschl RP. Tendinosis of the elbow (tennis elbow). Clinical features and findings of histological, immunohistochemical, and electron microscopy studies. J Bone Joint Surg Am 1999;81:259–78.
20. Coonrad RW, Hooper WR. Tennis elbow: its course, natural history, conservative and surgical management. J Bone Joint Surg Am 1973;55:1177–82.
21. Alfredson H, Ljung BO, Thorsen K, et al. In vivo investigation of ECRB tendons with microdialysis technique: no signs of inflammation but high amounts of glutamate in tennis elbow. Acta Orthop Scand 2000;71(5):475–9.

22. Nirschl RP, Pettrone FA. Tennis elbow: the surgical treatment of lateral epicondylitis. J Bone Joint Surg Am 1979;61:832–9.
23. Bales CP, Placzek JD, Malone KJ, et al. Microvascular supply of the lateral epicondyle and common extensor origin. J Shoulder Elbow Surg 2007;16:497–501.
24. Chen J, Wang A, Xu J, et al. In chronic lateral epicondylitis, apoptosis and autophagic cell death occur in the extensor carpi radialis brevis tendon. J Shoulder Elbow Surg 2010;19:355–62.
25. Howard TM, Shaw JL, Phillips JP. Physical examination of the elbow: the sports medicine resource manual. In: Seidenberg PH, Beutler AI, editors. The Sports Medicine Resource Manual. Philadelphia: Saunders; 2008. p. 75–8.
26. Magee DJ. Elbow. Orthopedic physical assessment. 5th edition. Philadelphia: WB Saunders; 2002. p. 361–95.
27. Callaway GH, Field LD, Deng XH, et al. Biomechanical evaluation of the medial collateral ligament of the elbow. J Bone Joint Surg Am 1997;79(8):1223–31.
28. Radunovic G, Vlad V, Micu MC, et al. Ultrasound assessment of the elbow. Med Ultrasound 2012;14(2):141–6.
29. Lubahn JD, Cermak MB. Uncommon nerve compression syndromes of the upper extremity. J Am Acad Orthop Surg 1998;6(6):378–86.
30. Ng GY, Chan HL. The immediate effects of tension of counterforce forearm brace on neuromuscular performance of the wrist extensor muscles in subjects with lateral humeral epicondylosis. J Orthop Sports Phys Ther 2004;34(2):72–8.
31. Groppel JL, Nirschl RP. A mechanical and electromyographical analysis of the effects of various joint counterforce braces on the tennis player. Am J Sports Med 1986;14(3):195–200.
32. Garg R, Adamson GJ, Dawson PA, et al. A prospective randomized study comparing a forearm strap brace versus a wrist splint for the treatment of lateral epicondylitis. J Shoulder Elbow Surg 2010;19(4):508–12.
33. Paoloni J, Appleyard R, Nelson J, et al. Topical nitric oxide application in the treatment of chronic extensor tendinosis at the elbow: a randomized, double-blinded, placebo-controlled clinical trial. Am J Sports Med 2003;31:915–20.
34. McCallum S, Paoloni J, Murrell G. Five-year prospective comparison study of topical glyceryl trinitrate treatment of chronic lateral epicondylitis at the elbow. Br J Sports Med 2011;45:416–20.
35. Paoloni JA, Murrell GA, Burch RM, et al. Randomized, double-blind, placebo-controlled clinical trial of a new topical glyceryl trinitrate patch for chronic lateral epicondylosis. Br J Sports Med 2009;43:299–302.
36. Stanish WD, Rubinovich RM, Curwin S. Eccentric exercise in chronic tendinitis. Clin Orthop Relat Res 1986;(208):65–8.
37. Ljung BO, Alfredson H, Forsgren S. Neurokinin 1-receptors and sensory neuropeptides in tendon insertions at the medial and lateral epicondyles of the humerus. Studies on tennis elbow and medial epicondylalgia. J Orthop Res 2004; 22(2):321–7.
38. Gaujoux-Viala C, Dougados M, Gossec L. Efficacy and safety of steroid injections for shoulder and elbow tendonitis: a meta-analysis of randomised controlled trials. Ann Rheum Dis 2009;68:1843–9.
39. Hay EM, Paterson SM, Lewis M, et al. Pragmatic randomised controlled trial of local corticosteroid injection and naproxen for treatment of lateral epicondylitis of elbow in primary care. BMJ 1999;319:964–8.
40. Smidt N, Van der Windt DA, Assendelft WJ, et al. Corticosteroid injections, physiotherapy, or a wait-and-see policy for lateral epicondylitis: a randomised controlled trial. Lancet 2002;359:657–62.

41. Krogh TP, Bartels EM, Ellingsen T, et al. Comparative effectiveness of injection therapies in lateral epicondylitis: a systematic review and network meta-analysis of randomized controlled trials. Am J Sports Med 2013;41(6):1435–46.

42. Goosens T, Peerbooms JC, van Laar W, et al. Ongoing positive effect of platelet-rich plasma versus corticosteroid injection in lateral epicondylitis: a double-blind randomized controlled trial with 2-year follow-up. Am J Sports Med 2001;39: 1200–8.

43. Edwards SG, Calandruccio JH. Autologous blood injections for refractory lateral epicondylitis. J Hand Surg Am 2003;28:272–8.

44. Suresh SP, Ali KE, Jones H, et al. Medial epicondylitis: is ultrasound guided autologous blood injection an effective treatment? Br J Sports Med 2006;40: 935–9.

45. Mishra A, Pavelko T. Treatment of chronic elbow tendinosis with buffered platelet-rich plasma. Am J Sports Med 2006;34:1774–8.

46. Peerbooms JC, Sluimer J, Bruijn DJ, et al. Positive effect of an autologous platelet concentrate in lateral epicondylitis in a double-blind randomized controlled trial: platelet-rich plasma versus corticosteroid injection with a 1-year follow-up. Am J Sports Med 2010;38:255–62.

47. Wadsworth TG. Lateral epicondylitis (tennis elbow). Lancet 1972;1:959–60.

48. Baumgard SH, Schwartz DR. Percutaneous release of the epicondylar muscles for humeral epicondylitis. Am J Sports Med 1982;10:233–6.

49. Placzek R, Drescher W, Deuretzbacher G, et al. Treatment of chronic radial epicondylitis with botulinum toxin A: a double-blind, placebo-controlled, randomized multicenter study. J Bone Joint Surg Am 2007;89:255–60.

50. Mense S. Neurobiological basis for the use of botulinum toxin in pain therapy. J Neurol 2004;251(Suppl 1):1–7.

51. Morre HH, Keizer SB, van Os JJ. Treatment of chronic tennis elbow with botulinum toxin. Lancet 1997;349:1746.

52. Keizer SB, Rutten HP, Pilot P, et al. Botulinum toxin injection versus surgical treatment for tennis elbow: a randomized pilot study. Clin Orthop Relat Res 2002;(401):123–31.

53. Wong SM, Hui AC, Tong PY, et al. Treatment of lateral epicondylitis with botulinum toxin: a randomized, double-blind, placebo-controlled trial. Ann Intern Med 2005;143:793–7.

54. Hayton MJ, Santini AJ, Hughes PJ, et al. Botulinum toxin injection in the treatment of tennis elbow. A double-blind, placebo-controlled trial. Ann Intern Med 2005;143:793–7.

55. Kalichman L, Bannuru RR, Severin M, et al. Injection of botulinum toxin for treatment of chronic lateral epicondylitis: systematic review and meta-analysis. Semin Arthritis Rheum 2001;40:532–9.

56. Thiel M. Application of shock waves in medicine. Clin Orthop Relat Res 2001;(387):18–21.

57. McCall BR, Pettrone FA. Extracorporeal shock wave therapy without local anesthesia for chronic lateral epicondylitis. J Bone Joint Surg Am 2005;87(6): 1297–304.

58. Spacca G, Necozione S, Cacchio A. Radial shock wave therapy for lateral epicondylitis: a prospective randomised controlled single-blind study. Eura Medicophys 2005;41:17–25.

59. Speed CA, Nichols D, Richards C, et al. Extracorporeal shock wave therapy for lateral epicondylitis: a double blind randomised controlled trial. J Orthop Res 2002;20:895–8.

60. Melikyan EY, Shahin E, Miles J, et al. Extracorporeal shock-wave treatment for tennis elbow. A randomized double-blind study. J Bone Joint Surg Br 2003; 85:852–5.
61. Buchbinder R, Green SE, Youd JM, et al. Systematic review of the efficacy and safety of shock wave therapy for lateral elbow pain. J Rheumatol 2006;33: 1351–63.
62. Jensen KT, Rabago DP, Best TM, et al. Response of knee ligaments to prolotherapy in a rat injury model. Am J Sports Med 2008;36(7):1347–57.
63. Rabago D, Slattengren A, Zgierska A. Prolotherapy in primary care practice. Prim Care 2010;37(1):65–80.
64. Rabago D, Yelland M, Patterson J, et al. Prolotherapy for chronic musculoskeletal pain. Am Fam Physician 2011;84(11):1209–10.
65. Scarpone M, Rabago D, Zgierska A, et al. The efficacy of prolotherapy for lateral epicondylosis: a pilot study. Clin J Sport Med 2008;18(3):248–54.

The Injured Runner

George G.A. Pujalte, MD[a,b,*], Matthew L. Silvis, MD[a,b]

KEYWORDS

- Running • Injury • Lower extremity • Medial tibial stress syndrome
- Compartment syndrome • Stress fractures • Achilles tendinopathy

KEY POINTS

- As more individuals participate in running-related activities to improve their health, clinicians need to be increasingly aware of common injuries.
- Training errors leading to overuse are the most common cause of running-related injuries.
- Obtaining a detailed history and performing a focused examination leads to most running-related diagnoses, with imaging reserved to differentiate among diagnoses with similar clinical presentations or to determine the degree of injury.

INTRODUCTION

Exercise is recognized as a fundamental aspect of good health. The risks of being sedentary are numerous, highlighted by the ever-increasing prevalence of obesity in the United States. Approximately 36% of adults in the United States are obese, and an additional 33% are overweight.[1] Clinicians are increasingly recommending aerobic exercise, particularly running, for the health benefits.

The American College of Sports Medicine recommends that all healthy adults 18 to 65 years of age participate in moderate-intensity aerobic (endurance) physical activity for a minimum of 30 minutes, 5 days each week, or vigorous-intensity aerobic physical activity for a minimum of 20 minutes, 3 days each week.[2] Adults older than 65 years have similar recommendations with modification of intensity depending on the person's overall health and recommendations to focus additionally on flexibility and balance.[3]

RUNNING
Introduction

In the past, running was mostly considered an elite sporting activity for competitive men in the United States.[4] However, 10% to 20% of Americans now run regularly.[5]

The authors have no disclosures.
[a] Department of Family and Community Medicine, Penn State Milton S. Hershey Medical Center, 500 University Drive, Hershey, PA 17033, USA; [b] Department of Orthopaedics and Rehabilitation, Penn State Milton S. Hershey Medical Center, 500 University Drive, Hershey, PA 17033, USA
* Corresponding author. Departments of Family and Community Medicine, and Orthopaedics and Rehabilitation, Penn State Milton S. Hershey Medical Center, H154, 500 University Drive, Hershey, PA 17033.
E-mail address: gpujalte@hmc.psu.edu

Med Clin N Am 98 (2014) 851–868
http://dx.doi.org/10.1016/j.mcna.2014.03.008
0025-7125/14/$ – see front matter © 2014 Elsevier Inc. All rights reserved.

Throughout communities within the United States, recreational road races and long-distance running comprise a significant percentage of sports activities. There has been a major increase in the number of road races linked to community celebrations, weight loss programs, memorial events, and charitable fundraising. As many as 30% of Americans participate in these events, and around 20% run regularly for fitness.[6]

The benefits of running are numerous, and they include lower risks of early death, coronary artery disease, cerebrovascular disease, hyperlipidemia, hypertension, type 2 diabetes mellitus, metabolic syndrome, colon cancer, and breast cancer. Additional benefits of running include weight loss, prevention of weight gain, prevention of falls, and improved mood.[7] Vigorous exercise in middle and older ages has been linked to reduced disability later in life as well as a notable survival advantage.[8]

However, running can be a hazardous sport. Every year, 19% to 79% of runners are injured.[9] Fifty percent of runners experience an injury that takes them out of running for a period of time during any year, and 25% of runners are injured at any given time.[5] The patterns of injuries that affect runners as well as the overall demographic of the running community have been changing.[10] No longer are marathons run by predominantly male participants. In 1980, women accounted for 10% of marathon participants. In 2005, 40% of all marathoners were women.[11] In addition, marathons and half-marathons are now run by individuals who do not have the typical body habitus of a competitive marathon runner. Heavier runners are affected by impact injuries at shorter distances compared with elite runners. However, only total running distance (more than 65 km [40 miles] per week) and a history of previous injury have shown strong statistical correlations with the prediction of running injuries.[10,12–15]

Most running-related injuries are caused by overuse. Risk factors for running-related injuries are numerous and generally are classified into 4 categories[16]:

1. Systemic (gender, weight, knee alignment, arch type, flexibility)
2. Running/training related (training frequency, alterations, terrain, race distance, running experience, shoe age, and running pace)
3. Health (previous injuries, medical problems)
4. Lifestyle (sedentary work, tobacco, cross training)

Injury frequencies per anatomic site based on a compilation of running studies suggests that, in order of increasing involvement, runners present with injuries of the (1) lower back, (2) hip and pelvis, (3) upper leg, (4) ankle, (5) foot, (6) lower leg, and (7) knee.[10] In a study of more than 2000 running-related injuries, the most common leg injuries included medial tibial stress syndrome (MTSS), Achilles tendinopathy, and tibial stress fracture.[17] However, the differential diagnosis for leg pain in a runner is broad (**Table 1**).[18]

Table 1	
Differential diagnosis of leg pain in runners	
Body System	**Possible Diagnosis**
Skeletal	MTSS, stress fracture
Musculotendinous	Tendinitis, tendinopathy, calf strain
Vascular	Exertional compartment syndrome, popliteal entrapment, venous thrombosis
Neurologic	Nerve entrapment, lumbosacral radiculopathy, neurogenic claudication
Infectious	—
Neoplastic	—

As more individuals participate in running-related activities to improve their health, clinicians must be increasingly aware of the common injuries encountered. This article focuses on the evaluation and management of common running-related injuries.

Evaluation of an Injured Runner

History

A thorough history is critical for the evaluation of the injured runner. Details such as the location, duration, onset, course, quality, and intensity of symptoms should be reviewed. Timing of symptoms can assist in determining the underlying cause (eg, at rest, or during or after a run). Self-treatments, prior medical treatments, previous diagnostic tests, and exacerbating and ameliorating factors should be reviewed. Sometimes forgotten is obtaining a history of prior surgeries, confounding medical issues, and developmental abnormalities. The clinician should also take note of any medications or supplements the runner has been using. Nutrition plays a role in running injuries as well, especially in female runners diagnosed with the female athlete triad.[19]

A complete history should include review of the injured runner's training habits. Most running injuries occur during a specific change in training, such as running volume, intensity, or equipment.[20] Too much, too far, too often is frequently the problem.[21] Asking questions in regard to weekly distance; changes in training intensity/duration; changes in running surface; surface grade; age of footwear; and recent change in footwear, orthotics, and/or running gait (barefoot/minimalist running) can often help determine the underlying cause of the injury.[16,22]

Physical examination

Clinicians should use comprehensive and focused examinations on injured runners as needed. However, the examination must reach beyond the site of injury. Most runners arrive at the clinic already knowing their diagnosis from previous experiences, from discussions with other runners, or from reading magazines/Web sites. The presenting injury is frequently the result of an inability to compensate for a primary dysfunction at another site.[20] Functional limitations and biomechanical risk factors may be identified through physical examination.

In general, the musculoskeletal examination is best performed with a sequential method that becomes focused when an abnormal finding is noted.[19] Both comprehensive and focused examinations begin with a screening gait evaluation and then observing the runner while standing, seated, lying supine, and lying on one side. A thorough site-specific examination is then performed beginning with active range of motion, followed by passive (when unlikely to cause harm), and then resisted range of motion. Palpation of anatomic structures and specialized tests specific to each body part are then conducted.[21]

Gait analysis

There are 3 phases of running gait: stance, swing, and float. For most runners, running gait begins with lateral heel strike followed by foot pronation during midstance and then foot supination during push-off.[23,24] Proper running gait is critical to absorb the impact of striking the ground, with excessive pronation and/or supination increasing the transmitted force of ground strike through the kinetic chain (muscles, ligaments, tendons, bones) of the lower extremities.[24]

Although running gait is highly variable, certain abnormalities have been associated with injury.[23] Observational gait analysis (eg, patient walking in the hallway) can provide useful information, whereas multiplanar videotape observational gait analysis provides the truest picture of running form.[21] Although gait analysis may help identify underlying biomechanical abnormalities, it remains to be seen whether correction of these factors helps prevent or treat running injuries.

Imaging and additional testing
An appropriately detailed history and physical examination are usually all that is needed to diagnose and treat many running-related injuries. Imaging is sometimes used to assist in differentiating among diagnoses with similar clinical presentations or to determine the degree of injury.[25] Imaging modalities and ancillary tests, such as compartment pressure testing, are discussed later in this article with regard to specific running-related injuries.

SPECIFIC ORTHOPEDIC CONDITIONS ENCOUNTERED IN RUNNERS
Lower Back, Hip, and Thigh Injuries

Introduction
Many competitive runners have hamstring injuries.[26] Running gait is stabilized by the hip rotators and abductors. Leg pain may be referred from the back, and, in runners, it may be caused by degenerative joint disease of the lumbar spine or it may have discogenic causes.

Cause
The mechanism of back pain is commonly related to fatigue and muscle inflexibility. Training that includes a lot of hill running may lead to piriformis, hip flexor, and quadriceps injuries. Biomechanics studies show greater stress on the hip flexors and quadriceps muscles during uphill running. Fast downhill runs may lead to impact forces on the legs that are 4 to 6 times body weight and, as such, may contribute to many leg injuries. Lower extremity running injuries have been associated with hip abductor and flexor weakness. Gluteus medius weakness has also been thought to increase the stress on, and the likelihood of injuries to, the hip rotators and piriformis with running.[10]

Clinical presentation
Muscle strains are the most common injuries in the back, hip, and thigh. These strains usually present as severe pain following a definable event. An overuse event has a gradual onset of pain preventing running or other activities.[27] Vague groin pain affects many runners, and may be caused by a sports hernia, conjoint tendinitis, or osteitis pubis (presents with direct tenderness over the symphysis pubis).

Physical examination
Mechanical back pain presents most commonly in runners, and is characterized by paraspinal muscle tenderness, no bony tenderness, and back pain with passive knee-to-chest stretch, with a negative discogenic examination.[28] The most common thigh injuries in runners are muscle strains, and these present as tenderness at the musculotendinous junction, made worse with active contraction of the muscle.[27]

Work-up
Radiographs may be helpful when diagnosing osteitis pubis, although they are normal in sports hernia and conjoint tendinitis. Running injuries that are not easily diagnosed after history and physical examination may need further diagnostic work-up. Obscure entities such as popliteal artery and nerve entrapments may be in this category.[10]

Treatment
Rest usually helps, and ice massage may help. Nonsteroidal antiinflammatory drugs (NSAIDs) are often used, as well as muscle relaxants.[27,28] The treatment of running

injuries requires a rehabilitation program that focuses on eccentric strengthening of weak muscles related to hip stabilization.

Iliotibial Band Syndrome

Introduction

Patellofemoral syndrome has been surpassed in the latest studies by iliotibial band syndrome (ITBS) as the most common knee problem in runners.[10,29] Lateral knee pain in a runner should make a clinician first think of ITBS, but lateral meniscal injuries, vastus lateralis strain, and popliteus tendinopathy are possibilities as well. The iliotibial band (ITB) is stabilized primarily by the gluteus medius, which blocks dynamic genu valgus and stabilizes foot strike in the stance phase of the running gait.[10,29,30]

Cause

Correction of biomechanical issues such as excess pronation; avoidance of running on cambered surfaces; training changes, including variable paced running; correction of leg length inequality; friction massage of the ITB; and ITB stretches are some of the usual treatments used to address ITBS and address underlying predisposing factors.[10] The overall risk of injuries to the lower extremities in runners seems also to be associated with hip flexion and abduction weakness.

Clinical presentation

Runners present complaining of lateral knee, thigh, and/or hip pain worsened by squatting, jumping, and/or running.[31] The pain is usually described as aching. Many runners notice worsening pain when running down hills and may notice discomfort when ascending/descending stairs.

Physical examination

There may be swelling and marked tenderness along the course of the ITB, especially where it crosses the femoral condyle. Tightness of the ITB is demonstrated when the runner is placed on the side and the affected hip is flexed and extended and the knee does not fall to the table (Ober sign).[31] The Noble test may also be used in diagnosing this condition. Here, the patient lies supine and the examiner places a thumb over the patient's lateral epicondyle as the patient repeatedly flexes and extends the affected knee. Pain elicited especially when the knee is flexed at a 30° angle indicates a positive finding.[31]

Treatment

Physical therapy to help correct hip abductor weakness has the strongest evidence of resolving ITBS symptoms (within 3 months in one study).[30] Foam rollers, ITB stretches, and ice may be beneficial. Running modifications to address risk factors as stated earlier may be of benefit. Corticosteroid injections and/or referral for surgery are rarely required for treatment.

Patellofemoral Pain Syndrome

Introduction

The most common running injury has traditionally been thought to be patellofemoral pain syndrome (PFPS). Beginners and young runners in particular most have this condition. Although PFPS can explain most anterior knee pain cases, suprapatellar and infrapatellar bursitis, plica syndrome, quadriceps and patellar tendinopathy, and partial tears are other possibilities.[31]

Cause

The cause is not known, but the most accepted hypothesis is that the pain arises from articular cartilage degradation secondary to increased stress on the patellofemoral joint.[32] PFPS is associated with lower extremity malalignment (such as from cavus feet) or imbalance (such as from vastus medialis weakness), and weakness of the hip abductors.[16,33–35]

Clinical presentation
Runners who recently altered distance or shoes may be affected within 30 to 60 days of the change. Pain is commonly described as being behind or around the kneecap. Sitting with the knee flexed for a long period of time (theater sign), climbing stairs, and/or running may exacerbate the pain. There may be popping, snapping, or grinding sensations under the kneecap. Minimal swelling may occur. Runners sometimes describe instability or a sensation of the knee giving way.[36]

Physical examination
There may be a small effusion, mild swelling, and peripatellar tenderness. Vastus medialis oblique muscle atrophy may be apparent.[16] The insertion of the patellar tendon may be too lateral, resulting in an increased Q angle.[16] The kneecap may have a lateral J-shift with active knee extension (lateral tracking of the patella as the quadriceps contracts). Applying pressure to the proximal patella while the runner actively uses the quadriceps muscle may cause pain and crepitus (positive patellar grind test).[16,36]

Work-up
On a sunrise radiograph view, a lateral patellar tilt may be noted. A more extensive work-up may reveal other conditions that may lead to anterior knee pain, such as systemic medical conditions, patellofemoral arthritis, patellar dislocation or subluxation, or osteochondral lesions.[36]

Treatment
Addressing factors such as Q angles, pronation, and hamstring tightness to treat PFPS is controversial.[10] There is strong evidence to support using orthotics to treat PFPS.[37] Improved function and pain reduction in PFPS have been observed with physical therapy (PT) and heat-molded orthotics, although there did not seem to be an additive effect of benefits from the two interventions.[38] Weakness of the gluteus medius and the vastus medialis should be addressed with physical therapy. Both closed-chain and open-chain rehabilitation programs are supported by excellent evidence.[39] The use of a patellar knee sleeve may also be helpful.[36]

Meniscal Injuries

Introduction
More recent studies indicate an increasing number of meniscal injuries comprising knee pain problems in runners.[10] Meniscal injuries seem to be the fourth most common problem in runners (mostly in male runners).[17] Runners who continue to run with meniscal injuries have not been extensively studied. Significant meniscal cartilage loss or meniscectomy decreases the knee's ability to dissipate impact. More studies are needed to determine whether osteoarthritis occurs earlier with meniscal injuries treated nonoperatively or after meniscectomies. Studies suggest that runners continue to run in spite of meniscal injuries, although intuition suggests that repetitive weight-bearing activities such as running are unadvisable after such injuries.[10]

Cause
No specific or major event may be recalled that caused the injury. Knee hyperflexion, hyperextension, varus or valgus strain, or twisting with the foot planted are all possible causes.[40]

Clinical presentation

There may be mild to moderate swelling of the knee, joint line pain, pain with extension or flexion, and/or locking and catching of the knee.[40]

Physical examination

There may be an effusion, joint line tenderness, and pain with passive range-of-motion testing. The McMurray test may be positive: with the patient supine, the hip is flexed, the knee maximally flexed, and the examiner internally or externally rotates the tibia while exerting a varus or a valgus force, feeling for a painful pop. With the patient supine, the knee has pain at 90° of flexion when the tibia is axially loaded as it is internally and externally rotated (Apley compression test).[40] The Thesaly test may also be used for diagnosis. Here, the clinician supports the patient by holding the patient's outstretched hands. The patient then rotates the affected knee and body, internally and externally, 3 times, keeping the knee flexed at 20°. A meniscal tear leads to joint line discomfort.[41]

Treatment

Rest, ice, compression, and elevation (RICE) are appropriate initially. Short-term crutch use may be helpful as well. As symptoms resolve, low-intensity, short runs without turns or hills may be started, with no cutting or twisting allowed. Failed conservative methods after 12 weeks or a mechanically locked knee may require surgical intervention.[40]

Stress Fractures in Runners

Stress fractures seem to comprise about 10% of running injuries.[10] Distance runners may have stress fractures of the sacrum, pelvis, fibula, femoral shaft, femoral neck, tibia, and foot. A stress fracture should be a consideration when a runner presents with groin pain. Diagnosis can be made with magnetic resonance imaging (MRI).

Treatment of all stress fractures involves decreasing bone impact by reducing training. Stress fractures have also been shown by a Cochrane Review to be preventable by shock-absorbing insoles.[42]

Low-level running can be resumed after 10 to 14 days of rest with low-risk stress fractures, such as of the distal third of the tibia and the fibula.[10] The injured bone may also be rested while cross-training occurs. However, non–weight bearing with crutches for at least 6 weeks allows healing of femoral neck stress, which is a high-risk injury. Healing may take longer for femoral neck stress fractures on the superior side (tension sided), and may require orthopedic surgery consult for possible pinning. Training for most runners with sacral stress fractures usually resumes only after at least 12 weeks of rest. At least 6 weeks of rest may be required for stress fractures of the femoral shaft and pelvic bones.[10]

High risk

The femoral neck is a high-risk stress fracture when on the tension side. Long distances lead to this injury, but moderate distances can still lead to stress fractures in inexperience runners. A prior stress fracture confers the highest risk for a new fracture.[43]

The so-called female athlete triad is composed of osteopenia, amenorrhea, and eating disorders, collectively increasing the risk for stress fractures in women. The date of last menstrual period, regularity, and age at menarche are important to obtain in female runners. There is an increased risk of stress fractures in women, presumably because of decreased body mass index, increased foot pronation, and wider pelvic width.[44–46]

Studies show a rate of stress fracture occurrence in female runners that is more than twice that of male runners.

The risk for a stress fracture in female cross-country runners doubles with a decrease of 1 standard deviation from normal bone mineral density and a prior stress fracture (relative risk [RR] = 5).[43]

Table 2 enumerates stress fractures in runners that have poor healing potential and are considered high risk.[16]

Low risk
African Americans are at lesser risk compared with white people.[47]

The risk factors for stress fractures were shown to have decreased by 27% when female US Navy basic trainees were given 800 IU of vitamin D and 2000-mg calcium supplementation.[48]

Table 2 enumerates stress fractures in runners that have excellent healing potential given adequate rest and conservative treatment (low risk).[16]

Stress Fractures of the Tibia

Introduction
The middle third of the medial tibia is the most common site of tibial stress fractures, especially in male runners.[49]

Cause
Some known causes are a change to a different or harder running surface, change in training shoes, worn running shoes, and increases in running intensity or distance.[49]

Table 3 enumerates factors that may predispose runners to stress fractures.[18,50]

Clinical presentation
Shin pain in a runner should raise a concern for a tibial stress fracture as a possible diagnosis. The pain usually occurs after activity, progressing to pain during activity. Swelling may be present.[51]

Physical examination
Hopping, tuning fork vibration, percussion, and direct palpation over a focal area may reproduce pain.[51] Swelling, erythema, and/or warmth may be evident over the stress fracture.[16] Muscle imbalances, leg length discrepancy, a high longitudinal arch, excessive forefoot varus, genu valgus/varum, and femoral anteversion may be noted on examination as well.[49,52,53]

Work-up
During the first 2 to 3 weeks, radiographs may not show a stress fracture. Periosteal thickening and callus formation may be seen on radiographs. Bone scans are no longer used frequently, because they are nonspecific, take too much time, and expose

Table 2	
Stress fracture risk based on healing potential	
High Risk	**Low Risk**
Femoral neck	Sacrum
Anterior tibia	Pubic ramus
Medial malleolus	Femoral shaft
Navicular	Tibia (except anterior)
Proximal fifth metatarsal	Fibula
Sesamoids	Metatarsal shaft

Table 3
Stress fracture risk factors

Intrinsic Risk Factors	Extrinsic Risk Factors
Poor preparticipation conditioning	Rapid increase in training program
Female gender	High weekly training distance
Menstrual imbalance	Irregular or angled surface
Decreased bone mineral density	Poor footwear
Genu valgus/varum	Running shoes >6 mo old
Leg length discrepancy	Low-fat diet
	Decreased calcium and vitamin D intake
	Tobacco use

patients to too much radiation. Although false-positives can occur, MRI is sometimes used to prognosticate and grade stress fractures.

MRI may be helpful in grading stress fractures and providing prognostic information, but false-positives can occur.[54]

Treatment
Conservative treatment and careful follow-up are required to ensure healing of stress fractures of the medial malleolus, tibial plateau, anterior tibia, and tibial metaphysis, because these heal poorly. Return to training from a tibial stress fracture may be accelerated by using long air splints.[42,55] Getting the patient pain free with regular ambulation is usually the initial goal in runners. This goal may require casting, using a walking boot (controlled ankle movement), with or without crutches. Runners may cross-train during this time. The goal of treatment is to progress the runner to weight-bearing exercise before resumption of running. Running may be initiated at 50% of the runner's usual distance and intensity, increasing this by no more than 10% weekly in terms of distance or intensity. This strategy allows adequate healing with activity, while lessening the risk of reinjury.

Chronic Exertional Compartment Syndrome

Introduction
Chronic exertional compartment syndrome (CECS) is common in runners or those who participate in sports requiring running. Ischemia results from exercise-induced soft tissue swelling in the limited volume of fascial compartments.[56]

Cause
This is an overuse injury in runners that is related to repetitive impact. Increased pressure leads to reversible ischemia within a closed fibro-osseous space. This ischemia leads to decreased blood flow and ischemic pain.[57,58]

Clinical presentation
Lower leg or persistent shin pain with exertion in a runner who does not report any trauma to the leg should lead a clinician to consider compartment syndrome. If noted in experienced runners, such symptoms should lead to a higher index of suspicion. The runner may have a squeezing, aching, or sharp pain with running, relieved by rest. The pain usually recurs within the same distance of running. There may be nerve or muscle dysfunction. The anterior leg may be tense and swollen.[56]

Table 4 enumerates the structures found in each compartment of the leg. The symptoms that arise depend on the compartment affected and correlate with the structures within each compartment.

Table 4
Leg compartments and structures affected by CECS

Anterior (45% of cases)	Tibialis anterior muscle
	Extensor hallucis longus muscle
	Extensor digitorum longus muscle
	Peroneus tertius muscle
	Deep peroneal nerve
	Anterior tibial artery and vein
Posterior, deep (40%)	Tibialis posterior muscle
	Extensor hallucis longus muscle
	Extensor digitorum longus muscle
	Posterior tibial nerve
	Posterior tibial artery and vein
Posterior, superficial (5%)	Gastrocnemius muscle
	Soleus muscle
	Sural nerve
Lateral (10%)	Peroneus longus muscle
	Peroneus brevis muscle
	Superficial peroneal nerve

Physical examination
There is tenderness over the involved compartment. There may be decreased sensation in the first web space of the foot, and even slight foot drop.

Work-up
Diagnostic compartment testing should be performed in runners who have persistent or frequent symptoms associated with foot numbness or leg weakness.

Treatment
Rest, PT, and orthotics are appropriate initial treatments. However, surgical compartment release may be needed for those who fail conservative management.[10]

MTSS

Introduction
Young runners are particularly affected by medial shin pain. This pain may occur in jumping sports as well. Stress along the medial fascial insertion of the soleus muscle has been implicated.[59]

Cause
A sudden increase in training intensity, especially in deconditioned runners, may lead to this condition.[59] The causes and risk factors for MTSS are the same as those for stress fractures (discussed earlier) and are enumerated in **Table 3**.

Clinical presentation
Shin splints are classically bilateral. The posterior medial border of the tibia is usually the part noted to have pain. There may be pain with resisted plantar flexion and inversion.[59]

Physical examination
The runner may have pronated feet. There may be pain when the runner tiptoes on tiptoe. Tenderness is elicited along the posteromedial border of the distal tibia.[59]

Work-up
Radiographs are usually normal in MTSS, or may show some periosteal thickening. MRI may show periosteal changes, and a bone scan may show linear uptake, but physical examination is usually all that is needed to reach the diagnosis.

Treatment
Activity modification, stretching, ice, and NSAIDs are used to treat MTSS. Shock-absorbing insoles have some evidence-based usefulness in preventing or reducing the risk of developing shin splints.[42,60,61] Shock-absorbing custom orthotics or insoles have also been shown to help with the treatment of MTSS.[60,62]

Gastrocnemius-Soleus Strain/Rupture

Introduction
Older runners are prone to calf injuries. Calf injuries have been shown to be the most common injury in runners more than 40 years old.[63] A tear at the musculotendinous insertion of the medial head of the gastrocnemius muscle (tennis leg) is particularly common in runners. Because the toe-off phase of gait occurs with most of the force directed along the medial aspect of the leg, the lateral head of the gastrocnemius is less likely to get injured.[10]

Cause
Overtraining, hill running, and excess speed work may lead to calf injuries. The risk may be increased by inflexible Achilles-calf complexes and cavus feet. However, more evidence is needed to support these observations. Excess training may lead to tears in the plantaris tendon and the intersection of the 2 heads of the gastrocnemius. Runners training at a distance too great for their fitness may get this source of chronic soleus pain, related to the soleus being a slow-twitch muscle, used more in repetitive training than in explosive movements.[64]

Clinical presentation
Runner may complain of sudden, sharp pain in the middle of the posteromedial leg, requiring them to decrease or stop their running. Runner may have felt a pop. Even walking may lead to intense pain.[64]

Physical examination
There is tenderness with stretching or local pressure. In tears, a local defect may be palpable, especially a few hours after injury. Within 1 to 2 days, ecchymosis and swelling may appear. Soleus syndrome should be considered if a runner presents with pain deep to the gastrocnemius on squeezing of the calf's medial and lateral aspects.[64]

Treatment
RICE for the first 48 hours may be helpful, along with crutches. A walking boot may be used for more severe cases. Neoprene sleeves may help support the leg. In 2 weeks, passive, then active, stretching may be started. When walking, a heel pad may help provide some comfort.[64]

Achilles Tendinopathy

Introduction
Runners with more than 10 years of experience, elite runners, and master runners are most commonly affected by Achilles tendinopathy.[65,66] Fifty-two percent of elite male runners experience Achilles tendinopathy in their lives.[26] Two areas on the Achilles tendon are prone to injuries: the insertion onto the heel and the avascular zone. The

tendon fibers at the insertion point may separate from the bone (enthesopathy). Runners who injure this part of the Achilles tendon may take longer to heal. The avascular zone is where the substance of the tendon forms from the interweaving of fibers from the soleus and the gastrocnemius, about 2 to 5 cm above the insertion.

Cause
Runners do not usually get frank Achilles tendon ruptures or retrocalcaneal bursitis. However, secondary bursitis and/or heel contusions may occur in runners who use shoes with very firm heel counters. Maximal sprinting, which comes with high tensile stress in the effort to achieve speed in a short amount of time, may lead to complete Achilles ruptures in highly competitive sprinters.[67]

Table 5 lists the factors that may predispose a runner to developing Achilles tendinopathy.[16]

Clinical presentation
Running leads to pain over the Achilles tendon, usually 3 to 4 cm above its insertion onto the calcaneus. A recent change in training and/or shoes usually coincides with the symptoms.[67]

Physical examination
There may be focal crepitus, swelling, and/or tenderness on the tendon. In chronic cases, there may be nodularity and thickening of the tendon. Overpronation may be noted, as well as gastrocnemius-soleus and hamstring inflexibility.[67]

Treatment
Eccentric exercise protocols seem to be the most evidence-based treatment of Achilles tendinopathy.[68] Patients with noninsertional injuries seem to benefit the most. The pathologic changes of tendinopathy have been shown by MRI and ultrasonography to resolve in patients who undergo eccentric exercise protocols.[69,70] More treatment failures and slower healing times have been noted when eccentric protocols are used on patients with insertional Achilles tendinopathy.

Eccentric rehabilitation protocols may be used for the treatment of soleus and gastrocnemius injuries as well.[65] Stretching, heel lifts, and ice massage are often used for treatment as well, although the evidence for these is less robust. Wearing custom orthotics along with 4 weeks of PT has been shown to significantly decrease pain from Achilles tendinopathy.[71] Significant reduction in pain has also been noted with the use of low-dose topical nitroglycerine patches combined with an eccentric rehabilitation protocol, compared with the protocol alone.[72] There is strong evidence suggesting that, in general, chronic tendinopathies benefit from the use of topical nitroglycerin.[73]

Table 5 Risk factors for Achilles tendinopathy	
Intrinsic Risk Factors	**Extrinsic Risk Factors**
Regional hypovascularity	Overuse
Endocrine/metabolic disorders	Poor flexibility
Genetic factors	Training errors
	Excessive lateral heel strike
	Hip muscle weakness
	Cycling position
	Incorrect bike fit

Plantar Fasciitis

Introduction

Plantar fasciitis is the most common cause of heel pain in runners. Plantar fasciitis is a traction periostitis at the origin of the plantar fascia over the medial tuberosity of the anterior calcaneus, with subsequent tearing and degeneration. The condition tends to get worse over time.[74]

Cause

A tight Achilles tendon, excessive training, hyperpronation, and a cavus foot are known causes.[74]

Clinical presentation

The first few steps after a long rest or in the morning may be described as most painful. Prolonged activity may also lead to the pain. The onset is usually insidious.[74]

Physical examination

The longitudinal arch may be tender. However, point tenderness over the calcaneal medial tubercle is more common.[74]

Treatment

At first, NSAIDs may be helpful. Stretching of the heel cord is the mainstay of treatment. Cross-friction massage as well as various PT modalities has been shown to help. Arch supports, heel cups, and arch taping have led to varying success in studies. Barefoot walking and weight bearing may need to be limited in the beginning. Night splints, cortisone injections, and short leg walking casts have been shown to be helpful as well.[75]

RUNNING SHOES, BAREFOOT RUNNING, ORTHOTICS, AND STRETCHING

Humans have been running barefoot or with minimalist footwear for millennia. The beginning of the end for the barefoot era occurred more than 30,000 years ago when protective footwear became commonplace to protect against acute injury, such as stepping on a sharp rock or scorching hot sand.[76] Footwear eventually evolved beyond a protective role and gained cultural respect as a status symbol (eg, wedges to increase height).[77] Despite these early modifications in shoe design, it was not until the running boom of the 1970s that shoe manufacturers really began to alter shoe designs. At present, with between 3 and 6 million American runners, running shoe manufacturing is a multibillion dollar industry.[5]

Although initial running shoe designs were little more than standard tennis shoes, footwear companies began marketing cushioned, waffled soles to increase comfort and decrease the physical stresses of running. Advances in running shoe technology continue to focus on injury reduction. Three common recommendations are (1) motion control shoes for low arches, (2) cushioned running shoes for high arches, and (3) stability shoes for neutral arches.[78,79]

Although these modifications have become popular within the running community as a means to reduce injury, there are limited data to suggest that these measures based on arch type or foot shape can reduce injury rates, which have remained stable over the past few decades.[80–83]

Biomechanical research and popular books such as Born to Run[84] have recently led to an interest in barefoot or minimalist running.[85] Barefoot runners land on their forefoot or midfoot instead of the heel, resulting in smaller impact forces at foot strike. No clinical studies have shown that this running style reduces the risk of injury, with some researchers concerned that barefoot running may alter the type, not incidence, of running injuries.[86]

The role of orthotics in the treatment and prevention of running-related injuries is equally debated. The overall risk for lower extremity injuries may be decreased with the use of orthotics.[87] An injured runner may recover faster. Injuries may be prevented, and the time to muscle fatigue may be increased by cushioning the feet and correcting biomechanical disorders with over-the-counter or personalized orthotics.[87]

Flexibility describes the range of motion present in a joint or group of joints that allows normal and unimpaired function.[88] Stretching is commonly used to increase a person's maximal functional range of motion or flexibility. Of the 4 types of stretching (ballistic, passive, static, and proprioceptive neuromuscular facilitation), static stretching is the most popular and likely the safest. Static stretching applies a steady force for 15 to 60 seconds. As with any form of exercise, stretching can be dangerous and may result in injury if performed incorrectly.[89]

Running injuries seem not to be preventable by stretching, at least based on current evidence.[90,91] Preexercise stretching does not seem to prevent sports injuries in general.[92] However, stretching is still highly favored by most sports practitioners.[5] There remains a prevailing belief among coaches that there are no drawbacks to stretching and that injuries may be decreased by preexercise stretching.[93] Based on the peer-reviewed literature, plantar fasciitis is the condition that seems to be most benefited by stretching.[94,95] Conflicting evidence shows stretching as being beneficial for other musculoskeletal conditions.[5] As for timing of stretching, it seems that stretching after, rather than before, activity may offer injury protection, at least for hamstring injuries.[96] In addition, stretching too vigorously before an athletic event has been shown to impair performance by resulting in an acute loss of strength. The injury prevention role of stretching in a runner has to be balanced against this consideration on an individualized basis.[89]

REFERENCES

1. Centers for Disease Control and Prevention. Prevalence of obesity in the United States, 2009-2010. Available at: http://www.cdc.gov/nchs/fastats/overwt.htm. Accessed February 18, 2013.
2. Haskell W, Lee I, Pate R, et al. Physical activity and public health: updated recommendation for adults from the American College of Sports Medicine and the American Heart Association. Med Sci Sports Exerc 2007;39(8):1423–34.
3. Nelson M, Rejeski W, Blair S, et al. Physical activity and public health in older adults: recommendations from the American College of Sports Medicine and the American Heart Association. Med Sci Sports Exerc 2007;39(8):1435–45.
4. Chalufour M. How demographics are affecting the racing scene. Running Times 2010. Available at: http://www.runnersworld.com/rt-columns/how-demographics-are-affecting-racing-scene?page. Accessed February 19, 2013.
5. Fields KB, Sykes JC, Walker KM, et al. Prevention of running injuries. Curr Sports Med Rep 2010;9:176–82. Accessed October 6, 2013.
6. Running USA. Running USA's annual marathon report [Internet]. 2011. Available at: http://www.runningusa.org/index.cfm?fuseaction=news.details&ArticleId= 332. Accessed October 6, 2013.
7. Larson O, Katovsky B. Tread lightly: form, footwear, and the quest for injury free running. New York: Skyhorse; 2012.
8. Chakravarty E, Hubert H, Lingala V, et al. Reduced disability and mortality among aging runners: a 21 year longitudinal study. Arch Intern Med 2008; 168(15):1638–46.

9. Van Gent RN, Siem D, van Middelkoop M, et al. Incidence and determinants of lower extremity running injuries in long distance runners: a systematic review. Br J Sports Med 2007;41:469–80.

10. Fields KB. Running injuries: changing trends and demographics. Curr Sports Med Rep 2011;10(5):299–303.

11. Wilder R. Preface: the runner. Clin Sports Med 2010;29:xv–xvi.

12. Boven AM, Janssen GM, Vermeer HG, et al. Occurrence of running injuries in adults following a supervised training program. Int J Sports Med 1989; 10(Suppl 3):S186–90.

13. Hootman JM, Macera CA, Ainsworth BE, et al. Predictors of lower extremity injury among recreationally active adults. Clin J Sport Med 2002;12:99–106.

14. Jacobs SJ, Berson BL. Injuries to runners: a study of entrants to a 10,000 meter race. Am J Sports Med 1986;14:151–5.

15. Walter SD, Hart LE, McIntosh JM, et al. The Ontario study of running related injuries. Arch Intern Med 1989;149:2561–4.

16. Oser S, Oser T, Silvis M. Evaluation and treatment of biking and running injuries. Prim Care 2013;40:969–86.

17. Taunton JE, Ryan MB, Clement DB, et al. A retrospective case-control analysis of 2002 running injuries. Br J Sports Med 2002;36:95–101.

18. Gallo R, Plakke M, Silvis M. Common leg injuries of long-distance runners: anatomical and biomechanical approach. Sports Health 2012;4(6):485–95.

19. Meininger AK, Koh JL. Evaluation of the injured runner. Clin Sports Med 2012; 31:203–15.

20. Magrum E, Wilder R. Evaluation of the injured runner. Clin Sports Med 2010;29: 331–45.

21. Plastaras CT, Rittenberg JD, Rittenberg KE, et al. Comprehensive functional evaluation of the injured runner. Phys Med Rehabil Clin N Am 2005;16(3):623–49.

22. Hreljac A. Impact and overuse injuries in runners. Med Sci Sports Exerc 2004; 36(5):845–9.

23. Dugan SA, Bhat KP. Biomechanics and analysis of running gait. Phys Med Rehabil Clin N Am 2005;16:603–21.

24. Fields KB, Bloom OJ, Priebe D, et al. Basic biomechanics of the lower extremity. Prim Care 2005;32:245–51.

25. Bresler M, Mar W, Toman J. Diagnostic imaging in the evaluation of leg pain in athletes. Clin Sports Med 2012;31:217–45.

26. Witvrouw E, Danneels L, Van Tiggelen D, et al. Open versus closed kinetic chain exercises in patellofemoral pain: a 5-year prospective randomized study. Am J Sports Med 2004;32:1122–30.

27. Clanton TO, Coupe KJ. Hamstring strains in athletes: diagnosis and treatment. J Am Acad Orthop Surg 1998;6:237–48.

28. van Tulder MW, Koes BW, Bouter LM. Conservative treatment of acute and chronic nonspecific low back pain: a systematic review of randomized controlled trials of the most common interventions. Spine 1997;22:2128–56.

29. McKean KA, Manson NA, Stanish WD. Musculoskeletal injury in the masters runners. Clin J Sport Med 2006;16:149–54.

30. Fredericson M, Weir A. Practical management of iliotibial band friction syndrome in runners. Clin J Sport Med 2006;16:261–8.

31. Lavine R. Iliotibial band friction syndrome. Curr Rev Musculoskelet Med 2010; 3(1–4):18–22.

32. Collado H, Fredericson M. Patellofemoral pain syndrome. Clin Sports Med 2010; 29(3):377–98.

33. Cichanowski HR, Schmitt JS, Johnson RJ, et al. Hip strength in collegiate female athletes with patellofemoral pain. Med Sci Sports Exerc 2007;39:1227–32.
34. Duffey MJ, Martin DF, Cannon DW, et al. Etiologic factors associated with anterior knee pain in distance runners. Med Sci Sports Exerc 2000;32:1825–32.
35. Ireland ML, Willson JD, Ballantyne BT, et al. Hip strength in females with and without patellofemoral pain. J Orthop Sports Phys Ther 2003;33:671–6.
36. Papagelopoulos PJ, Sim FH. Patellofemoral pain syndrome: diagnosis and management. Orthopedics 1997;20:148–57.
37. Barton CJ, Munteanu SE, Menz HB, et al. The efficacy of foot orthoses in the treatment of individuals with patellofemoral pain syndrome: a systematic review. Sports Med 2010;40:377–95.
38. Collins N, Crossley K, Beller E, et al. Foot orthoses and physiotherapy in the treatment of patellofemoral pain syndrome: randomised clinical trial. Br J Sports Med 2009;43:169–71.
39. Witvrouw E, Mahieu N, Roosen P, et al. The role of stretching in tendon injuries. Br J Sports Med 2007;41:224–6.
40. Messner K, Gao J. Review: the menisci of the knee joint. Anatomical and functional characteristics, and a rationale for clinical treatment. J Anat 1998;193:161–78.
41. Harrison BK, Abell BE, Gibson TW. The Thessaly test for detection of meniscal tears: validation of a new physical examination technique for primary care medicine. Clin J Sport Med 2009;19(1):9–12.
42. Rome K, Handoll HH, Ashford RL. Interventions for preventing and treating stress fractures and stress reactions of bone of the lower limbs in young adults. Cochrane Database Syst Rev 2005;(2):CD000450.
43. Kelsey JL, Bachrach LK, Procter-Gray E, et al. Risk factors for stress fracture among young female cross-country runners. Med Sci Sports Exerc 2007;39:1457–63.
44. Beck TJ, Ruff CB, Shaffer RA, et al. Stress fracture in military recruits: gender differences in muscle and bone susceptibility factors. Bone 2000;27(3):437–44.
45. Bijur PE, Horodyski M, Egerton W, et al. Comparison of injury during cadet basic training by gender. Arch Pediatr Adolesc Med 1997;151(5):456–61.
46. Korpelainen R, Orava S, Karpakka J, et al. Risk factors for recurrent stress fractures in athletes. Am J Sports Med 2001;29(3):304–10.
47. Milner CE, Ferber R, Pollard CD, et al. Biomechanical factors associated with tibial stress fracture in female runners. Med Sci Sports Exerc 2006;38:323–8.
48. Lappe J, Cullen D, Haynatzki G, et al. Calcium and vitamin D supplementation decreases incidence of stress fractures in female navy recruits. J Bone Miner Res 2008;23:741–9.
49. Matheson GO, Clement DB, McKenzie DC, et al. Stress fractures in athletes: a study of 320 cases. Am J Sports Med 1987;15:46–58.
50. McCormick F, Nwachukwu B, Provencher M. Stress fractures in runners. Clin Sports Med 2012;31:291–306.
51. Kortebein PM, Kaufman KR, Basford JR, et al. Medial tibial stress syndrome. Med Sci Sports Exerc 2000;32:27–33.
52. Barnes A, Wheat J, Milner C. Association between foot type and tibial stress injuries: a systematic review. Br J Sports Med 2008;42:93–8.
53. Jones B, Bovee M, Harris J, et al. Intrinsic risk factors for exercise-related injuries among male and female army trainees. Am J Sports Med 1993;2(5):705–10.

54. Bergman A, Fredericson M, Ho C, et al. Asymptomatic tibial stress reactions: MRI detection and clinical follow-up in distance runners. AJR Am J Roentgenol 2004;183:635–8.
55. Gillespie WJ, Grant I. Interventions for preventing and treating stress fractures and stress reactions of bone of the lower limbs in young adults. Cochrane Database Syst Rev 2000;(2):CD000450.
56. Blackman PG. A review of chronic exertional compartment syndrome in the lower leg. Med Sci Sports Exerc 2000;32(Suppl 3):S4–10.
57. Wanich T, Hodgkins C, Columbier JA, et al. Cycling injuries of the lower extremity. J Am Acad Orthop Surg 2007;15(12):748–56.
58. George C, Hutchinson M. Chronic exertional compartment syndrome. Clin Sports Med 2012;31:307–19.
59. Burne S, Khan K, Boudville P, et al. Risk factors associated with exertional medial tibial pain: a 12 month prospective clinical study. Br J Sports Med 2004;38(4):441–5.
60. Moen MH, Tol JL, Weir A, et al. Medial tibial stress syndrome: a critical review. Sports Med 2009;39:523–46.
61. Thacker SB, Gilchrist J, Stroup DF, et al. The prevention of shin splints in sports: a systematic review of literature. Med Sci Sports Exerc 2002;34:32–40.
62. Loudon JK, Dolphino MR. Use of foot orthoses and calf stretching for individuals with medial tibial stress syndrome. Foot Ankle Spec 2010;3:15–20.
63. Marti B, Vader JP, Minder CE, et al. On the epidemiology of running injuries. The 1984 Bern Grand-Prix Study. Am J Sports Med 1988;16:285–94.
64. Brewster CE. Acute tears of the medial head of the gastrocnemius. Foot Ankle Int 1985;5:186–90.
65. Kingma JJ, de Knikker R, Wittink HM, et al. Eccentric overload training in patients with chronic Achilles tendinopathy: a systemic review. Br J Sports Med 2007;41:e3.
66. Knobloch K, Yoon U, Vogt PM. Acute and overuse injuries correlated to hours of training in master running athletes. Foot Ankle Int 2008;29:671–6.
67. Alfredson H, Cook J. A treatment algorithm for managing Achilles tendinopathy: new treatment options. Br J Sports Med 2007;41(4):211–6.
68. Alfredson H, Pietila T, Jonsson P, et al. Heavy-load eccentric calf muscle training for the treatment of chronic Achilles tendinosis. Am J Sports Med 1998;26:360–6.
69. Grigg NL, Wearing SC, Smeathers JE. Eccentric calf muscle exercise produces a greater acute reduction in Achilles tendon thickness than concentric exercise. Br J Sports Med 2009;43:280–3.
70. Shalabi A, Kristoffersen-Wilberg M, Svensson L, et al. Eccentric training of the gastrocnemius-soleus complex in chronic Achilles tendinopathy results in decreased tendon volume and intratendinous signal as evaluated by MRI. Am J Sports Med 2004;32(5):1286–96.
71. Mayer F, Hirschmuller A, Muller S, et al. Effects of short-term strategies over 4 weeks in Achilles tendinopathy. Br J Sports Med 2007;41:e6.
72. Paoloni JA, Appleyard RC, Nelson J, et al. Topical glyceryl trinitrate treatment of chronic noninsertional Achilles tendinopathy. A randomized, double-blind, placebo-controlled trial. J Bone Joint Surg Am 2004;86A:916–22.
73. Gambito ED, Gonzalez-Suarez CB, Oquinena TI, et al. Evidence on the effectiveness of topical nitroglycerin in the treatment of tendinopathies: a systematic review and meta-analysis. Arch Phys Med Rehabil 2010;91:1291–305.
74. Coady CM, Gow N, Stanish W. Foot problems in middle-aged patients: keeping active people up to speed. Phys Sportsmed 1998;26(5):31–42.

75. Goff JD, Crawford R. Diagnosis and treatment of plantar fasciitis. Am Fam Physician 2011;84(6):676–82.

76. D'Aout K, Pataky T, Clercq D, et al. The effects of habitual footwear use: foot shape and function in native barefoot walkers. Footwear Sci 2009;1:81–94.

77. Stewart S. Footgear – its history, uses, and abuses. Clin Orthop Relat Res 1972; 88:119–30.

78. Asplund CA, Brown DL. The running shoe prescription: fit for performance. Phys Sportsmed 2005;33:17–24.

79. Butler RJ, Hamill J, Davis I. Effect of footwear on high and low arched runners' mechanics during a prolonged run. Gait Posture 2007;26:219–25.

80. Ferber R, Hreljac A, Kendall K. Suspected mechanisms in the cause of overuse running injuries: a clinical review. Sports Health 2009;1:242–6.

81. Knapik JJ, Brosch LC, Venuto M, et al. Effect on injuries assigning shoes based on foot shape in air force basic training. Am J Prev Med 2010;38:S197–211.

82. Knapik JJ, Trone D, Swedler D, et al. Injury reduction effectiveness of assigning running shoes based on plantar shape in Marine Corps basic training. Am J Sports Med 2010;38:1759–67.

83. Richards CE, Magin PJ, Callister R. Is your prescription of distance running shoes evidence based? Br J Sports Med 2009;43:159–62.

84. McDougall C. Born to run: a hidden tribe, superathletes, and the greatest race the world has never seen. New York: Vintage Books; 2009.

85. Rixe JA, Gallo RA, Silvis ML. The barefoot debate: can minimalist shoes reduce running related injuries. Curr Sports Med Rep 2012;11(3):160–5.

86. Guiliani J, Masini B, Alitz C, et al. Barefoot-simulating footwear associated with metatarsal stress injury in 2 runners. Orthopedics 2011;34:e320–3.

87. Franklyn-Miller A, Wilson C, Bilzon J, et al. Foot orthoses in the prevention of injury in initial military training: a randomized controlled trial. Am J Sports Med 2011;39(1):30–7.

88. Subotnick SI. Foot orthotics. In: O'Connor FG, Wilder RP, Nirschl R, editors. Textbook of running medicine. New York: McGraw-Hill; 2001. p. 595–603.

89. Corbin CB. Flexibility. Clin Sports Med 1984;3:101–17.

90. Jenkins J, Beazell J. Flexibility for runners. Clin Sports Med 2010;29:365–77.

91. Yeung EW, Yeung S. Interventions for preventing lower limb soft tissue injuries in runners. Cochrane Database Syst Rev 2001;(3):CD001256.

92. Thacker SB, Gilchrist J, Stroup DF, et al. The impact of stretching on sports injury risk: a systematic review of the literature. Med Sci Sports Exerc 2004; 36:371–8.

93. Shehab R, Mirabelli M, Gorenflo D, et al. Pre-exercise stretching and sports related injuries: knowledge, attitudes and practices. Clin J Sport Med 2006; 16:228–31.

94. DiGiovanni BF, Nawoczenski DA, Lintal ME, et al. Tissue specific plantar fascia-stretching exercise enhances outcomes in patients with chronic heel pain. J Bone Joint Surg 2003;85:1270–7.

95. DiGiovanni BF, Nawoczenski DA, Malay DP, et al. Tissue specific plantar fascia-stretching exercise improves outcomes in patients with chronic heel pain: a prospective clinical trial with two-year follow-up. J Bone Joint Surg 2006;88: 1775–81.

96. Verrall GM, Slavotinek JP, Barnes PG. The effect of sports specific training on reducing the incidence of hamstring injuries in professional Australian Rules football players. Br J Sports Med 2005;39:363–8.

The Physical Therapy Prescription

Cayce A. Onks, DO, MS, ATC[a,b],*, John Wawrzyniak, MA, ATC, PT, CSCS[c]

KEYWORDS

- Physical therapy • Visit • Prescription • Indications

KEY POINTS

- Physical therapists are licensed health care professionals who maintain, restore, and improve movement, activity, and health, enabling individuals of all ages to have optimal functioning and quality of life.
- The advent of evidence-based medicine over the past 30 years allows patients to benefit from interventions that are scientifically sound and, when appropriately provided, produce cost-effective outcomes.
- Patient entrance into physical therapy in most cases starts with a referral from a health care provider. In musculoskeletal medicine common referrals include pain, weakness, and instability leading to loss of motion, strength, and function.
- The physical therapy referral should include the diagnosis, frequency, and duration of therapy services in addition to any precautions or protocol considerations.
- After a comprehensive musculoskeletal evaluation, the physical therapist will structure a clinical and home treatment program, allowing patients to overcome physical limitations and maximize function.

INTRODUCTION TO PHYSICAL THERAPY

The history of physical therapy can be traced to Ancient Greek culture and the use of massage and hydrotherapy by Hippocrates.[1] Physical therapy as a profession dates to 1894, when 4 nurses in England formed the Society of Trained Masseuses, later to become known as the Chartered Society for Physiotherapy.[2] In the United States "reconstruction aides" were educated at Walter Reed Hospital in Washington, DC in an effort to help manage the injuries suffered by soldiers in World War I.[3]

No disclosures for either author.
[a] Department of Family and Community Medicine, Penn State Milton S. Hershey Medical Center, 30 Hope Drive, Hershey, PA 17033-0859, USA; [b] Department of Orthopaedics and Rehabilitation, Penn State Milton S. Hershey Medical Center, 30 Hope Drive, Hershey, PA 17033-0859, USA; [c] Department of Orthopaedics and Rehabilitation, Therapy Services, Penn State Milton S. Hershey Medical Center, Mail Code EC 130, 30 Hope Drive, PO Box 859, Hershey, PA 17033-0859, USA
* Corresponding author. Penn State Hershey Medical Group, Mail Code HP21, 3025 Market Street, Camp Hill, PA 17011.
E-mail address: conks@hmc.psu.edu

By 1921 the first physical therapy research articles were published in *The PT Review*. The Physical Therapy Association was founded later to become known as the American Physical Therapy Association (APTA). The APTA is still in existence today, and is the governing body of physical therapy in the United States. The APTA sets educational standards, and oversees the 213 institutions offering physical therapy education programs and the 309 institutions offering physical therapy assistant education programs to students across the United States.[1]

In the 1940s wounded World War II veterans and the outbreak of poliomyelitis (polio) marked an increase in the need for physical therapists and their services. Practice in the 1950s continued to be influenced by the Korean War.[4] The development of the Salk vaccine brought an end to the polio epidemic, and by the early 1960s the profession began to focus on other disabilities. The 1960s saw the development of neurologic techniques for treatment of patients with stroke, cerebral palsy, and other disorders of the central nervous system.[3] The cardiopulmonary area of physical therapy also developed with the advancement of open heart surgery.[3] Development of total joint replacements in the 1960s created an additional need for postoperative physical therapy.[3] The period of time between 1950 and 2000 gave rise to technological advances in modalities and methodology, allowing physical therapists to expand practice and the types of diseases and conditions that they could positively influence.[1]

For the last 100 years, physical therapy education has evolved from early training programs for reconstruction aids to its current status as the doctor of physical therapy (DPT) degree.[1] After graduation, candidates must pass a licensure examination. Licensure is managed by individual states. Physical therapists then become licensed health care professionals who maintain, restore, and improve movement, in addition to overall activity levels, thus enabling individuals of all ages to strive toward optimal functioning and quality of life.[1]

By way of a significant push to expanding physical therapy toward evidence-based practice, patients benefit from interventions that are scientifically sound and, when appropriately provided, produce cost-effective outcomes.[1] Within the profession of physical therapy, specializations have been developed to better serve patients (**Box 1**).

Reimbursement of physical therapy services from Medicare and third-party payers has traditionally, and in most cases still requires, a referral from a health care provider. The professional training and expertise that characterize physical therapists has been recognized by 48 states and the District of Columbia. These states have removed provisions requiring a referral by a health care provider for physical therapy evaluation and

---

Box 1
Physical therapy specializations

Cardiovascular and pulmonary

Clinical electrophysiology

Geriatrics

Neurology

Orthopedics

Pediatrics

Sports

Women's health

treatment, from their statutes[5]; this is known as direct access. Provisions for direct access and reimbursement are controlled by each individual state board of physical therapy and vary from state to state. Individual insurance companies establish provisions and reimbursement rates for direct access to physical therapy services, and in some cases do not provide payment for service unless referred by a health care provider.

THE PHYSICAL THERAPY VISIT

The patient's admission to physical therapy most often starts with seeing a licensed physician. The patient is then referred to physical therapy for evaluation and treatment of the problem. The purpose of the initial physical therapy visit is to establish a clinical and home program that will lead to resolution of the patient's symptoms.

The physical therapist first conducts a detailed review of the patient's history (**Box 2**), followed by a thorough physical examination (**Box 3**) including biomechanical analysis, range of motion, strength evaluation, and special tests. Integrating information from the history and physical examination, the physical therapist is able to set goals and formulate a treatment plan. This plan will include the frequency of physical therapy visits and the expected duration for a successful outcome.

Because of the changing landscape of health care delivery, the physical therapist must take into consideration any health plan or financial restraints of the patient when developing the treatment plan. This approach may include a limited number of physical therapy visits allowed by the patient's health care plan, copays for physical therapy services, and work, time, and family restraints. The physical therapy plan is a blueprint for the patient to achieve rehabilitation goals, and provides the basis for a home program to prevent reoccurrence of injury.

Physical therapists use a combination of therapeutic modalities, manual therapy techniques, and exercise to reduce pain, restore mobility, strengthen, and ultimately

---

Box 2
Patient history

Age

Occupation

Leisure activities

Postural stresses

Functional disability core

Health status

When the problem started

What brought on the symptoms

Location of symptoms

Symptoms constant or intermittent

What makes symptoms better/worse

Previous episodes

Previous treatment

Medications

Imaging

Box 3
Physical examination

Observation

Baseline measurements: pain/function

Active movements

Passive movements

Resisted movements

Neurologic: sensory/motor

Repeated movements/static tests

Special tests

---

restore patients to the highest level of function possible. Common therapeutic modalities are listed in **Box 4**. The physical therapist decides which modalities are best suited to treat the patient and his or her condition. The physical therapist will make a clinical judgment, taking into account individual patient's problems in addition to indications and contraindications of use.

The physical therapy plan must be comprehensive and focus on the individual as a whole, not merely the injured site. This approach will ensure a safe return to work and activity while preventing injury to other parts of the body. The selection of therapeutic exercise for the patient's particular problem is determined from the physical examination and the patient's response to exercise during the initial clinical visit. The physical therapist must then determine which exercises are appropriate, and the dosage (number of sets and repetitions) and frequency of the exercise program. Patients undergo ongoing reassessment to ensure they are progressing toward their goals. By following a simple red, yellow, and green light system (**Table 1**), patients will know how to safely progress with their exercise program.

The physical therapy program may include stretching and strengthening exercise, and joint and soft-tissue mobility techniques. Strengthening exercise may take the

---

Box 4
Therapeutic modalities

Ice pack

Ice massage

Ice immersion

Moist hot pack

Ultrasound

Diathermy

Whirlpool

Laser

Neuromuscular electrical stimulation (NMES)

Transcutaneous electrical nerve stimulation (TENS)

Traction

Vasopneumatic compression

Table 1		
Green light system		
Red light	Pain produced or increased with exercise and remains worse	Stop exercise
Yellow light	Pain with exercise but no worse after	Continue with caution
Green light	No pain during exercise or exercise abolishes pain	Continue and progress with exercise

form of isometric (no movement), concentric (shortening), and eccentric (lengthening) loading of the muscle to provide overload and facilitate strength gains.[6] Common forms of exercise include open kinetic chain exercise (exercises that are performed where the extremity is free to move) and closed kinetic chain exercise (performed where the extremity is fixed in space and cannot move).[6] For example, a closed chain exercise for the knee would be a squat, whereas an open chain exercise of the knee would be a straight leg raise. Common forms of resistance for strength training include body weight, bands, dumbbells, and barbells.

Aquatic exercise (**Fig. 1**) offers accommodating resistance that can help patients with strengthening in addition to regaining lost motion.[7] Because of buoyancy, patients who are non–weight bearing or partially weight bearing can begin early loading of the lower extremity to promote joint mobility, muscle strengthening, and a progressive pathway to full weight bearing following injury or fracture to the lower extremity.[6,7]

Manual stretching techniques such as hold-relax can be performed by the physical therapist to facilitate gains in flexibility and range of motion in joints.[8] These techniques are helpful, but must be accompanied by self-stretching techniques performed by the patient as part of the home exercise program.

Soft-tissue mobilization may include massage, or techniques such as active release therapy (ART) and Graston. The Graston technique is a form of instrument-assisted soft-tissue mobilization that uses 6 patented stainless-steel instruments to evaluate and treat soft-tissue restrictions. This technique has expanded on the concept of transverse tissue massage originally made popular by James Cyriax. The stainless-steel instruments amplify the feel of soft-tissue restrictions, aiding in the detection of restrictions at the injury site and along the kinetic chain. By using various strokes, varying pressure, and incorporating muscle activity and joint movement during

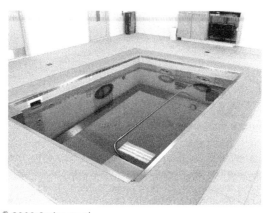

Fig. 1. Hydroworx® 2000 Series pool.

treatment, the clinician can release scar tissue and myofascial restrictions. Physiologically, the Graston technique also recreates the normal inflammatory response, leading to a more aggressive healing response including fibroblastic proliferation.

Self soft-tissue mobilization may include use of a foam roller (**Fig. 2**) or stick roller (**Fig. 3**). These techniques are commonly used by clinicians and reportedly inhibit muscle spasm, providing pain relief while allowing greater flexibility and joint mobility. Research with these techniques is limited, and further research is needed to determine the underlying physiology associated with the proposed benefits.

As the patient recovers and progresses toward established goals, the physical therapist must prepare the patient for discharge. Clinical tools include functional testing to ensure the patient is ready for return to work or sport. Work-hardening programs can provide patients with job-simulation scenarios over a full day to ensure that they are ready to safely return to the vigorous demands of their employment.

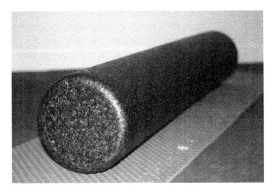

Fig. 2. Foam roller.

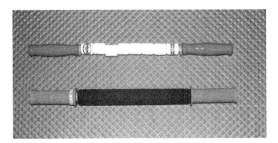

Fig. 3. Stick roller.

INDICATIONS AND EVIDENCE FOR PHYSICAL THERAPY REFERRAL

Physical therapy has become much more rigorous in its attempt to validate the field since the advent of evidence-based medicine some 30 years ago. As a result, evidence-based clinical practice guidelines were developed and defined as a systematically developed statement to help practitioners and clients with decisions about appropriate health care for specific clinical circumstances.[9] The Cochrane collaboration has also made significant contributions to the rehabilitation field, and is considered the international highest standard for evidence-based medicine.[10]

Because of the increasing body of clinically relevant evidence for physical therapy, there are many treatment options in several areas within medicine for practitioners to choose. Some examples include neurologic and musculoskeletal disabilities, in addition to cardiopulmonary, oncology, burn, perisurgical, deconditioned or disabled, and developmental issues. In musculoskeletal medicine the indication for physical therapy may be based on a symptom rather than a confirmed diagnosis. As a result, referral decisions can be made for several reasons that include physical examination abnormalities, symptoms, or a diagnosis.

EXAMINATION-BASED REFERRALS

Many times in musculoskeletal medicine there may not be an obvious diagnosis when the patient initially presents to the clinic. The practitioner may recognize that the patient could benefit from physical therapy because of the deficiencies noted during the examination (**Box 5**), a common situation whereby referrals are warranted.

Physical therapists will not only treat these deficiencies, but often can provide objective information that can help a practitioner determine potential causes of the deficiency.

SYMPTOM-BASED REFERRALS

Patient symptoms, the most common of which is pain, may also be an indication for referral; this is particularly true in the setting of an acute musculoskeletal injury. Other examples of symptoms would be a feeling of joint instability and overall weakness. In a 2012 Cochrane review, low- to moderate-quality evidence for flexibility and strengthening for patients who have chronic neck pain was identified.[11] Another review demonstrated that exercise therapy (strengthening of the abdominal and hip muscles) in athletes with groin pain improves short-term outcomes in pain in comparison with passive modalities.[12] These examples take a problem that could have multiple causes and apply general physical therapy principles to treat patients' symptoms (**Box 6**).

DIAGNOSIS-BASED REFERRALS

Physical therapy consultations are also requested based on diagnosis. Most of the evidence that supports physical therapy focuses on a specific diagnosis or problem area. Some of the most common examples in musculoskeletal medicine include muscle strains, ligament sprains, osteoarthritis, and tendinopathy.

It may be counterintuitive that increasing the use of a joint will improve the symptoms of osteoarthritis, but this seems to be the case. A 2008 Cochrane review suggested that therapeutic exercise at least provides short-term benefit for decreasing knee pain and increasing physical function in patients with osteoarthritis of the

---

Box 5
Examination-based physical therapy referral

Decreased range of motion

Loss of flexibility

Decrease in strength

Decrease in neuromuscular control

Loss of function

| Box 6 |
| Symptom-based physical therapy referral |
| Pain |
| Instability |
| Weakness |

knee.[13] Another systematic review showed that exercise was superior to no exercise in osteoarthritis, and that combining exercises that increase strength, flexibility, and aerobic capacity is likely to contribute to management of osteoarthritis.[14] Ultrasound may also proffer benefit to pain relief and function.[15] Physical therapists can implement these modalities and provide a noninvasive starting point in the treatment of osteoarthritis.

Physical therapy has also been shown to be beneficial in patients with rheumatoid arthritis. One Cochrane review found that electrical stimulation may have a clinically beneficial effect on grip strength and fatigue resistance for rheumatoid arthritis patients with muscle atrophy.[16] Another Cochrane study showed that therapeutic ultrasound may have an effect on grip strength and morning stiffness, and reduce the number of painful, swollen joints.[17] Occupational therapy was also shown to have a positive effect on functional ability in patients with rheumatoid arthritis (Table 2).[18]

Tendinopathy is a common complaint in musculoskeletal medicine, in contrast to tendonitis. Tendinopathy was found in a histologic analysis of 88 patients with lateral epicondylitis. The analysis identified immature fibroblasts and vascular infiltration in surgical tissue samples.[19] This finding was confirmed by other studies and led to a change in thinking regarding the treatment of epicondylitis, which is really a chronic noninflammatory condition. Therapies such as strengthening have become popular treatment options as a result. A recent systematic review found that there was moderate evidence for stretching and strengthening of epicondylopathy versus ultrasound plus friction massage.[20] There was also moderate evidence for add-on cervical and thoracic manipulation to concentric and eccentric strengthening for treatment of the wrist and forearm.[20] Another review suggested that the initial nonoperative treatment of tendinopathy in sport should include eccentric strengthening, or lengthening of the muscle fibers during contraction, which should represent the cornerstone of treatment.[21] A systematic review looking specifically at Achilles tendinopathy also concluded that the evidence supports the use of eccentric exercises.[22] A physical therapy referral can help to evaluate and initiate these treatment options for patients.

Radiculopathy is another common musculoskeletal complaint in the primary care setting. Peripheral nerve root irritation from foraminal encroachment or a herniated nucleus pulposus can be seen in the cervical and lumbar spine.[23] Physical therapy treatment options have been studied extensively for pain relief related to these complaints. A systematic review looking at manual therapy in the treatment of cervical

| Table 2 | |
Common diagnosis-based referral	
Osteoarthritis	Patient deconditioning
Rheumatoid arthritis	Perioperative
Tendinopathy	Ligament injury/sprain
Radiculopathy	Muscle injury/strain

radiculopathy concluded that manual therapy in conjunction with therapeutic exercise was effective in regard of improving active range of motion and function while decreasing pain and disability.[24] Another review studied whether manipulation or mobilization for neck pain improved outcomes, and found evidence of short-term or intermediate-term changes in pain and function.[25]

Patient deconditioning or disability is also a common reason for referral to physical therapy. The benefits of physical activity, management, and treatment of chronic disease and disability have been well documented, and the choice of therapy should be tailored to the patient's disability.[26] Chronic diseases such as heart disease, stroke, diabetes, lung disease, Alzheimer dementia, hypertension, and cancer have increasing morbidity related to lack of physical activity.[27] Lack of physical activity and poor dietary habits also significantly contribute to obesity.[27] Referrals for physical therapy to address these disabilities are valuable potential treatment options.

The perioperative physical therapy referral is common, especially in patients wishing to return to physical activity or sport. General recommendations have been made regarding the need for quantification of muscle strength, stability, neuromuscular control, and function in patients who desire to return to athletics following an anterior cruciate ligament reconstruction.[28] There has been no consensus, however, for the optimal rehabilitation program and time to return to sport.[29] Physical therapy has also been evaluated other clinical areas. For patients who will be undergoing elective cardiac surgery, small trials have suggested that physical therapy reduces postoperative pulmonary complications (atelectasis, pneumonia) and decreases the length of stay in hospital.[30]

These indications for physical therapy are only a few of those based on physical examination, symptoms, and specific diagnoses in musculoskeletal medicine. There are many other examples not mentioned in this article. The body of evidence supporting physical therapy services is growing as clinical scientists become more adept at developing clinically relevant, outcome-based research protocols.

WRITING A PHYSICAL THERAPY PRESCRIPTION

When physically writing a prescription for physical therapy, the practitioner must include several components. First there needs to be a diagnosis. As discussed earlier, this may be an actual diagnosis such as lateral epicondylopathy or may be a symptom or examination finding such as knee pain or knee instability. The prescription should ask the physical therapist to evaluate and treat the patient for the diagnosis that the practitioner has established. The next component is a recommendation for the number of times per week the practitioner considers the patient can benefit from the therapy. A health care provider might make this decision based on goals of the patient (ie, regain range of motion and decrease pain), whether the patient has time to go to the sessions, the nature of the condition (acute, subacute, and chronic), and whether insurance will pay for the requested number of visits. For most practitioners the initial prescription is a baseline recommendation that can be modified as per recommendations from the physical therapist or in response to how well the patient benefits from the therapy. The practitioner should also list any specific protocols to be provided by the physical therapist. For example, in the diagnosis of tendinopathy, if a provider considers that the patient could benefit from eccentric strengthening, this should be specifically asked for. Another example would be perioperative protocols that are frequently used by orthopedic surgeons. Most rehabilitation protocols will be left to interpretation by the treating physical therapist based on the indication for referral. The prescription should include any limitations such as the patient's weight-bearing

---

Box 7
Components of a physical therapy prescription

Patient name and date

Diagnosis

Frequency and duration

Specific instructions

Safety precautions

Signature

---

status. Finally, as with every physician order, the prescription for the order to be performed must be signed and dated (**Box 7**).

SUMMARY AND DISCUSSION

The use of physical therapy has been reported since the time of Hippocrates, and has evolved most notably since World War I. The training has become more rigorous over the years and has culminated in the DPT degree that has been established in recent years. With the advancement of training, there has also been advancement in the scientific evidence for the use of physical therapy. Therapeutic modalities will continue to require research, as there is a continuing need to prove the proposed physiologic effects. Studies have been historically difficult to perform because of the hands-on therapy provided to the patient, and can be operator dependent. For this reason, a close working relationship should exist between the physician and physical therapist with the goal of providing patient care that leads to clinically relevant outcomes. The physical therapist should provide a dynamic care plan to the patient depending on the patient's response to therapy.

The initial physical therapy visit includes a comprehensive history and physical examination with emphasis on biomechanical analysis, range of motion, strength, and special testing. The physical therapist then creates a rehabilitation plan taking into consideration manual techniques, modalities, and exercises that will maximize the patient's potential for complete recovery. The therapist also prognosticates at that time regarding the anticipated duration and number of visits needed, taking into account the clinical and socioeconomic situation of the patient. All of this is typically initiated after a referral from a health care provider and a written prescription has been provided. The physical therapy referral imparts a useful option to the care plan of clinicians, particularly for musculoskeletal ailments.

REFERENCES

1. A comprehensive review of a 21st century health care profession. American Physical Therapy Association; 2011. Available at: www.apta.org/uploadedFiles/APTAorg/Practice_and_Patient_Care/PR_and_Marketing/Market_to_Professionals/TodaysPhysicalTherapist.pdf. Accessed November 1, 2013.
2. History of the chartered society of physiotherapy. 1. Chartered Society of Physiotherapy. Available at: http://www.csp.org.uk/about-csp/history/csp-history. Accessed November 1, 2013.
3. Moffat M. The history of physical therapy practice in the United States. J Phys Ther Educ 2003;17:15–25.

4. Murphy W. Healing the generations: a history of physical therapy and the American Physical Therapy Association. Lyme (CT): Greenwich Publishing Group Inc; 1995.
5. Direct access to PT services: overview. American Physical Therapy Association. Updated October 27, 13. Available at: http://www.apta.org/StateIssues/DirectAccess/Overview. Accessed November 1, 2013.
6. GL H, Leaver-Dunn D. Physical rehabilitation of the injured athlete. Philadelphia: W.B. Saunders; 1998.
7. Fuller C. Physical rehabilitation of the injured athlete. Philadelphia: W.B. Saunders; 1998.
8. Gribble PA, Guskiewicz KM, Prentice WE, et al. Effects of static hold-relax stretching on hamstring range of motion using the Flexability LE 1000. J Sport Rehabil 1999;8:195–208.
9. Philadelphia panel evidence-based clinical practice guidelines on selected rehabilitation interventions: overview and methodology. Phys Ther 2001;81(10):1629–40.
10. Cochrane reviews. Available at: http://www.cochrane.org/cochrane-reviews. Accessed November 16, 2013.
11. Kay TM, Gross A, Goldsmith CH, et al. Exercises for mechanical neck disorders. Cochrane Database Syst Rev 2012;(8):CD004250.
12. Almeida MO, Silva BN, Andriolo RB, et al. Conservative interventions for treating exercise-related musculotendinous, ligamentous and osseous groin pain. Cochrane Database Syst Rev 2013;(6):CD009565.
13. Fransen M, McConnell S. Exercise for osteoarthritis of the knee. Cochrane Database Syst Rev 2008;(4):CD004376.
14. Uthman OA, van der Windt DA, Jordan JL, et al. Exercise for lower limb osteoarthritis: systematic review incorporating trial sequential analysis and network meta-analysis. BMJ 2013;347:f5555.
15. Rutjes AW, Nuesch E, Sterchi R, et al. Therapeutic ultrasound for osteoarthritis of the knee or hip. Cochrane Database Syst Rev 2010;(1):CD003132.
16. Brosseau LU, Pelland LU, Casimiro LY, et al. Electrical stimulation for the treatment of rheumatoid arthritis. Cochrane Database Syst Rev 2002;(2):CD003687.
17. Casimiro L, Brosseau L, Robinson V, et al. Therapeutic ultrasound for the treatment of rheumatoid arthritis. Cochrane Database Syst Rev 2002;(3):CD003787.
18. Steultjens EM, Dekker J, Bouter LM, et al. Occupational therapy for rheumatoid arthritis. Cochrane Database Syst Rev 2004;(1):CD003114.
19. Nirschl RP, Pettrone FA. Tennis elbow. The surgical treatment of lateral epicondylitis. J Bone Joint Surg Am 1979;61(6A):832–9.
20. Hoogvliet P, Randsdorp MS, Dingemanse R, et al. Does effectiveness of exercise therapy and mobilisation techniques offer guidance for the treatment of lateral and medial epicondylitis? A systematic review. Br J Sports Med 2013;47:1112–9.
21. Ackermann PW, Renstrom P. Tendinopathy in sport. Sports Health 2012;4(3):193–201.
22. Sussmilch-Leitch SP, Collins NJ, Bialocerkowski AE, et al. Physical therapies for Achilles tendinopathy: systematic review and meta-analysis. J Foot Ankle Res 2012;5(1):15.
23. Onks CA, Billy G. Evaluation and treatment of cervical radiculopathy. Prim Care 2013;40(4):837–48.
24. Boyles R, Toy P, Mellon J Jr, et al. Effectiveness of manual physical therapy in the treatment of cervical radiculopathy: a systematic review. J Man Manip Ther 2011;19(3):135–42.
25. Gross A, Miller J, D'Sylva J, et al. Manipulation or mobilisation for neck pain: a Cochrane review. Man Ther 2010;15(4):315–33.

26. Chodzko-Zajko WJ, Proctor DN, Fiatarone Singh MA, et al. American College of Sports Medicine position stand. Exercise and physical activity for older adults. Med Sci Sports Exerc 2009;41(7):1510–30.
27. Elsawy B, Higgins KE. Physical activity guidelines for older adults. Am Fam Physician 2010;81(1):55–9.
28. Barber-Westin SD, Noyes FR. Factors used to determine return to unrestricted sports activities after anterior cruciate ligament reconstruction. Arthroscopy 2011;27(12):1697–705.
29. Yabroudi MA, Irrgang JJ. Rehabilitation and return to play after anatomic anterior cruciate ligament reconstruction. Clin Sports Med 2013;32(1):165–75.
30. Hulzebos EH, Smit Y, Helders PP, et al. Preoperative physical therapy for elective cardiac surgery patients. Cochrane Database Syst Rev 2012;(11):CD010118.

Durable Medical Equipment: Types and Indications

Bret C. Jacobs, DO, MA[a,b,]*, Justin A. Lee, MD[c]

KEYWORDS

- Brace • Durable medical equipment • Counterforce brace • Cock-up brace
- Pneumatic brace • Ankle stirrup • Lace-up brace • Patellar strap

KEY POINTS

- Durable medical equipment (DME) is useful for treating various upper and lower extremity orthopedic conditions.
- DME is divided into three types: prophylactic, functional, and rehabilitative or postoperative.
- Proper diagnosis is essential when selecting type of DME for orthopedic conditions.
- Clinicians should have a basic understanding of braces that are available for various conditions but it is not necessary to know every type of brace for each possible injury.

INTRODUCTION

The treatment of common musculoskeletal conditions includes medications, physical therapy, surgery, and durable medical equipment (DME), including braces and splints. Treatment often requires a combination of these items to achieve the desired outcome. At times, it may seem difficult and daunting to decide the best treatment, especially when dealing with DME.

There are various types of DME to treat musculoskeletal conditions. In simple terms, DME is medical equipment that is used for specific treatment of a medical condition, illness, or injury. The equipment should be reusable and considered nondisposable.[1] Examples of DME include braces or orthosis, wheelchairs, walkers, canes, hospital beds, and similar supplies.[2] There are various other types of DME that meet this definition; however, the types of DME most useful for musculoskeletal conditions include braces, orthoses, and mobility devices.

Disclosures: The authors have nothing to disclose.
[a] Department of Family & Community Medicine, Penn State Milton S. Hershey Medical Center, 500 University Drive, Mail Code HP 06, Hershey, PA 17033, USA; [b] Department of Orthopaedics & Rehabilitation, Penn State Milton S. Hershey Medical Center, 500 University Drive, Mail Code HP 06, Hershey, PA 17033, USA; [c] Department of Family Medicine, Brody School of Medicine, East Carolina University, 101 Heart Drive, Mail Stop 654, Greenville, NC 27834, USA
* Corresponding author.
E-mail address: bjacobs@hmc.psu.edu

Med Clin N Am 98 (2014) 881–893
http://dx.doi.org/10.1016/j.mcna.2014.03.010
0025-7125/14/$ – see front matter © 2014 Elsevier Inc. All rights reserved.

Various terms refer to musculoskeletal-related DME products. Terms such as brace, orthotic device, orthosis, and splint are often used interchangeably and can refer to the same device, depending on the context. In Greek, orthosis means "making straight." As defined by Merriam-Webster Dictionary, an orthosis is "a device for supporting, immobilizing, or treating muscles, joints, or skeletal parts which are weak, ineffective, deformed, or injured."[3] Brace is an accepted term to mean orthosis or orthotic device. For simplicity, it is used throughout this article to refer to orthosis.

General Considerations in DME Use

If the various terms referring to DME are not confusing enough, there are a myriad of devices that are applied to each part of the body. It is important to realize that proper diagnosis is essential when selecting the type of DME. The same area of the body can be treated with different types of DME, depending on the condition being treated and the needs of the patient.

TYPES OF BRACES

Braces are divided into three broad groups: prophylactic, functional, and rehabilitative or postoperative. Prophylactic braces are intended to prevent or reduce the severity of injury. Functional braces are used to provide stability and enhance function to an injured area to allow participation in activities. Rehabilitative or postoperative braces are used for short periods of time (days to weeks) after acute injury or surgery. Rehabilitative or postoperative braces allow controlled range of motion and provide protection during the rehabilitative period.[4] Some braces are used for all of these functions. Choice of brace depends on the injury being treated and the goal of treatment (**Table 1**).

All braces are effective in helping patients with musculoskeletal injuries. There are four basic stages of rehabilitation following musculoskeletal injury: (1) preventing further injury and controlling pain and swelling; (2) improving strength and flexibility; (3) improving strength, endurance, and proprioception until near-normal function is achieved; and (4) returning to activities and sporting activities. Braces are adjuncts to help with this process and achieve desired effects through various mechanisms. Some restrict motion whereas others augment movement. Some braces provide cushion and support to damaged and injured tissues and others promote proprioception and performance. Whatever the mechanism of action, the goal is to achieve adequate function and performance.[5]

PROPER PRESCRIBING PRACTICES

Before any brace or rehabilitation plan is prescribed, the clinician must have a firm understanding of the diagnosis and the needs of the patient. Is the goal for the patient to

Table 1 Basic DME brace types	
Brace Type	**Goal of Brace**
Functional brace	Provide stability Enhance function
Prophylactic brace	Prevent injury or decrease severity of possible injury
Rehabilitative or postoperative brace	Allow controlled range of motion Help limit swelling

return to athletics or work, or simply to be functional and pain free? Selecting the correct brace for the desired application is as important as the long-term goal of treatment. It is also important to understand that a brace or DME can cause pain or further injury if not properly fitted or if used incorrectly. The clinician must understand these consequences and appropriately educate patients.

Clinicians should have a basic understanding of the braces that are available for various conditions. Clinicians do not necessarily know every single type of brace for each possible injury, nor is it practical for an office to stock several different braces for the same condition. Instead, it is advisable to have a good understanding of one to two braces that are suitable for certain conditions and to have these in the office available for patients. This will allow better familiarity with specific braces and products. There are times when common braces are not suitable or available. In these cases, it is useful to have access to an orthotist. An orthotist specializes in braces, both off-the-shelf and custom-made, and is a valuable resource to help treat patients.

DME FOR THE UPPER EXTREMITY
Elbow

Lateral epicondylitis, also known as tennis elbow, is a common condition causing pain and discomfort along the lateral aspect of the elbow at attachment of the common extensor tendon origin of the lateral epicondyle. The extensor carpi radialis brevis is one of the most commonly affected tendons. This pain is often aggravated by active wrist extension, supination, and power grip.[6] The incidence in general practice is approximately 4 to 7 per 1000 patients per year with an annual incidence of 1% to 3% in the general population.[7] Duration of symptoms can range from 6 months to 2 years if untreated. Lateral epicondylitis can lead to loss of work or activity for several weeks or months if not properly managed. Risk factors for lateral epicondylitis, along with other overuse injuries, include age more than 35 years, high activity level (sport or occupation), high-demand work, and inadequate fitness level.[8]

The most common brace for lateral epicondylitis is the elbow strap or elbow band, which is commonly referred to as a counterforce brace (**Fig. 1**). The brace is placed on the elbow one to two finger breadths distal to the lateral epicondyle over the common extensor tendon. The brace should fit snugly but should not cause increased pain or numbness of the fingers or hand, which is a sign that the brace is too tight. The proposed mechanism of the brace is that it applies pressure along the proximal forearm, reduces forces on the common extensor tendon, and distributes forces to noninjured tissues thus reducing pain during activities.[9]

In 2004, Struijs and colleagues[9] completed a study comparing physical therapy with bracing for tennis elbow. A counterforce brace increased daily activity levels

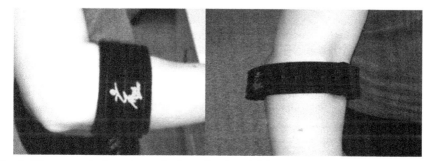

Fig. 1. Elbow counterforce brace for lateral epicondylitis.

compared with physical therapy alone. Physical therapy was found superior to bracing for decreasing pain, improving disability, and patient satisfaction after 6 weeks but not at long-term follow-up. A combination of physical therapy and bracing was superior to a brace alone or physical therapy alone at 6 weeks but not at long-term follow-up. A Cochrane review and a systematic review by Bisset and colleagues,[10] in 2005, failed to show effectiveness of the counterforce brace for treatment of lateral epicondylitis.[7]

The literature does not clearly support the use of a counterforce brace for lateral epicondylitis but more research is needed. From the existing research, the use of a counterforce brace early in treatment in conjunction with physical therapy that focuses on progressive strengthening and eccentric exercises seems ideal. A counterforce brace is safe and relatively inexpensive. If not used properly, the brace can lead to increased pain in the elbow, nerve compression of the radial nerve or anterior interosseous nerve, or venous congestion; therefore, it is essential to counsel patients on proper fit and usage.

Wrist

Carpal tunnel syndrome is the most common peripheral nerve compression syndrome with a prevalence of 2.7% to 5.8% in the general population. Carpal tunnel syndrome is more common in female patients and often occurs in those more than 30 years of age. Carpal tunnel syndrome involves compression of the median nerve at the level of the wrist.[11,12] Symptoms include pain and paresthesia along the thumb, index finger, and middle finger. Other symptoms may include nighttime pain and radiation of symptoms into the forearm. With advanced disease, muscle atrophy and muscle weakness can also be present.

Treatment is divided into nonsurgical and surgical options. Nonsurgical treatment is indicated for initial treatment in patients with intermittent symptoms and those without signs of muscle weakness or muscle atrophy. These splints can also be used for those awaiting surgical intervention. Wrist splinting with a cock-up or neutral wrist splint are most often used. The splint is used mainly as a rehabilitative brace but it can also act as a functional brace. Wrist splints work by immobilizing the wrist and limiting compression of the median nerve, which occurs in both flexion and extension.[11,13]

Limited evidence indicates that bracing can improve symptoms during the first 2 to 3 weeks of use.[14] Nighttime splint use is often recommend, although the literature shows that full-time splinting throughout the day is more effective (Level of Evidence: A, based on systematic review by Goodyear-Smith and Arroll).[11] Even though full-time splinting is supported in the literature, nighttime use is often more tolerable and accepted by patients. A Cochrane review demonstrated limited evidence that, in the short term, a splint worn at night is more effective than no treatment.[13]

Cock-up wrist splints (**Fig. 2**) are commonly used to treat carpal tunnel syndrome, although neutral wrist splints are also an option. Some studies have shown neutral splinting is superior to cock-up splinting (20° extension).[11] Cochrane reviews have demonstrated limited evidence that neutral wrist-splinting results are superior overall and for nocturnal symptom relief when compared with cock-up splinting. These reviews also show limited evidence that one splint type is more effective than are others.[13,14]

Based on these findings, the literature seems to favor neutral wrist splinting instead of cock-up wrist splinting. Although full-time use of wrist splints seems the most effective, nocturnal use will still offer some benefit and likely be more accepted by patients.

Hand

Fingertip injuries are common in athletes and the general population. The distal phalanx is a common site of injury and is the most commonly fractured bone in the hand.[15]

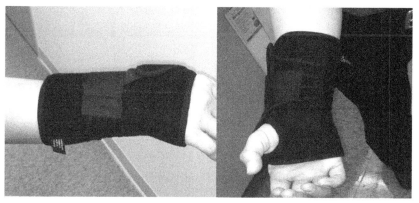

Fig. 2. Cock-up wrist splint.

A mallet finger is a flexion deformity of the distal interphalangeal (DIP) joint caused by a disruption of the extensor tendon mechanism. This is the result of forcefully flexing the DIP joint when it is fully extended. There are two forms of a mallet finger including a bony mallet: an avulsion fracture of the distal phalanx and a soft-tissue mallet involving only the extensor tendon. In either case, the patient will present with inability to fully extend the DIP joint.

Mallet finger responds well to nonoperative treatment; however, injuries involving one-third or more of the articular surface of the distal phalanx may require surgery and these cases should be referred. The treatment of choice is splinting the finger in full extension for a period of 6 to 8 weeks. This may be accomplished with an aluminum, stack, or similar splint, which keeps the DIP joint in full extension (**Fig. 3**). The DIP joint should never be allowed to flex during the treatment period, a key point for patients. When changing the splint, the patient must support the finger on a flat surface and slide the splint off the finger with splint replacement while keeping the finger in extension.[15] If the finger is allowed to flex, the treatment period restarts from the beginning.[5] A Cochrane review demonstrated that the type of splint used is not as important as patient compliance for a successful outcome.[16] Adverse effects from splinting of a mallet finger may include skin necrosis if the DIP joint is over extended

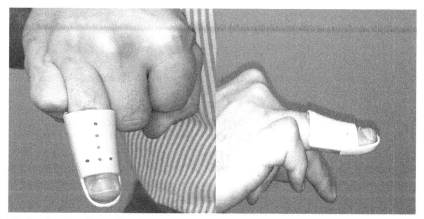

Fig. 3. Stack splint for mallet finger injury.

during splinting, maceration of the skin from being in splint for a prolonged period of time, and skin blanching from having the finger in a position of hyperextension.[5]

DME FOR THE LOWER EXTREMITY
Knee

Knee injuries are common among athletes and the general population. These injuries may be related to trauma, overuse, or accumulated effects of osteoarthritis. These injuries lead to lost time from work, sports, and academics, and can account for substantial effects on quality of life.

Knee osteoarthritis
Osteoarthritis is a growing epidemic in the United States and across the globe. An estimated 50 million Americans have been diagnosed with osteoarthritis and this number is continuing to grow. Osteoarthritis is characterized by erosion of the articular cartilage, formation of osteophytes along bone margins, and subchondral sclerosis.[17] Osteoarthritis is the leading cause of disability in the United States and affects 34% of people more than 65 years of age. Eighty percent of patients with knee osteoarthritis have mobility issues and 25% cannot perform major activities of daily living.[18]

Treatment of knee osteoarthritis may include medications, physical therapy, exercise, weight loss, the use of braces or orthotic devices, and surgery. Nonsteroidal anti-inflammatory drugs have long been the mainstay of arthritis treatment, although they are starting to undergo more scrutiny due to increasing rates of adverse effects. Therefore, conservative, nonmedication therapies for arthritis are becoming more important.[19]

Various DME devices are helpful for the treatment of knee osteoarthritis, including assistive walking devices (eg, cane, crutch, walker), knee braces, and shoe orthotic inserts. A cane can help patients be more mobile and studies have shown a cane helps reduce intraarticular loading forces in the knee by more than 10%. Canes are most effective for medial and lateral compartment knee osteoarthritis but are not as useful for patellofemoral osteoarthritis.[19] Proper cane fitting is completed by having the patient stand with the cane on the contralateral side of the body (opposite the joint with osteoarthritis) with ground contact just lateral to the lateral malleolus. The handle of the cane should be at the approximate level of the superior tip of the greater trochanter. The patient should have their arm in approximately 20° to 30° of elbow flexion while using the cane to walk. During ambulation, the cane will move forward along with the affected leg.[19]

Unloader Braces
In addition to walking aids, knee braces and shoe orthotics help to decrease pain and improve physical function, and in some cases slow disease progression. Unloader braces, which work as functional braces, are designed to reduce loading on a specific compartment of the knee. Unloader braces can be designed as a medial unloader brace for medical compartment osteoarthritis or lateral unloader brace for lateral compartment osteoarthritis. These braces are designed to improve bony alignment of the tibia and femur.[19,20] Several studies have shown up to 50 percent improvement in pain and function with an unloader brace.[20] A recent Cochrane review demonstrated effectiveness of treating unicompartmental osteoarthritis with a brace, especially osteoarthritis of the medial compartment.[21] Patients were able to walk longer distances, indicating improved level of function. The improved mobility may allow arthritic patients to increase their level of activity, leading to weight loss and improved muscle strength, both of which can help with osteoarthritis treatment.[5]

Patient compliance may be an issue with unloader braces. These braces may have some benefit with regular activities of daily living (ADLs). Patients should be encouraged to primarily wear them with physical or sporting activities. Possible adverse effects from unloader braces include low back pain, posterior knee pain, skin irritation, poor fit, and leg pain.[21] All of these fctors may contribute to overall compliance.

Ligamentous knee injuries

Braces for ligamentous knee injuries are prophylactic, rehabilitative, or functional. Prophylactic braces primarily prevent injury to the medial collateral ligament (MCL) from excessive valgus force to the knee. The incidence of MCL injuries is approximately 24 per 100,000 athletes per year in the United States and 2.1 injuries per 1000 athletes in the National Collegiate Athletic Association.[22] Studies have shown that prophylactic knee braces may provide greater than 10% to 30% greater MCL resistance to valgus stress compared with the unbraced knee.[4,23] These braces are commonly seen in football, but the American Academy of Orthopedic Surgeons and the American Academy of Pediatrics state there is insufficient evidence to routinely recommend the use of prophylactic knee braces in football. Multiple studies have shown trends that these braces can be helpful in certain high-risk situations. Nevertheless, overall, prophylactic braces do not prevent or decrease the severity of MCL injuries.[4,24]

Functional knee braces are designed to enhance knee stability following ligamentous and/or meniscus injuries. The goal is to prevent further injury. Functional knee braces typically have a hinged design or other sturdy material for lateral stability, such as a plastic composite (**Fig. 4**). Studies have shown little difference when comparing custom functional braces to off-the-shelf versions.[4] It is often routine practice for physicians to prescribe a functional knee brace to athletes following an anterior cruciate ligament (ACL) reconstruction. Up to 87% of orthopedic surgeons prescribe a functional brace after ACL reconstruction.[25] There is lack of evidence that these braces are helpful at high levels of athletic participation; however, they often perform well in low-force conditions.[5] A study by Risberg and colleagues[26] showed functional knee braces lead to increased thigh atrophy and decreased quadriceps strength but do not have significant effect on joint laxity, pain, or patient satisfaction. These braces supply additional support to the knee but should not replace a

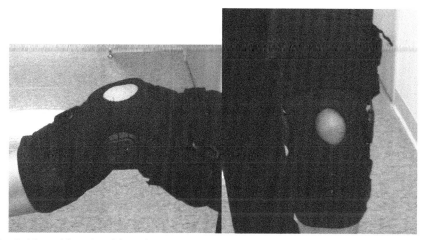

Fig. 4. Hinged functional knee brace.

solid rehabilitation program that focuses on core strength, lower extremity strength, and flexibility.

Rehabilitative knee braces are used immediately after injury and sometimes in the postoperative period. A common example of a rehabilitative knee brace is the knee immobilizer, which is a brace consisting of a foam liner and multiple straps that extend from the middle of the thigh to the ankle. This brace is designed to prevent knee flexion or range of motion (**Fig. 5**). Knee immobilizers are typically applied in the emergency department or office setting immediately following an injury, although it is rare that they are truly indicated. Knee immobilizers should be used only if there is concern for a patellar dislocation, patellar fracture, or multiligamentous injury before definitive treatment. In the acute period, knee immobilizers help decrease swelling and pain but can predispose patients to significant knee stiffness or quadriceps atrophy, especially if the patient does not comply with regular office follow-up intervals. An adjustable, hinged knee brace has the ability to adjust the amount of flexion and extension allowed by the knee. These braces are helpful when trying to allow controlled range of motion.

Braces for the patella

Anterior knee pain related to patellofemoral syndrome and patellar tendinitis is a common complaint in the office. These patients complain of pain that is often worse with ascending or descending the stairs, after prolonged sitting, and during squatting activities. Two common functional knee braces used for these conditions include a knee sleeve (**Fig. 6**) and patellar strap (**Fig. 7**). Knees sleeves are generally composed of an elastic or neoprene type material that applies compression to the knee. A central cutout for the patella is advisable for added comfort. The patellar strap is placed below the patella where it slightly elevates the knee cap with flexion and extension while decreasing traction forces across the patellar tendon.[4,27] Evidence on the effect of either brace is limited and a Cochrane review was unable to recommend for or against the use of these functional braces.[27] Again, a thorough rehabilitation program focusing on strengthening and flexibility should be used. Knee sleeves and patellar straps can be a useful second-line therapy. They are relatively inexpensive and have no real

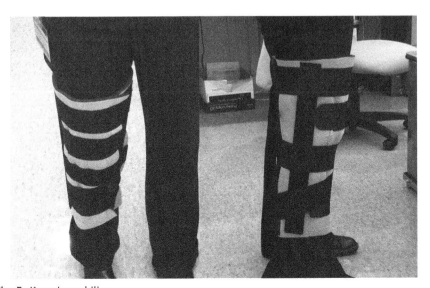

Fig. 5. Knee immobilizer.

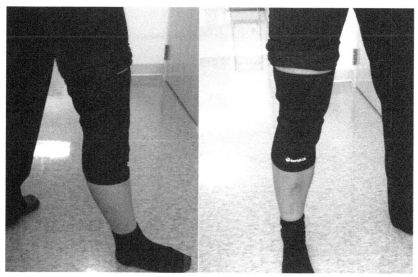

Fig. 6. Knee sleeve.

contraindications. If a patient has been using these devices and fails to notice any improvement, stopping their use is recommended.

Lower Leg: Tibia and Fibula

Lower extremity stress fractures are injuries common in active individuals, especially runners. The tibia is the most common area for a stress fracture, accounting for 24% of all stress fractures.[28] Runners averaging more than 25 miles per week are at increased risk but other athletes are at risk as well. Healing time for tibial stress fractures ranges from 4 to 12 weeks or longer. A pneumatic leg brace can be used to aid in treatment and provide a quicker recovery. Several studies have shown that, after proper diagnosis, treatment of tibial stress fractures is facilitated by activity restriction and a pneumatic leg brace.[29,30] Athletes using a pneumatic brace can return to activities 3 to 4 weeks before those treated without a pneumatic brace.[31] A Cochrane review also confirmed quicker recovery with the use of a pneumatic brace but did indicate further studies are needed.

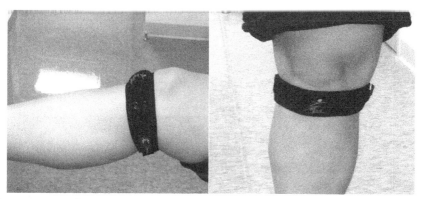

Fig. 7. Knee patellar strap.

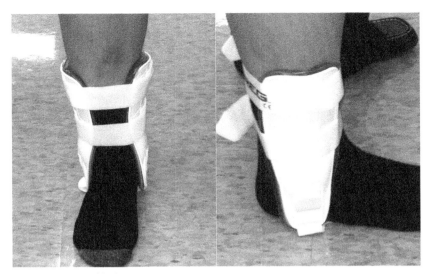

Fig. 8. Pneumatic ankle brace.

In clinical practice, one of the most important factors for lower extremity stress fracture healing is activity restriction. Pneumatic leg braces are often helpful for athletes who have some pain as they start to advance activities of daily living and sporting activities. These braces help to stabilize the fracture site and redistribute loading forces throughout the lower leg.[29]

Ankle Injuries

Ankle sprains are common among athletes and nonathletes. They account for many office visits with an overall incidence of 2.15 per 1000 person-years.[32] The greatest risk factor for sustaining an ankle sprain is a previous ankle sprain. DME for ankle sprains are divided into functional, rehabilitative, and prophylactic, similar to braces for other parts of the body. Following an acute ankle sprain, a patient may benefit from the use of a rigid, stirrup-type brace, such as a pneumatic ankle brace (**Fig. 8**), or a controlled ankle motion (CAM) or fracture boot (**Fig. 9**). Both braces limit range of motion and help decrease swelling. A pneumatic ankle brace functions as a

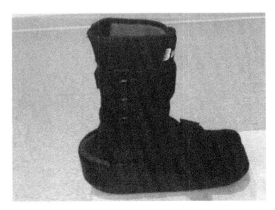

Fig. 9. Cam boot.

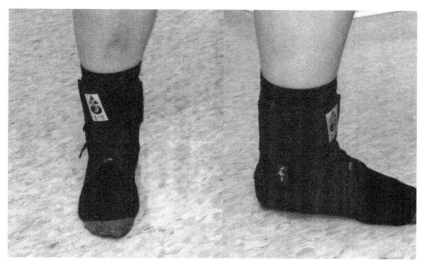

Fig. 10. Lace-up ankle brace for ankle sprain.

functional and rehabilitative brace; however, it tends to be too rigid. A semirigid, lace-up ankle brace is preferred when a patient is returning to activity. Lace-up braces may have elastic straps that cross the ankle for some additional support (**Fig. 10**).

Multiple studies have demonstrated a decreased incidence of recurrent ankle sprains with the use of ankle braces.[33,34] These braces provide mechanical support and stability to the ankle and also improve proprioception. Several reviews, including a Cochrane review, recommend the use of a semirigid, lace-up ankle brace to prevent ankle sprains during high-risk sporting activities that pose a risk for inversion ankle sprain, such as soccer, basketball, volleyball.[34,35] Braces decrease the risk of an ankle sprain by approximately 69%.[32] It is recommended that athletes wear some type of ankle brace with activity for at least 12 months after injury because this is the approximate length of time for ligaments to completely heal. Again, the brace is not a replacement for a proper rehabilitation program that includes strengthening and proprioceptive training.

SUMMARY

Various types of DME exist, all of which provide a specific goal and function depending on the body area being treated. The broad categories of prophylactic, functional, and rehabilitative provide an indication of the goal of a brace. At this time, there is limited research and literature focusing on the use of various DME. Therefore, many of the braces used in practice have only anecdotal support at best. More research needs to be completed to assess the overall effectiveness of DME products.

REFERENCES

1. United Healthcare. Durable medical equipment, orthotics, ostomy supplies, medical supplies, and repairs/replacements. 2012. Available at: https://www.united healthcareonline.com/ccmcontent/ProviderII/UHC/en-US/Assets/ProviderStaticFiles/ProviderStaticFilesPdf/Tools%20and%20Resources/Policies%20and%20Protocols/Medical%20Policies/Medical%20Policies/DME_CD.pdf. Accessed November 9, 2013.

2. U.S. Department of Health and Human Services – Centers for Medicare & Medicaid Services. Your medicare benefits. 2013. Available at: http://www.medicare.gov/Publications/Pubs/pdf/10116.pdf. Accessed November 9, 2013.
3. Merriam-Webster Online Dictionary: definition of "orthotic." 2013. Available at: http://www.merriam-webster.com/dictionary/orthotic?show=0&t=1384042618. Accessed November 9, 2013.
4. Martin TJ, Committee on Sports Medicine and Fitness. Technical report: knee brace use in the young athlete. Pediatrics 2001;108(2):503–7.
5. Leggitt JC, Jarvis CG. Proper indications and uses of orthopedic braces. In: Seidenberg PH, Beutler AI, editors. The sports medicine resource manual. Philadelphia: Saunders; 2008. p. 483–94.
6. Garg R, Adamson GJ, Dawson PA, et al. A prospective randomized study comparing a forearm strap brace versus a wrist splint for the treatment of lateral epicondylitis. J Shoulder Elbow Surg 2010;19:508–12.
7. Struijs PA, Smidt N, Arola H, et al. Orthotic devices for the treatment of tennis elbow. Cochrane Database Syst Rev 2002;(1):CD001821. http://dx.doi.org/10.1002/14651858.CD001821.
8. Nirschl RP. Elbow tendinosis/tennis elbow. Clin Sports Med 1992;11:851–70.
9. Struijs PA, Kerkhoffs GM, Assendelft WJ, et al. Conservative treatment of lateral epicondylitis: brace versus physical therapy or a combination of both-a randomized controlled trial. Am J Sports Med 2004;32(2):462–9.
10. Bisset L, Paungmali A, Vicenzino B, et al. A systematic review and meta-analysis of clinical trials on physical interventions for lateral epicondylalgia. Br J Sports Med 2005;39:411–22.
11. Goodyear-Smith F, Arroll B. What can family physicians offer patients with carpal tunnel syndrome other than surgery? A systematic review of nonsurgical management. Ann Fam Med 2004;2(3):267–73.
12. LeBlanc KE, Cestia W. Carpal tunnel syndrome. Am Fam Physician 2011;83(8): 952–8.
13. Page MJ, Massy-Westropp N, O'connor D, et al. Splinting for carpal tunnel syndrome. Cochrane Database Syst Rev 2012;(7):CD010003. http://dx.doi.org/10.1002/14651858.CD010003.
14. O'connor D, Marhsall S, Massy-Westropp N. Non-surgical treatment (other than steroid injection) for carpal tunnel syndrome. Cochrane Database Syst Rev 2012;(7):CD003219. http://dx.doi.org/10.1002/14651858.CD003219.
15. Wang QC, Johnson BA. Fingertip injuries. Am Fam Physician 2001;63(10): 1961–6.
16. Handoll HH, Vaghela MV. Interventions for treating mallet finger injuries. Cochrane Database Syst Rev 2008;(3):CD004574. http://dx.doi.org/10.1002/14651858.CD004574.pub2.
17. Ringdahl E, Pandit S. Treatment of knee osteoarthritis. Am Fam Physician 2011; 83(11):1287–92.
18. Center for Disease Control and Prevention. Osteoarthritis. 2009. Available at: http://www.cdc.gov/arthritis/basics/osteoarthritis.htm. Accessed November 11, 2013.
19. Gross KD. Device use: walking aids, braces, and orthoses for symptomatic knee osteoarthritis. Clin Geriatr Med 2010;26:479–502.
20. Hunter DJ, Lo GH. The management of osteoarthritis: an overview and call to appropriate conservative treatment. Med Clin North Am 2009;93:127–43.
21. Brouwer RW, van Raaij TM, Jakma TT, et al. Braces and orthoses for treating osteoarthritis of the knee. Cochrane Database Syst Rev 2009;(1):CD004020. http://dx.doi.org/10.1002/14651858.pub2.

22. Morelli V, Bright C, Fields A. Ligamentous injuries of the knee: anterior cruciate, medial collateral, posterior cruciate, and posterolateral corner injuries. Prim Care 2013;40:335–56.
23. Najibi S, Albright JP. The use of knee braces, part 1: prophylactic knee braces in contact sports. Am J Sports Med 2005;33(4):602–11.
24. Salata MJ, Gibbs AE, Sekiya JK. The effectiveness of prophylactic knee bracing in American football: a systematic review. Sports Health 2010;2(5):375–9.
25. Albright JC, Crepeau AE. Functional bracing and return to play after anterior cruciate ligament reconstruction in the pediatric and adolescent patient. Clin Sports Med 2011;30:811–5.
26. Risberg MA, Holm I, Steen H, et al. The effect of knee bracing after anterior cruciate ligament reconstruction. A prospective, randomized study with two years' follow-up. Am J Sports Med 1999;27(1):76–83.
27. D'hondt NE, Struijs PA, Kerkhoffs GM, et al. Orthotic devices for treating patellofemoral pain syndrome. Cochrane Database Syst Rev 2008;(2):CD002267. http://dx.doi.org/10.1002/14651858.CD002267.
28. Patel DS, Roth M, Kapil N. Stress fractures: diagnosis, treatment, and prevention. Am Fam Physician 2011;83(1):39–46.
29. Swenson EJ, DeHaven KE, Sebastianelli WJ, et al. The effect of a pneumatic leg brace on return to play in athletes with tibial stress fractures. Am J Sports Med 1997;25(3):322–8.
30. Whitelaw GP, Wetzler MJ, Levy AS, et al. A pneumatic leg brace for the treatment of tibial stress fractures. Clin Orthop Relat Res 1991;270:301–5.
31. Rome K, Handoll HH, Ashford RL. Interventions for preventing and treating stress fractures and stress reactions of bone of the lower limbs in young adults. Cochrane Database Syst Rev 2009;(1):CD000450. http://dx.doi.org/10.1002/14651858.CD000450.pub2.
32. Tiemstra JD. Update on acute ankle sprains. Am Fam Physician 2012;85(12):1170–6.
33. Stasinopoulos D. Comparison of three preventative methods in order to reduce the incidence of ankle inversion sprains among female volleyball players. Br J Sports Med 2004;38:182–5.
34. Handoll HH, Quinn KM, de Bie R. Interventions for preventing ankle ligament injuries. Cochrane Database Syst Rev 2008;(4):CD000018. http://dx.doi.org/10.1002/14651858.CD000018.
35. Thacker SB, Stroup DF, Branche CM, et al. The prevention of ankle sprains in sports. A systematic review of the literature. Am J Sports Med 1999;27(6):753–60.

Musculoskeletal Imaging
Types and Indications

Peter H. Seidenberg, MD[a],*, Allyson H. Howe, MD[b]

KEYWORDS

- Musculoskeletal imaging • Radiology • Injury evaluation • Radiographs
- Magnetic resonance imaging • Computed tomography
- Musculoskeletal ultrasonography • Nuclear medicine

KEY POINTS

- No imaging modality can surpasses the value of a well performed history and physical examination. Radiographs are indicated to evaluate suspected fracture, dislocation, or arthritis. The history and physical examination will guide as to which views are required.
- Magnetic resonance imaging (MRI) is an effective tool in the evaluation of soft tissue disorders. However, its use is contraindicated in patients with pacemakers, defibrillators, and spinal stimulators.
- Ultrasonography is effective in examining tendons, cysts, and peripheral nerves. Tears, tenosynovitis, and tendinosis are readily differentiated on sonograms. Dynamic evaluation is helpful in confirming the severity of the tendon injury.
- Computed tomography (CT scan) is able to reconstruct images in both two and three dimensional images. This can assist in the evaluation of complex fractures. However, caution is advised in overuse of this imaging modality due to the high dose of radiation utilized.

INTRODUCTION

Musculoskeletal imaging has come a long way since the discovery of x-rays by Wilhelm Conrad Röntgen in 1895.[1] Today, in addition to conventional radiographs, clinicians have numerous options available to assist in the care of their patients. However, knowing which modality is best for evaluating the presenting complaint is of upmost importance to the physician wishing to practice efficient and cost-effective medicine. This article reviews the indications for common musculoskeletal imaging modalities to assist in the evaluation of acute and chronic musculoskeletal pathology.

Radiographs are most advantageous in the evaluation of bony abnormalities such as fractures, dislocations, and osteoarthritis. Radiography is the least expensive imaging modality, but its drawbacks include difficulty evaluating complex fractures, stress fractures, and soft-tissue structures. In addition, radiographs require the use of low levels

[a] Penn State Sports Medicine, Penn State University, State College, 1850 East Park Avenue, Suite 112, PA 16803, USA; [b] University of Southern Maine, Portland, ME, USA
* Corresponding author.
E-mail address: pseidenberg@hmc.psu.edu

Med Clin N Am 98 (2014) 895–914
http://dx.doi.org/10.1016/j.mcna.2014.04.003
0025-7125/14/$ – see front matter
medical.theclinics.com

of ionizing radiation to produce an image. In skeletally immature patients, contralateral views should be obtained to increase the detection of growth-plate injuries.

By contrast, computed tomography (CT) scans use much higher doses of radiation. However, this technology is able to produce high-resolution images in both 2 and 3 dimensions, compensate for overlapping structures, and provide finer cuts of the area of interest.[2] CT is useful in the evaluation of stress fractures and complex fractures or dislocations. It can also evaluate ligaments, masses, and fluid collections.

Bone scintigraphy (bone scan) is a nuclear medicine study used in the investigation of stress fractures, occult fractures, and bone tumors or infections.[3] The procedure requires intravenous injection of a radioactive material that is taken up by metabolically active bone. Because bone metabolism is increased in pathologic conditions, abnormalities will appear as "hot spots" on the images acquired by the gamma camera. The modality also uses radiation, and requires the patient to return after the injection at specified times for the different phases of the scan. Each phase can take from 20 to 70 minutes to complete. The radiation exposure is higher than for radiography but lower in comparison with CT.

Magnetic resonance imaging (MRI) carries no risk of radiation exposure, as it uses magnetic coils to produce pictures. It is typically used in the evaluation of soft-tissue disorders involving ligaments, tendons, cartilage, intervertebral discs, and masses. In addition, MRI is effective in further characterizing bony injuries, including subtle fractures and contusions. However, because of the magnetic field, the modality is contraindicated in patients with metallic implants such as pacemakers, defibrillators, and spinal stimulators.[4] The study time is approximately 30 minutes, which can be difficult for patients with claustrophobia. To combat this, open MRI scanners have been developed. However, in general, open scanners have poorer resolution in comparison with closed units.

Musculoskeletal ultrasonography (US) uses sound waves to produce images. US carries no radiation risk, is relatively low in cost, and is able to evaluate structures dynamically. It is effective in evaluation of effusions (joint and paratenon), cysts, ligaments, muscles, and tendons.[5] US readily demonstrates the disorganized connective tissue of the tendinosis in distinct contrast to the normal fibrillar pattern of healthy tendon.[6] Calcium deposits within the tendon (calcific tendinosis) may also be demonstrated. With the use of power Doppler, neovascularization can also be identified. In addition to its diagnostic benefits, US is used to guide aspirations and injections. However, this modality is limited by the body habitus of the patient and the skill of the sonographer.

Although the aforementioned modalities are available to clinicians, it must be emphasized that musculoskeletal imaging does not replace a thorough history and physical examination. Instead, radiologic studies should be regarded as methods to confirm the suspected diagnosis.

NECK

When cervical spine injury is suspected, radiographs should be obtained. The series should include anteroposterior (AP), lateral, odontoid, and bilateral oblique views. **Fig. 1** demonstrates common lines used to assist in interpreting the films.[7] In nonemergent settings, if no fracture is seen but the history suggests radicular symptoms that are positional in nature, lateral flexion and extension views should be obtained.[8] A CT scan can demonstrate more subtle fractures and ligament injuries, and is often used in emergency cases. The sensitivity for detecting acute cervical spine injury for plain radiographs and CT imaging is 52% and 98%, respectively.[9]

MRI is reserved for the evaluation of radicular symptoms that have not responded to conservative therapy, and can demonstrate nerve-root impingement caused by disc

LATERAL CERVICAL SPINE LANDMARKS

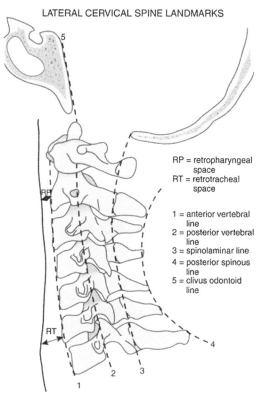

RP = retropharyngeal
        space
RT = retrotracheal
        space

1 = anterior vertebral
        line
2 = posterior vertebral
        line
3 = spinolaminar line
4 = posterior spinous
        line
5 = clivus odontoid
        line

Fig. 1. Radiographic lines on lateral view of the cervical line. (*From* Seidenberg PH. Radiographic lines and angles. In: Seidenberg PH, Beutler AI, editors. The sports medicine resource manual. Philadelphia: Saunders-Elsevier; 2008. p. 164; with permission; and *Adapted from* Greenspan A. Orthopedic radiology: a practical approach. 3rd edition. Philadelphia: Lippincott Williams & Wilkins; 2000.)

herniation and/or arthritis. MRI is also indicated acutely for suspected cervical cord injury. In those unable to undergo MRI, CT is used. Bone scan and US are not commonly used in cervical spine injury.

SHOULDER

Radiographs are used to evaluate suspected shoulder fracture, dislocation, or arthritis. The history and physical examination will guide as to which views are required. If dislocation of the glenohumeral joint (GHJ) is suspected, AP, AP with internal rotation, West Point axillary, and scapular Y views are required. The AP with internal rotation enhances visualization of a Hill-Sachs lesion (compression fracture of the posterolateral humeral head), whereas the West Point axillary view assists in identification of a Bankhart fracture (avulsion of the anterior-inferior glenoid). Both of these findings are common with anterior shoulder dislocation. Posterior GHJ dislocation is often overlooked on standard AP view, but with the addition of the scapular Y view it can be readily identified.[10]

With rotator-cuff impingement, outlet views are helpful in looking for a hooked acromion (**Fig. 2**). If acromioclavicular joint (ACJ) injury is present, bilateral ACJ views are obtained with and without weights. For possible clavicle fracture, AP and AP with caudal tilt views are beneficial.

ANATOMIC SPECIMEN

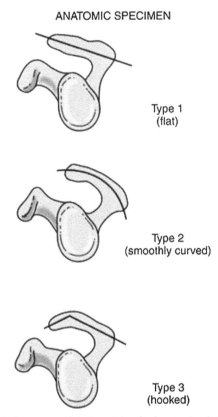

Type 1
(flat)

Type 2
(smoothly curved)

Type 3
(hooked)

Fig. 2. Acromion morphology on outlet view. A hooked acromion is thought to contribute to supraspinatus impingement during overhead movement. (*From* Greenspan A. Upper limb I: shoulder girdle and elbow. In: Orthopedic radiology: a practical approach. 3rd edition. Philadelphia: Lippincott Williams & Wilkins; 2000. p. 102; and Seidenberg PH. Radiographic lines and angles. In: Seidenberg PH, Beutler AI, editors. The sports medicine resource manual. Philadelphia: Saunders-Elsevier; 2008, with permission; and *Adapted from* Greenspan A. Orthopedic radiology: a practical approach. 3rd edition. Philadelphia: Lippincott Williams & Wilkins; 2000.)

MRI is indicated for suspected rotator-cuff rupture, rotator-cuff tendinosis that is not responding to conservative therapy, and labral abnormality. In addition, following dislocation MRI will demonstrate Hill-Sachs and Bankhart lesions, if present, and allow evaluation of the anterior glenohumeral ligaments. Intra-articular contrast improves recognition of rotator-cuff, labral, and glenohumeral ligament tears.[11]

US is helpful in the evaluation of rotator-cuff injury (**Fig. 3**).[6] Several studies have demonstrated sensitivity and specificity equivalent to those of MRI for diagnosis of rotator-cuff tears.[12,13] Dynamically, US can demonstrate subacromial impingement and subluxation of the biceps tendon out of the bicipital groove (**Fig. 4**). CT and bone scans are not commonly used in the evaluation of shoulder injury.

ELBOW

In the setting of acute trauma, elbow radiographs are used to evaluate for fractures and/or dislocation. Initially a fracture may not appear obvious; however, clues that one is present can be seen by evaluating for intra-articular effusion. A lucency anterior

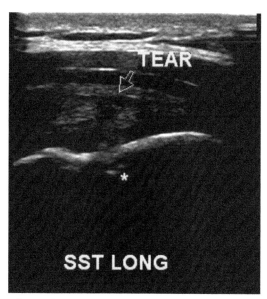

Fig. 3. Ultrasonographic evaluation of supraspinatus tear. A longitudinal view of the supraspinatus tendon demonstrates absence of signal in the area of the tear (*outlined*). Note the cortical irregularity of the greater tuberosity of the humerus that is commonly associated with full-thickness or articular surface supraspinatus tears (*asterisk*). Arrow indicates tear. SST, supraspinatus tendon.

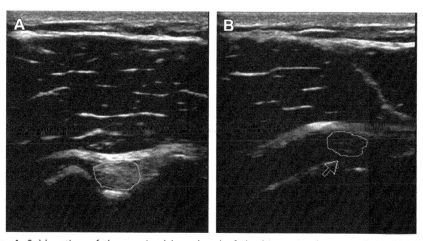

Fig. 4. Subluxation of the proximal long head of the biceps tendon out of the bicipital groove. The long head of the biceps is well situated within the bicipital groove (*outlined in A*). However, during dynamic examination with external rotation of the shoulder (*B*), the long head of the biceps is seen to sublux out of the groove (*arrow*). With return to neutral rotation of the shoulder, the biceps returned to its normal position. This figure demonstrates an advantage of ultrasonography over other imaging modalities, namely, dynamic evaluation.

to the distal humerus (a sail sign) may be a normal finding, but will be more pronounced in fractured joints owing to the presence of hemarthrosis. However, a posterior fad pad is never considered normal, and if seen, an occult intra-articular fracture should be suspected. In addition, the anterior humeral and radiocapitellar lines are also used to detect subtle fractures (**Figs. 5** and **6**). In skeletally immature patients with acute or chronic pain, contralateral elbow films should be obtained to investigate for subtle apophyseal injury, which may be overlooked if only the injured elbow is imaged.

MRI is used to evaluate for tendon or ligament ruptures. The most common tendon rupture is the distal biceps, for which confirmation is important because the treatment is surgical repair. Intra-articular contrast can make ligament tears more apparent and can also assist in the investigation of suspect loose bodies within the joint.

US is increasing in popularity in the evaluation of elbow injury. Its most common use is in the evaluation of epicondylitis.[14,15] However, US is also helpful in the investigation of olecranon bursitis, loose bodies, and tendon or ligament tears.[14,16] On dynamic examination, subtle tendon tears can become more apparent with muscle contraction. The anterior band of the ulnar collateral ligament can be easily imaged in both rest and stress views (**Fig. 7**).[17,18]

Bone scans of the elbow may assist in the evaluation of occult fractures, bursitis, and tumors but, because of low specificity, are not commonly used. CT scans are ordered by musculoskeletal specialists during the evaluation of complex fractures.

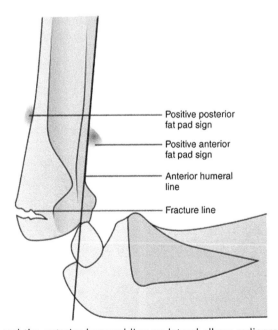

Fig. 5. Fat pads and the anterior humeral line on lateral elbow radiographs. The anterior humeral line is drawn along the anterior humerus through the lateral epicondyle. The line normally passes through the middle third of the condyle. If it does not, a supracondylar fracture is suspected. An anterior fat pad may be a normal finding. However, a posterior fat pad is always considered pathologic and suggests an occult intra-articular fracture. (*From* Seidenberg PH. Radiographic lines and angles. In: Seidenberg PH, Beutler AI, editors. The sports medicine resource manual. Philadelphia: Saunders-Elsevier; 2008, with permission; and *Adapted from* Greenspan A. Orthopedic radiology: a practical approach. 3rd edition. Philadelphia: Lippincott Williams & Wilkins; 2000.)

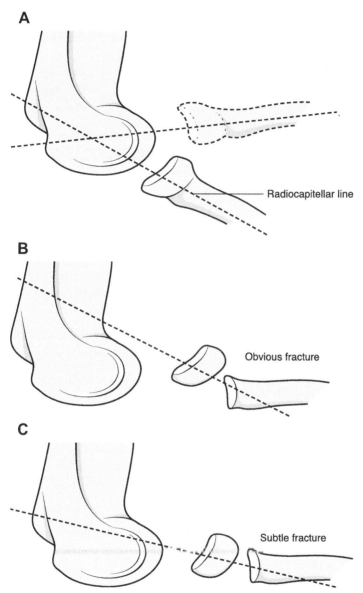

Fig. 6. (*A–C*) The radiocapitellar line on lateral elbow radiographs. A line is drawn bisecting the long axis of the radius and radial head. It should intersect with the capitellum, regardless of the degree of elbow flexion. If it does not, a fracture of the proximal radius or distal humerus is suspected. (*Adapted from* Simon RR, Koenigsknecht SJ. Proximal humerus. In: Emergency orthopedics. East Norwalk (NJ): Appleton & Lange; 1987. p. 103.)

WRIST

Radiographs are commonly used for acute trauma of the wrist. AP, lateral, and oblique views should always be obtained. Fractures and dislocations are often easily identified. Knowledge of radiographic lines should be used to identify ligamentous disruption. A volar intercalated segment instability (VISI) or dorsal intercalated segment

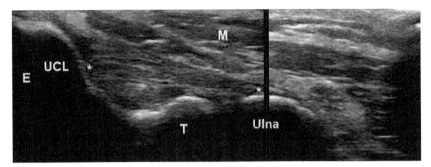

Fig. 7. Ultrasonographic evaluation of the anterior band of the ulnar collateral ligament. Panoramic image of the anterior band of the ulnar collateral ligament in a longitudinal plane to the ligament. Two still images were combined to make the panoramic image. The ligament can also be imaged during valgus stress as part of the dynamic examination. Asterisks indicate ulnar collateral ligament. E, medial epicondyle; M, medial elbow; T, trochlea.

instability (DISI) of the wrist can be identified on lateral films by examining the scapho-lunate angle (**Fig. 8**). An angle less than 30° indicates a VISI deformity; an angle greater than 60° indicates a DISI deformity. An abnormal capitolunate angle (>30°) further confirms carpal instability.[7] The addition of a clenched-fist view will help pinpoint scapho-lunate ligament tears (**Fig. 9**).[7]

If snuff-box or scaphoid tubercle tenderness is present on examination, a scaphoid view should be added. However, scaphoid fractures may not be obvious on plain films for up to 2 weeks after injury. As such, repeat films are often necessary. Bone scan or MRI can identify the fracture more quickly if diagnostic confirmation cannot wait 2 weeks. MRI is preferred over bone scan, as it is also able to identify ligamentous injury. MRI is also used to evaluate triangular fibrocartilage complex tears and complicated ganglion cysts. CT is used to investigate occult fractures and to follow fracture healing in high-risk injuries.

US is effective in examining tendons, cysts, and carpal tunnel syndrome (**Fig. 10**).[19] Tears, tenosynovitis, and tendinosis are readily differentiated on US.[5] Dynamic evaluation is helpful in confirming the severity of the tendon injury.

HAND

Hand and finger injuries are well suited to radiographs. AP, lateral, and oblique views should always be obtained. Joint congruency should be examined, and loss of the normal contour increases the suspicion of fracture. CT is reserved for the evaluation of complex fractures. Bone scan can confirm occult fracture but is rarely used in the hand. MRI is helpful in suspected flexor tendon rupture and in tears of the ulnar collateral ligament of the first metacarpophalangeal joint (gamekeeper's thumb). US can confirm tendon injury, especially during dynamic evaluation. Likewise, dynamic sonographic stress views are useful in the evaluation of ligament tears (**Fig. 11**).

LUMBAR SPINE

Lumbar back pain is a common complaint in primary care, and most humans will have back pain at some time during their lives. For many, the first episode of back pain occurs between the ages 20 and 40 years, and may be one of the first reasons they present to a doctor as an adult.[20] Back pain can be severe and debilitating even when the cause is benign. It commonly causes significant anxiety, and fear of a dangerous etiology.

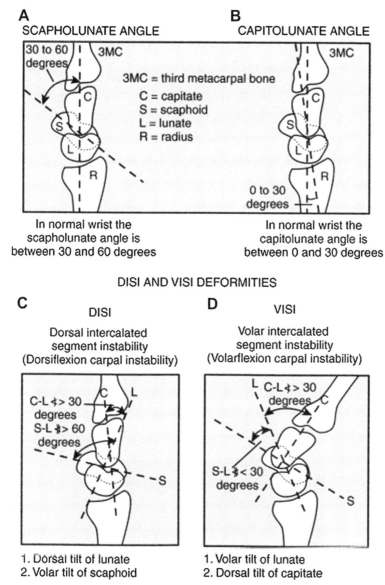

A
SCAPHOLUNATE ANGLE

30 to 60 degrees

3MC

3MC = third metacarpal bone
C = capitate
S = scaphoid
L = lunate
R = radius

In normal wrist the
scapholunate angle is
between 30 and 60 degrees

B
CAPITOLUNATE ANGLE

3MC

0 to 30 degrees

In normal wrist the
capitolunate angle is
between 0 and 30 degrees

DISI AND VISI DEFORMITIES

C
DISI

Dorsal intercalated
segment instability
(Dorsiflexion carpal instability)

C-L ∢ > 30 degrees
S-L ∢ > 60 degrees

1. Dorsal tilt of lunate
2. Volar tilt of scaphoid

D
VISI

Volar intercalated
segment instability
(Volarflexion carpal instability)

C-L ∢ > 30 degrees

S-L ∢ < 30 degrees

1. Volar tilt of lunate
2. Dorsal tilt of capitate

Fig. 8. (A–D) Scapholunate and capitolunate angles demonstrating DISI and VISI deformities. (*From* Seidenberg PH. Radiographic lines and angles. In: Seidenberg PH, Beutler AI, editors. The sports medicine resource manual. Philadelphia: Saunders-Elsevier; 2008. Fig. 17.24, with permission; and *Adapted from* Greenspan A. Orthopedic radiology: a practical approach. 3rd edition. Philadelphia: Lippincott Williams & Wilkins; 2000.)

Most episodes of acute low back pain do not require any imaging. The first 4 to 6 weeks of a new episode of back pain without red flags often results in resolution of the pain with or without imaging. In fact, when imaging modalities are used too quickly in the setting of a self-limiting problem, the results can often be difficult for the provider or the patient to interpret.[21]

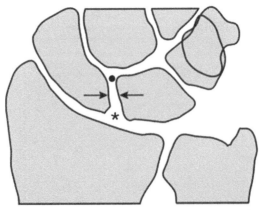

Fig. 9. Clenched-fist view. The normal gap is 2 mm or less. Greater than this suggests sca-pholunate ligament tear. dot, distal scapholunate space; asterisk, proximal scapholunate space; *arrow* notes where to measure the space (middle of the joint). (*Adapted from* Keats TE, Sistrom C. Upper extremity. In: Atlas of radiologic measurement. 7th edition. St Louis (MO): Mosby; 2001. p. 192; with permission.)

Imaging can be useful when the pain does not resolve or if there are certain concerns for a serious cause. When the primary diagnosis of concern is cancer, cauda equina, infection, or fracture, imaging should be used to help determine if these are present. Red-flag symptoms in the history of low back pain include significant trauma (motor vehicle crash or fall from a height), temperature greater than 38°C, unintentional weight loss, new back pain in a person older than 50 years, saddle anesthesia, or other nerve deficits such as new bowel or bladder incontinence, pain at rest, and a history of malignancy. If any of the red-flag symptoms are present in a patient with back pain, imaging studies are indicated (**Table 1**).

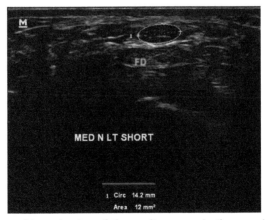

Fig. 10. Ultrasonographic evaluation of the median nerve in the carpal tunnel. Short-axis view of the median nerve in the volar wrist at the level of the carpal tunnel. A cross-sectional area greater than 10 mm^2 is considered abnormal. However, specificity is increased with a cutoff of 14 mm^2. FD, flexor digitorum tendon group; LT, left; MED N, median nerve. (*From* Lange J. Carpal tunnel syndrome diagnosed using ultrasound as a first-line examination by the surgeon. J Hand Surg Eur Vol 2012;38:627–32.)

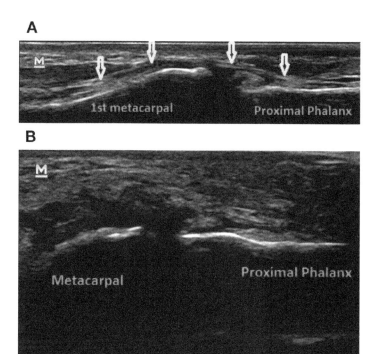

Fig. 11. Ultrasonogram of ulnar collateral ligament tear of the first metacarpophalangeal joint. (*A*) Intact ligament. Yellow arrows depict the ligament. (*B*) Ruptured ulnar ligament of the first metacarpophalangeal joint in the opposite hand of the same patient. The ends of the ligament are outlined. Intraoperatively, the patient was also found to have a Stener lesion.

Radiographs of the lumbar spine come with significant radiation exposure concerns to the unprotected gonads, and should be undertaken with a thoughtful approach to what advantage they might offer. Oblique films are relatively costly in terms of harm (radiation load) for the potential diagnostic assistance they can provide. Spondylolysis is a unilateral or bilateral pars defect that causes axial back pain, and occurs commonly in athletes who do repetitive back-extension movements within their sport or training. Spondylolisthesis occurs when there is a bilateral pars defect and a subsequent shift of the affected vertebrae anteriorly or posteriorly.

Herniated discs are common in humans. Repetitive flexion loads with twisting maneuvers (ie, rotation) can tear soft-tissue structures (annulus) and allow leakage of the nucleus pulposis substance that is irritating to surrounding nerves. The disc itself can extrude and irritate an exiting nerve root. Many people without pain have herniated discs on MRI of the lumbar spine, and often the location of a herniated disc does not correlate with the described pain the patient is feeling (**Table 2**).[21] It is important to approach the examination of someone with back pain with the goal of identifying the key location where the injury is suspected to be, as it correlates best with the location of the patient's discomfort (**Table 3**). If there are findings that correlate appropriately, the findings of the imaging test can be relied upon and the patient treated accordingly.

HIP

The first goal of an initial interview for hip pain should be to clarify where the pain occurs. The general term hip can mean the pain is in the lateral pelvis, anterior groin,

Table 1
Imaging of the lumbar spine

Type	How to Order	Limitations	When to Order	Considerations
Plain films	AP and lateral	Consider flexion and extension views. Oblique views not necessary	Evaluate for fracture, spondylolisthesis, spondylolysis (not very sensitive), fracture	Cannot evaluate soft tissues well
MRI	MRI of lumbar spine without contrast (unless evaluating for tumor, then contrast is helpful)	Cannot be ordered if the patient has a pacemaker or metal implants in the body	Evaluate for herniated nucleus pulposis, metastatic disease	Expensive and often overly sensitive, can be challenging to correlate MRI findings with patient's pain
CT lumbar spine	CT of lumbar spine without contrast if looking for fracture, with contrast if concerned for tumor or mass	Radiation load to the patient	Excellent for fracture	
SPECT scan	Single-photon emission CT scan; need to clarify specific body region (ie, lumbar spine)	Not available at all centers	Low radiation load, specific to the area that is being evaluated, ideal to diagnose presence and activity of a spondylolysis lesion	Need to inject radiotracer dye, cannot use in pregnant or breastfeeding women
Bone scan	Nuclear medicine 3-phase bone scan		Can help rule out infection or occult metastatic tumor	Highlights any area of increased metabolic activity, very sensitive but not specific

Table 2
Lumbar spine abnormalities on MR images of asymptomatic subjects

Finding	Patient Age in Years		
	20–39	40–59	60–80
Herniated disk	21	22	36
Spinal stenosis	1	0	21
Disk bulge	56	50	79
Disk degeneration	34	59	93

Values are percentages of total study group (67 patients).
Data from Boden SD, Wiesel SW. Lumbar spine imaging: role in clinical decision making. J Am Acad Orthop Surg 1996;4(5):238–48.

posterior gluteal region, or lower back. The location of pain when a patient is concerned about the hip can often lead to a proper differential and help determine the proper imaging techniques to be used.

Plain films of the hip are easy to obtain and cause minimal discomfort to patients. The most typical views to obtain are an AP of the pelvis, which allows visualization of both the femoral necks and heads and their articulation with the pelvic bones, and a cross-table lateral of the individual hip in question. The lateral film offers a view of the acetabulum and femoral head articulation.

CT of the hip is useful when a 3-dimensional view is needed. This view often becomes useful when there is concern for fracture of deeper pelvis structures such as the pubic rami or acetabulum.

MRI of the hip is the imaging technique of choice for soft-tissue concerns such as tendon tears or ruptures (ie, rectus femoris in a soccer player or proximal hamstring in a water skier). Often a femoral neck stress injury is best seen on MRI because of its ability to demonstrate edema in the bone before an actual fracture occurs.

Musculoskeletal US is used for direct visualization of the joint during intra-articular injections. Evaluation of the gluteal tendons, sometimes called the rotator cuff of the hip, is possible in a nonobese patient with lateral hip discomfort. Bursa around the hip can also be visualized, aiding accurate injection with cortisone to help resolve discomfort.

Table 3
Symptoms and examination findings based on level of lumbar disc herniation

Level of Herniation	Pain	Numbness	Weakness	Reflexes
L3–L4	Low back, hip, posterolateral thigh, anterior leg	Anteromedial thigh and knee	Quadriceps	Knee jerk diminished
L4–L5	Lateral thigh, lateral leg	Lateral lower leg and 1st web space	Dorsiflexion of great toe	Nothing significant
L5–S1	Sacroiliac joint, down lateral thigh into lateral leg	Posterior calf, lateral foot	Gastrocnemius (cannot walk on toes more than a few steps)	Ankle jerk diminished

Data from Madden CC, Putukian M, Young CC, et al. Netter's sports medicine. Philadelphia: Saunders/Elsevier; 2010.

Lateral hip pain is classically over the greater trochanter, iliotibial band, and attachment of the gluteal tendons on the trochanter. Often people will have a history of increased exertion (often simply walking or running) and may have pain with rolling onto the hip at night. With this classic presentation, many providers will administer a local corticosteroid injection to the trochanteric bursa to help with pain. If this does not work, or tendon injury at the gluteal tendons is suspected, MRI or bedside US can be helpful.

Plain radiographs should always be considered when anterior groin pain is present to help determine the general formation of the joint and whether there is significant joint-space narrowing. Rarely, bone tumors or lytic lesions can be seen on plain films, and will require additional imaging for further definition. Most often this imaging is with CT or MRI.

KNEE

Knee pain is a common presenting complaint. Three bones make up the 2 joints of the knee: the femur, the tibia, and the patella articulate to form the tibiofemoral and the patellofemoral joints. If imaging is needed, weight-bearing films of the knees will be most useful to determine joint-space narrowing and anatomic alignment (ie, of the patella). Weight-bearing knee films are superior to MRI in identifying the degree of joint-space narrowing because the films are taken with the patient standing, compared with MRI which is generally performed with the patient supine. A 3- or 4-view series is recommended to evaluate the 3 compartments of the knee: patellofemoral, medial tibiofemoral, and lateral tibiofemoral. The 4-view series usually includes a standing tunnel view (weight-bearing AP view with the knee flexed to 30°), which can help diagnose "bone-on-bone" arthritis when present.[22]

Stability of the knee comes from 4 main ligaments. The anterior cruciate ligament (ACL) and the posterior cruciate ligament are located in the center of the joint while the lateral collateral ligament and the medial collateral ligament are located outside of the tibiofemoral articulation. Together, these ligaments provide anteroposterior, mediolateral, and rotational stability. Between the tibia and the femur are 2 soft-tissue cartilaginous structures known as the medial and lateral meniscus, which provide shock absorption from axial loads.

Degenerative arthritis of the knee joint is fairly common. Plain films are easy to obtain, and provide adequate information to diagnose degenerative change in the knee. The 4 findings on plain films associated with degenerative change are: subchondral sclerosis, subchondral cystic change, osteophytes, and joint-space narrowing (which indicates loss of articular cartilage).[22] MRI is not generally as helpful in diagnosis of osteoarthritic changes in the knee, although subchondral lesions can be seen and, perhaps, better characterized at an earlier stage with the sensitivity afforded by MRI.

ACL injuries can happen with or without direct contact to the knee. Often the patient reports hearing a snap or a pop in the knee during a twisting event. There is usually a large effusion that develops over a matter of hours, and a feeling of instability in the knee that prevents the patient from return to normal athletic or twisting activities. There is no better imaging test to diagnose an ACL tear than an MRI. On MRI the knee is extended fully, and in this position the ACL should be held tight. A disturbance in the linear congruity of the ligament indicates a tear.

The menisci of the knee are recognized as having load-bearing function, and provide stabilization of the joint during flexion and extension movements.[23] Clinically a meniscus tear tends to present with medial or lateral joint-line knee pain, a feeling of instability, and a small knee effusion. There may be a history of a twisting knee injury, which puts an abnormal load on the menisci and can tear the structure. Many meniscus tears will improve with conservative treatment, and immediate imaging is not usually necessary. One setting whereby urgent consideration for advanced imaging is important is when a patient who is considered to have a meniscal tear lacks full extension of the knee joint, as this could mean that the torn meniscus has flapped back into the joint, thus blocking full extension (bucket-handle tear). Plain films and CT are not useful in determining whether a meniscus tear is present. Bedside US can identify an abnormally positioned meniscus (ie, extruded meniscus) that may be a sign of a meniscal tear, but lacks sensitivity for routine use. MRI is the optimal way to identify a tear. The criteria for a meniscus tear on MRI include abnormal meniscus shape and signal through the meniscus that extends to the superior and/or inferior articular surface. Meniscus extrusion or subchondral edema may also be seen, further supporting the diagnosis of tear.[23]

ANKLE

Ankle sprains are one of the most common musculoskeletal injuries encountered in primary care practice, especially among teenagers and young adults.[24,25] Use of the Ottawa ankle and foot rules have been shown to be very useful in determining who should have imaging at initial presentation. According to the Ottawa criteria, a radiograph should be obtained if the patient is unable to ambulate for 4 steps after the injury or at the point of medical provider evaluation; if there is pain in the midfoot zone; or if there is bony tenderness in the distal 6 cm of the posterior edge of the lateral or medial malleolus, base of the fifth metatarsal, or navicular bone. The Ottawa ankle rules are 100% sensitive in ruling out fracture in the adult population, and nearly 100% sensitive in children as young as 5 years.[25,26] An ankle series includes AP, lateral, and mortise views (oblique view) to better evaluate the tibiotalar joint in congruity. On the mortise view there should be a symmetric radiolucent area around the talus of equal width that generally measures less than 4 mm in total.[27]

Chronic ankle pain after lateral ankle sprain is not as common but, when present, imaging is often useful. Use of plain films to determine alignment and bone health (ie, to rule out an osteochondral defect [OCD]) is an important first step. OCD lesions in the ankle most commonly occur at the most superior portion of the talus, called the talar dome, following an ankle inversion injury. These injuries of the cartilage and underlying bone can result in a loose fragment in the joint if left untreated. Surgical exploration with consideration for microfracture surgery by an orthopedic surgeon is important to help maintain the integrity of the tibiotalar joint surface.[28] MRI of the ankle can be useful at grading these OCD lesions and for determining the presence of chronic ligament disturbance.[29] The anterior talofibular ligament and the calcaneofibular ligament are most commonly injured, and show sensitivity and specificity of 75%/86% and 50%/98%, respectively, in determining complete tears with the use of imaging alone compared with surgical exploration.

Tendon injuries in the foot and ankle are easily evaluated by musculoskeletal US techniques. One example of this is with Achilles tendinopathy, which is common and can take a long time to improve. When there is significant disability, swelling, or pain with an Achilles tendon injury, bedside musculoskeletal US is an ideal way to dynamically evaluate the tendon further. Partial tendon tears, underlying retrocalcaneal bursitis, and neovascularization of the tendon can be identified using US. MRI can identify the tendon anatomy but cannot provide dynamic input. Plain films and CT scans are not helpful in the evaluation of the Achilles tendon. Moreover, US is excellent for the evaluation of the posterior tibialis and peroneal tendons. In addition, dynamic examination can be used to demonstrate peroneal subluxation secondary to superior retinaculum disruption.

FOOT

The etiology of foot pain and the identification of an injured structure is critical to decreasing the chance of further injury from continued weight bearing. Often the initial imaging test of choice in the foot is a plain radiograph series. Weight-bearing plain films can be useful in identifying bony or ligamentous injury, particularly in the Lisfranc joint where widening can occur. It is critical to obtain a 3-view series (AP, lateral, and oblique) to ensure the ability to look at all areas of the foot, because the bony structures of the foot frequently overlap and make it difficult to identify individual structures in every film.

Musculoskeletal US has recently been used more frequently to provide a dynamic view of the soft tissues of the foot, but lacks the ability to accurately diagnose osseous injury. CT imaging of the foot can adequately define osseous injury and fracture, but does a poor job of identifying soft-tissue damage. The imaging modality of choice for the foot has become MRI, because of its sensitivity in aiding the identification of soft-tissue (ligament, tendon, nerve) and osseous abnormalities.[30]

Fracture of the metatarsal bones and phalanges of the forefoot are generally easy to discover on plain films. Midfoot and hindfoot fracture of the cuboid, cuneiform, navicular, talus, and calcaneus bones often need higher-level imaging with CT or MRI to identify a fracture. A fracture should be suspected if edema, ecchymosis, and severe pain with weight bearing are present. Plain films are generally the best first imaging test to order, followed by a CT if fracture is the main concern. MRI can identify fractures as well, and is often ordered when the differential includes something other than fracture, such as a tendon or ligament injury.

There are numerous joints in the foot where the bony/cartilage interface can be injured. Frequently plain films are normal in these cases, and persistent pain results in the need for further imaging. MRI can identify the health of hyaline cartilage and identify areas of cartilage and bony injury, which manifests as edema noted in the hyaline cartilage or subchondral bone. These findings signify osteochondral injury.

Most stress-fracture injury to bones will occur with a history of increased load compared with the inherent load tolerance of a particular body part. This disorder can occur in the setting of increased exercise resulting in fatigue of a particular bone (ie, training errors with excessive running) or from routine training in the setting of insufficient bone strength (ie, osteoporosis). If pain is present for more than 2 weeks, there may be abnormalities noted on plain films that identify the injury, including focal periosteal reaction, abnormal callous formation, dense sclerotic lines, or true fracture lines. Many times, however, the plain film is not sufficiently sensitive to identify bony edema consistent with stress injury. MRI can help identify stress reactions by showing varying degrees of marrow edema in the affected bone.[30] It is important to identify the spectrum of stress injury to stress fracture to avoid progression to stress fracture and nonunion.

Fracture of the fifth metatarsal in the proximal portion can occur with inversion injury of the foot. Plain films are often all that is needed to make the diagnosis (**Fig. 12**). The attachment of the peroneal tendons to this bone can cause a traction tug during an inversion event that can pull (or avulse) a piece of bone from the end of the fifth metatarsal. These avulsion fractures are oriented perpendicular to the bone itself (occur in a medial to lateral direction) and are proximal to the metaphyseal-diaphyseal junction at

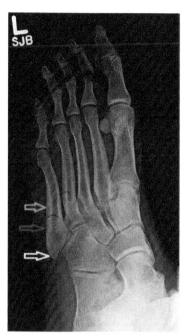

Fig. 12. Fifth metatarsal fracture classification. Oblique view of the left foot depicting transverse fractures of the fourth and fifth metatarsals. Metatarsal fractures are classified as shaft fractures (*green arrow*), Jones fractures (*red arrow* at the metaphyseal-diaphyseal junction), or styloid avulsion fractures (*yellow arrow*). The fifth metatarsal fracture shown here is just distal to the metaphyseal-diaphyseal junction and is therefore considered a shaft fracture.

the styloid process. Such injuries heal well with protected weight bearing and can be seen clearly on plain films. A fracture further distal on the bone at the metaphyseal-diaphyseal junction can result in nonunion because of the poor blood supply in the area. This type of fracture, known as a Jones fracture, needs many weeks of non–weight-bearing treatment to heal. Many active patients with a Jones fracture decide to undergo a surgical pinning to help stabilize the fracture and assist healing. For this reason, consultation with an orthopedic surgeon is prudent in the setting of a Jones fracture.

Injury at the tarsometatarsal joint, the Lisfranc joint, can lead to midfoot instability and chronic pain if not recognized or treated correctly. Injury can occur after high-velocity impact during a fall from height or motor vehicle accident, or during lower-velocity accidents during sporting events. In the lower-velocity instance, the injury occurs when the foot is forcibly plantarflexed, the metatarsophalangeal joints are concurrently dorsiflexed, and a downward force is placed on the heel of the foot.[31] In general, Lisfranc injuries can involve a fracture, dislocation, or sprain of the joint. Imaging of the foot should occur with a weight-bearing AP view alongside a non–weight-bearing view to discern if there is abnormal separation of the first and second metatarsals and medial and middle cuneiform bones (**Fig. 13**). It is also possible to take weight-bearing views of both feet concurrently for comparison. An MRI can clarify whether the Lisfranc ligament has intact or torn plantar and dorsal fibers. The Lisfranc ligament stabilizes the gap between the medial cuneiform and base of the second metatarsal.[30] Disruption of this ligament complex can lead to rapidly progressive osteoarthritis in the midfoot, leading to chronic pain and disability.

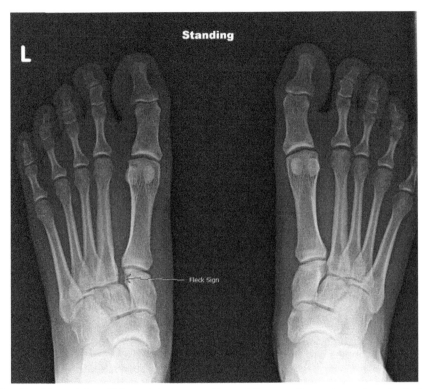

Fig. 13. Lisfranc injury. Lisfranc injuries are often subtle on radiographs, and are best visualized on weight-bearing views with comparison with the unaffected side. There is typically widening of the space between the first and second metatarsal bases. The disrupted ligament will often cause a small avulsion fracture, called a fleck sign (depicted on the left foot).

REFERENCES

1. History of radiography. NDT Resource Center. Iowa State University. Available at: http://www.ndt-ed.org/EducationResources/CommunityCollege/Radiography/Introduction/history.htm. Accessed November 16, 2013.
2. Buckwalter KA, Rydberg J, Kopecky KK, et al. Musculoskeletal imaging with multislice CT. AJR Am J Roentgenol 2001;176:979–86.
3. Wheeless CR. Triphasic bone scan. In: Wheeless' textbook of orthopaedics. Available at: http://www.wheelessonline.com/ortho/triphasic_bone_scan. Accessed November 16, 2013.
4. Magnetic resonance imaging. Wikipedia. Available at: http://en.wikipedia.org/wiki/Magnetic_resonance_imaging. Accessed November 16, 2013.
5. Yim ES, Corrado G. Ultrasound in athletes: emerging techniques in point-of-care practice. Curr Sports Med Rep 2012;11(6):298–303.
6. Martinoli C, Derchi LE, Pastorino C, et al. Analysis of echotexture of tendons with US. Radiology 1993;186:839–43.
7. Seidenberg PH. Radiographic lines and angles. In: Seidenberg PH, Beutler AI, editors. The sports medicine resource manual. Philadelphia: Saunders-Elsevier; 2008. p. 163–77.
8. White AA 3rd, Johnson RM, Panjabi MM, et al. Biomechanical analysis of clinical stability in the cervical spine. Clin Orthop Relat Res 1975;109:85–96.

9. Holmes JF, Akkinepalli R. Computed tomography versus plain radiography to screen for cervical spine injury: a meta-analysis. J Trauma 2005;58(5):902–5.

10. St. Pierre P, Gonzales R. Injuries of the shoulder and arm. In: Seidenberg PH, Beutler AI, editors. The sports medicine resource manual. Philadelphia: Saunders-Elsevier; 2008. p. 233–52.

11. Pavic R, Margetic P, Bensic M, et al. Diagnostic value of US, MR and MR arthrography in shoulder instability. Injury 2013;44(Suppl 3):S26–32.

12. de Jesus JO, Parker L, Frangos AJ, et al. Accuracy of MRI, MR arthrography, and ultrasound in the diagnosis of rotator cuff tears: a meta-analysis. AJR Am J Roentgenol 2009;192:1701–7.

13. Smith TO, Back T, Toms AP, et al. Diagnostic accuracy of ultrasound for rotator cuff tears in adults: a systematic review and meta-analysis. Clin Radiol 2011; 66(11):1036–48. http://dx.doi.org/10.1016/j.crad.2011.05.007.

14. Radunovic G, Vlad V, Micu MC, et al. Ultrasound assessment of the elbow. Med Ultrason 2012;14(2):141–6.

15. Poltawski L, Ali S, Jayaram V, et al. Reliability of sonographic assessment of tendinopathy in tennis elbow. Skeletal Radiol 2012;41(1):83–9.

16. Lobo Lda G, Fessell DP, Miller BS, et al. The role of sonography in differentiating full versus partial distal biceps tendon tears: correlation with surgical findings. AJR Am J Roentgenol 2013;200(1):158–62.

17. Smith W, Hackel JG, Goitz HT, et al. Utilization of sonography and a stress device in the assessment of partial tears of the ulnar collateral ligament in throwers. Int J Sports Phys Ther 2011;6(1):45–50.

18. Wood N, Konin JG, Nofsinger C. Diagnosis of an ulnar collateral ligament tear using musculoskeletal ultrasound in a collegiate baseball pitcher: a case report. N Am J Sports Phys Ther 2010;5(4):227–33.

19. Chen SF, Lu CH, Huang CR, et al. Ultrasonographic median nerve cross section areas measured by 8-point "inching test" for idiopathic carpal tunnel syndrome: a correlation of nerve conduction study severity and duration of clinical symptoms. BMC Med Imaging 2011;11:22.

20. Casazza BA. Diagnosis and treatment of acute low back pain. Am Fam Physician 2012;85(4):343–50.

21. Boden SD, Wiesel SW. Lumbar spine imaging: role in clinical decision making. J Am Acad Orthop Surg 1996;4(5):238–48.

22. Johnson TR, Steinbach LS. Essential of musculoskeletal imaging. Rosemont (IL): American Academy of Orthopaedic Surgeons; 2004.

23. Ghosh P, Taylor TK. The knee joint meniscus. A fibrocartilage of some distinction. Clin Orthop Relat Res 1987;(224):52–63.

24. Schneck CD, Mesgarzadeh M, Bonakdarpour A, et al. MR imaging of the most commonly injured ankle ligaments. Radiology 1992;184:499–506.

25. Tiemstra JD. Update on acute ankle sprains. Am Fam Physician 2012;85(12): 1170–5.

26. Dowling S, Spooner CH, Liang Y, et al. Accuracy of Ottawa ankle rules to exclude fractures of the ankle and midfoot in children: a meta-analysis. Acad Emerg Med 2009;16(4):277–87.

27. Wheeless textbook of orthopaedics. Ankle frx: medial clear space vs lateral talar shift. Available at: www.wheelessonline.com/ortho/. Accessed December 1, 2013.

28. Femino JE, Amendola A. Ankle and leg injuries. In: Madden CC, Putukian M, Young CC, McCarty EC, editors. Netter's sports medicine. Philadelphia: Saunders-Elsevier; 2010. p. 429–37.

29. Park HJ, Cha SD, Kim SS, et al. Accuracy of MRI findings in chronic lateral ankle ligament injury: comparison with surgical findings. Clin Radiol 2012;67:313–8.
30. Burge AJ, Gold SL, Potter HG. Imaging of sports-related midfoot and forefoot injuries. Sports Health 2012;4(6):518–34.
31. Lattermann C, Goldstein JL, Wukich DK, et al. Practical management of Lisfranc injuries in athletes. Clin J Sport Med 2007;17(4):311–5.

Index

Note: Page numbers of article titles are in **boldface** type.

Med Clin N Am 98 (2014) 915–926
http://dx.doi.org/10.1016/S0025-7125(14)00085-6
0025-7125/14/$ – see front matter © 2014 Elsevier Inc. All rights reserved.

medical.theclinics.com

Printed and bound by CPI Group (UK) Ltd, Croydon, CR0 4YY

03/10/2024

01040488-0006